Evidence-Based Clinical Orthodontics

Evidence-Based
Clinical Orthodontics

Edited by

Peter G. Miles, BDSc, MDS

Senior Lecturer
Department of Orthodontics
University of Queensland School of Dentistry
Brisbane, Australia

Visiting Lecturer
Graduate Program in Orthodontics
Seton Hill University Center for Orthodontics
Greensburg, Pennsylvania

Daniel J. Rinchuse, DMD, MS, MDS, PhD

Professor and Associate Director
Graduate Program in Orthodontics
Seton Hill University Center for Orthodontics
Greensburg, Pennsylvania

Donald J. Rinchuse, DMD, MS, MDS, PhD

Professor and Program Director
Graduate Program in Orthodontics
Seton Hill University Center for Orthodontics
Greensburg, Pennsylvania

Quintessence Publishing Co, Inc

Chicago, Berlin, Tokyo, London, Paris, Milan, Barcelona,
Istanbul, Moscow, New Delhi, Prague, São Paulo, and Warsaw

Dedication

This book is dedicated to our families, teachers, mentors, students, and in particular to our patients. More importantly, this book is dedicated to you, the reader, the present and future of orthodontics.

Library of Congress Cataloging-in-Publication Data

Evidence-based clinical orthodontics / edited by Peter G. Miles, Daniel J. Rinchuse, Donald J. Rinchuse.
    p. ; cm.
  Includes bibliographical references and index.
  ISBN 978-0-86715-564-8
  I. Miles, Peter G. II. Rinchuse, Daniel J. III. Rinchuse, Donald Joseph.
  [DNLM: 1. Malocclusion--therapy. 2. Dental Bonding. 3. Evidence-Based Dentistry. 4. Orthodontics--methods. WU 440]

  617.6'43--dc23
                    2012017471

5 4 3 2 1

quintessence
books

© 2012 Quintessence Publishing Co Inc

Quintessence Publishing Co Inc
4350 Chandler Drive
Hanover Park, IL 60133
www.quintpub.com

Editor: Leah Huffman
Design: Ted Pereda
Production: Sue Robinson

Printed in China

Contents

In Memoriam

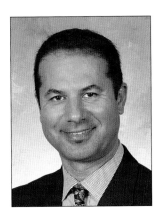

Dr Tiziano Baccetti (1966–2011)

Chapter 9 of this book, "The Effectiveness of Treatment Procedures for Displaced and Impacted Maxillary Canines," was written by Dr Tiziano Baccetti. This may well have been his last scholarly work; he completed this chapter just a few weeks before his untimely and tragic death on November 25, 2011, at the young age of 45. While posing for a photograph on a historic bridge in Prague, Czech Republic (he was the Keynote Speaker at the 9th International Orthodontic Symposium held November 24 to 26, 2011), he slipped on old stonework at the base of one of the saintly statues that decorate the bridge and fell 8 meters to the rocks below. It was the Charles Bridge—Ponte Carlo in Italian, the same name as Tizanio's beloved father, who knows that bridge well and for whom the picture was intended.

Tiziano authored over 240 scientific articles on diverse orthodontic topics. He has been described by those who knew him best as a "superman." This is supported by what he had accomplished in his short life. In 2011, Tiziano gave the Salzmann Lecture at the 111th Annual American Association of Orthodontists Session on "Dentofacial Orthopedics in Five Dimensions." In concluding his presentation, he explained how his grandfather in Italy had told him as a young boy that one day he would "find his America" and fulfill his dreams. Tiziano said at the end of his lecture, "I have found my America, fulfilled my dreams." Few, even with a long life, can say that they have fulfilled their dreams, their ambitions. We can be comforted that Tiziano did.

We feel fortunate that we can share Tiziano's excellent chapter with our readers.

Foreword

This text can serve as a reference guide for research and studies in many difficult clinical areas where there is a lack of evidence-based information. The distinguished editors are all involved in education, research, and practice, and they have invited other well-known experts and authorities to critically evaluate the literature and topics such as early treatment, extraction and nonextraction, Class III treatment, asymmetries, temporary skeletal anchorage devices (miniscrews), impacted canines, root resorption, temporomandibular disorders, retention, stability, and accelerated orthodontic tooth movement. These are all critical areas in the full scope of clinical orthodontic practice. I am sure that every orthodontist will learn from the enormous contributions provided so clearly in this text. The first chapter introduces and defines *evidence-based clinical practice*. Every other chapter provides evidence for and against each controversy and concludes with a summary and points to remember.

The topics are covered in detail with extensive illustrations, cases, diagrams, and references. All discussions are based on current research findings, and when evidence is not available, it is clearly stated as such. As the editors point out, the purpose of this book is to provide the orthodontist with an evidence-based perspective on selected important orthodontic topics and to stimulate practicing orthodontists to reflect on their current treatment protocols from an evidence-based view. In the future, clinical decisions should be based ideally on evidence rather than personal opinion, and treatment strategies should be proven to be both efficacious and safe.

I am very honored and privileged to have been asked to present this foreword because this text should be the evidence-based text for EVERY orthodontist and student.

Robert L. Vanarsdall, Jr, DDS
Assistant Dean for Advancement of Dental Specialties
Professor, Department of Orthodontics
University of Pennsylvania

Preface

The specialty of orthodontics has evolved from an apprenticeship to a learned profession requiring academic training. Nevertheless, many in our profession still cling to biased beliefs and opinions rather than embracing evidence-based practice. When evidence conflicts with what experience has taught, it becomes even more difficult for such practitioners to change their views. Hence, there is complacency and resistance within the profession to adopt evidence-based treatments.

Most orthodontists experience at least enough treatment success to support a practice. Yet treatment success does not necessarily equate with treatment efficacy or even verification of an appropriate diagnosis. This success can be the biggest obstacle to change. Clinical success may be associated with a multitude of appliances, strong belief in a particular philosophy, financial motivations (even unethical ones such as inappropriate phase I treatments), the difficulties involved in switching from an experience-based practice to an evidence-based practice, and a simple lack of understanding of evidence-based clinical practice (described in chapter 1). In our profession, therefore, treatment efficacy is currently evaluated broadly in relation to benefits, costs, risks, burden, and predictability of success with various treatment options.

No longer can the role of evidence-based decision making be shunned and ignored in favor of clinical experience alone. From both ethical and legal perspectives, sound clinical judgment must be based on the best evidence available. Today a paternalistic view, whereby the doctor knows what is best for the patient without soliciting patient input, is unacceptable. Patients have a right to autonomy and input into their treatment provided that it does no harm.

The 2001 Institute of Medicine report estimated that it takes an average of 17 years for new, effective medical research findings to become standard medical practice.[1] For example, there was a reemergence of the use of self-ligating brackets in the mid-1990s amid claims not only of faster ligation but also of quicker and more comfortable treatment. Several prospective clinical trials began to be published in 2005 and then two systematic reviews in 2010 concluded that in fact there was no difference in discomfort or treatment time when self-ligating brackets were used compared with conventional brackets. Yet despite the weight of evidence, these claims of faster treatment times and less discomfort are still made and supported by many orthodontists. As Dr Lysle Johnston, Jr, pointed out, our specialty tends to have a pessimistic attitude toward evidence and a minimal capacity to judge its quality. But what effect does this pessimism have on our patients? Can we as an orthodontic profession really wait 17 years to incorporate emerging quality evidence into our clinical practices?

With the exponential growth of information in today's world, how does the busy orthodontist evaluate evidence that will affect his or her practice? This book was conceived out of a need for evidence regarding relevant clinical topics and ongoing controversies in orthodontics such as early treatment, bonding protocols, treatment of Class II and Class III malocclusions, asymmetries, impacted canines, root resorption, retention, and accelerated tooth movement. We have done our best to incorporate the best evidence available regarding these topics, and hopefully this book will show you not only how to judge quality evidence but also why it is so important to implement it.

Reference

1. Institute of Medicine. Crossing the Quality Chasm: A New Health System for the 21st Century. Washington, DC: National Academies Press, 2001.

Acknowledgments

This book would not have been possible without the support of the publisher, Quintessence, and the tedious and dedicated work of our editor, Leah Huffman. We especially want to thank all of the contributing authors who have taken the time to write chapters in this book.

Contributors

Tiziano Baccetti, DDS, PhD*
Assistant Professor
Department of Orthodontics
University of Florence
Florence, Italy

Thomas M. Graber Visiting Scholar
Department of Orthodontics and Pediatric Dentistry
University of Michigan School of Dentistry
Ann Arbor, Michigan

William A. Brantley, PhD
Professor and Director
Graduate Program in Dental Materials Science
Division of Restorative, Prosthetic, and Primary Care
    Dentistry
College of Dentistry
The Ohio State University
Columbus, Ohio

Lam L. Cheng, BDSc, MDSc, MOrth RCS (ED),
    MRACD (Ortho)
Honorary Associate Professor
Department of Orthodontics
Faculty of Dentistry
The University of Sydney
Sydney, Australia

M. Ali Darendeliler, BDS, PhD, Dip Orth, Certif Orth,
    Priv Doc, MRACD (Ortho)
Professor and Chair
Department of Orthodontics
Faculty of Dentistry
The University of Sydney
Sydney, Australia

Theodore Eliades, DDS, MS, Dr Med, PhD
Professor and Director
Department of Orthodontics and Pediatric Dentistry
University of Zurich
Zurich, Switzerland

Sanjivan Kandasamy, BDSc, BSc Dent, Doc Clin
    Dent, MOrth RCS, MRACDS
Clinical Senior Lecturer
Department of Orthodontics
University of Western Australia
Perth, Australia

Adjunct Assistant Professor
Department of Orthodontics
University of Saint Louis
St Louis, Missouri

Eric Liou, DDS
Director
Department of Orthodontics and Craniofacial Dentistry
Chang Gung Memorial Hospital
Taipei, Taiwan

Program Director
Department of Orthodontics
Graduate School of Craniofacial Medicine
Chang Gung University
Taoyuang, Taiwan

*Deceased.

Peter G. Miles, BDSc, MDS
Senior Lecturer
Department of Orthodontics
University of Queensland School of Dentistry
Brisbane, Australia

Visiting Lecturer
Graduate Program in Orthodontics
Seton Hill University Center for Orthodontics
Greensburg, Pennsylvania

Private practice
Caloundra, Australia

Peter Ngan, DMD
Professor and Chair
Department of Orthodontics
West Virginia University School of Dentistry
Morgantown, West Virginia

James Noble, BSc, DDS, MSc, FRCD(C)
Visiting Lecturer
Division of Orthodontics
University of Manitoba
Winnipeg, Manitoba
Canada

Visiting Clinical Lecturer
Graduate Program in Orthodontics
Seton Hill University Center for Orthodontics
Greensburg, Pennsylvania

Nikolaos Pandis, DDS, MS, Dr med dent, MSc
Private practice
Corfu, Greece

Daniel J. Rinchuse, DMD, MS, MDS, PhD
Professor and Associate Director
Graduate Program in Orthodontics
Seton Hill University Center for Orthodontics
Greensburg, Pennsylvania

Donald J. Rinchuse, DMD, MS, MDS, PhD
Professor and Program Director
Graduate Program in Orthodontics
Seton Hill University Center for Orthodontics
Greensburg, Pennsylvania

John J. Sheridan, DDS, MSD
Clinical Associate Professor
School of Orthodontics
Jacksonville University
Jacksonville, Florida

Timothy Tremont, DMD, MS
Clinical Associate Professor
Department of Orthodontics
West Virginia University School of Dentistry
Morgantown, West Virginia

Private practice
White Oak, Pennsylvania

Nikolaos Pandis
DDS, MS, Dr med dent, MSc

Daniel J. Rinchuse
DMD, MS, MDS, PhD

Donald J. Rinchuse
DMD, MS, MDS, PhD

James Noble
BSc, DDS, MSc, FRCD(C)

CHAPTER

1

Introduction: Evidence-Based Clinical Practice

A quandary for the busy orthodontist in clinical practice is, "What knowledge and information should I be using in clinical decision making?" Some clinicians base their clinical decisions on their own unique observations and experiences, or perhaps even those of an "expert" currently on the lecture circuit, while other orthodontists base their clinical judgments on the available scientific evidence rather than anecdotal reports. Clinicians may also rotate back and forth between an experience-based and an evidence-based view. In recent years, it has been recognized that the ideal approach to decision making in health care should be based on scientific evidence rather than personal opinions.[1]

What is evidence-based dentistry? A recent *JADA* article by Ismail and Bader[2] defined *evidence-based dentistry* as "an unbiased approach to oral health care that follows a process of systematically collecting and analyzing scientific evidence with the objective of gaining useful decision-making information with minimal bias." So-called *evidence scientists* have prioritized each type of evidence according to the importance and weight it is accorded during decision making. At the low end of the hierarchy lies expert opinion, and at the high end lie high-quality meta-analyses and systematic reviews and randomized controlled trials (RCTs) with a very low risk of bias[3] (Table 1-1). Being ranked as low-level does not necessarily mean that evidence is false but rather that the priority given to decision making is low because the potential cost versus benefit might be highly unfavorable for large numbers of patients.[4] In fact, critical discoveries such as penicillin and DNA have emerged from lower levels of evidence. It should also be noted that although RCTs are considered the gold standard for assessing the effectiveness of treatment interventions, implementing them is not always feasible or ethical. For example, it would be unethical to randomize participants to smoking and nonsmoking groups with the objective to evaluate the effect of smoking on

lung cancer; in such circumstances, high-quality observational studies must be used to determine causality. Finally, predictive models (prognostic and diagnostic) are best developed using high-quality prospective cohort studies because they are most likely to simulate real-life scenarios.

The orthodontist's focus for clinical decision making should be on treatment protocols and strategies that are proven to be both efficacious and safe. To facilitate evidence-based decision making, a plethora of guidelines have been developed that aim at improving research methodology, reporting, appraisal, synthesis, and translation of scientific evidence into clinical practice. The EQUATOR Network website is an excellent source for accessing reporting guidelines.[5] Among the guidelines pertinent to orthodontics are the CONSORT (Consolidated Standards of Reporting Trials),[6] PRISMA (Preferred Reporting Items for Systematic Reviews and Meta-Analyses),[7] STROBE (Strengthening the Reporting of Observational Studies in Epidemiology),[8] MOOSE (Meta-analyses of Observational Studies in Epidemiology),[9] STARD (Standards for Reporting of Diagnostic Accuracy),[10] AMSTAR (Assessment of Multiple Systematic Reviews),[11] SORT (Strength of Recommendation Taxonomy),[12] and the Cochrane risk of bias tools.[13] These guidelines were developed and are continuously updated by evidence-based expert teams.

At the core of the Cochrane collaboration (www.cochrane. org) is a database that prepares, maintains, updates, and promotes systematic reviews. Since its inception in 1993, over 15,000 contributors from over 100 countries have been involved with the Cochrane collaboration, making it the largest organization related to this type of work.[13]

In the past, narrative reviews were the only form in which multiple studies on a particular topic were reported in peer-reviewed journals. Narrative reviews are associated with a high risk of bias because they offer no systematic, transparent method for searching for studies, including studies, appraising the studies that are included,

Table 1-1	Revised grading system for recommendations in evidence-based guidelines*
Level of evidence	**Description**
1++	High-quality meta-analyses, systematic reviews of RCTs, or RCTs with a very low risk of bias
1+	Well-conducted meta-analyses, systematic reviews of RCTs, or RCTs with a low risk of bias
1−	Meta-analyses, systematic reviews of RCTs, or RCTs with a high risk of bias
2++	High-quality systematic reviews of case-control or cohort studies *or* high-quality case-control or cohort studies with a very low risk of confounding, bias, or chance and a high probability that the relationship is causal
2+	Well-conducted case-control or cohort studies with a low risk of confounding, bias, or chance and a moderate probability that the relationship is causal
2−	Case-control or cohort studies with a high risk of confounding, bias, or chance and a significant risk that the relationship is not causal
3	Non-analytic studies (eg, case reports, case series)
4	Expert opinion

*Adapted from Harbour and Miller.[3]

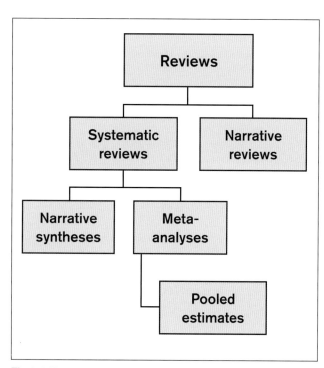

Fig 1-1 Types of reviews.

or conducting data abstraction and qualitative or quantitative (meta-analysis) synthesis (Fig 1-1). Recognition of these shortcomings opened the way to systematic reviews, which, if properly conducted, are more useful for resolving controversies and provide more accurate intervention effect estimates, thus powering the cycle of knowledge (Fig 1-2). As previously mentioned, systematic reviews require transparent and carefully controlled methodology in order

for their results to be valid because combining mismatched data may justify the well-known *GIGO (garbage in, garbage out)* label.[14] The main biases encountered with systematic reviews are selection bias (selective study inclusion), publication bias (studies with significant results are more likely to be published than studies with nonsignificant results), and heterogeneity of quality of included studies. The inclusion in systematic reviews of only a portion of the available studies, which are not sufficiently homogenous in quality, number of participants, interventions, and outcomes, impedes the generation of valid results.[13]

An important consideration is the translation of scientific evidence into clinical practice. Several tools have been developed to help clinicians make sense of and apply the published scientific evidence. One of the most recent initiatives aimed at bridging the gap between evidence and clinical practice is GRADE (Grading of Recommendations, Assessment, Development, and Evaluation),[15] which also has been incorporated into the Cochrane systematic reviews. The GRADE approach postulates that clinical practice guidelines should consider not only the quality of the available evidence but also the values and preferences of patients, its safety, and its cost[16] (Fig 1-3). This approach has only two recommendation levels: strong and weak. GRADE recognizes all outcomes and classifies them as either critical, important but not critical, or not important. The evidence is then graded for all outcomes and is assigned one of four ratings, as shown in Table 1-2. After deliberation, a recommendation—either strong or weak—is given, depending on the previous information and whether there is one approach accepted across the board (strong recommendation) or alternative options for the patient are available that he or she is likely to accept and follow. In other words, according to GRADE, based on the available evidence, if we are certain that the benefits clearly outweigh the risks and other burdens, then we are likely to

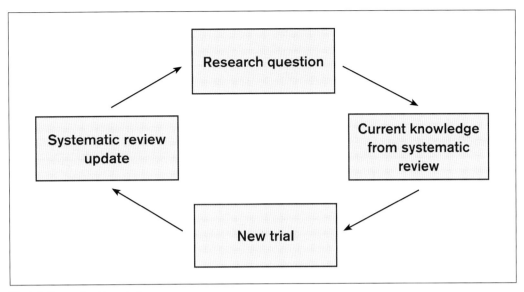

Fig 1-2 The cycle of knowledge.

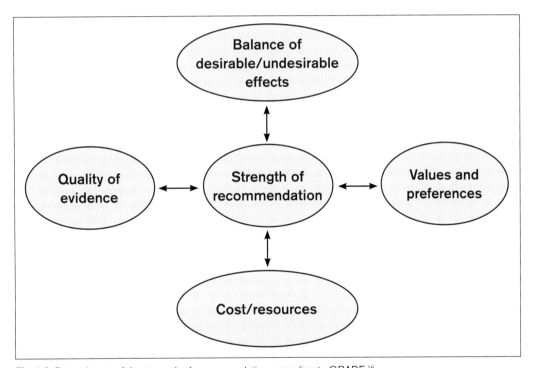

Fig 1-3 Determinants of the strength of recommendation according to GRADE.[16]

Table 1-2	Categories of quality of evidence according to GRADE[16]
Rank	**Description**
High	Further research is very unlikely to change our confidence in the estimate of effect.
Moderate	Further research is likely to have an important impact on our confidence in the estimate of effect and may change the estimate.
Low	Further research is very likely to have an important impact on our confidence in the estimate of effect and is likely to change the estimate.
Very low	Any estimate of effect is very uncertain.

make a strong recommendation regarding the intervention of interest. For example, when deciding between full orthodontic bonding and full banding from molar to molar, a strong recommendation for bonding may be given because the benefits of bonding compared with banding clearly outweigh the risks and other burdens. A myopic approach would be to consider only the fact that bands might have lower failure rates compared with brackets. A more appropriate approach would be to consider other associated outcomes, such as time required to band, patient discomfort, periodontal problems, decay under failing bands, patient esthetics, extra space required and increased probability for extractions, and cost.

However, if benefits and risks are balanced or if there is uncertainty about the benefits and risks, then a weak recommendation is likely. For example, when deciding between one-stage and two-stage orthodontic treatments in the absence of clear evidence favoring either approach, fully informed patients are likely to make different choices depending on their values and preferences. While a patient with a large overjet who is concerned about esthetics and potential damage of the maxillary front teeth might opt for early treatment, a more cost-conscious patient may choose the one-stage treatment approach.

Forrest and Miller[17] defined *evidence-based clinical practice* (EBCP) as "the integration of the best research evidence with clinical expertise and patient values." It integrates scientific or evidence-based orthodontics with patient preferences and patient autonomy, clinical or patient circumstances, and clinical experience and judgment. Pertinent to this paradigm is the dictum made by Dr Lawrence Jerrold[18]: "Never treat a stranger." Knowing the patient's chief complaint and obtaining a complete patient history (medical, dental, and social) are essential. According to Principle 1 of the American Association of Orthodontists' Principles of Ethics and Code of Professional Conduct,[19] "Members shall be dedicated to providing the highest quality orthodontic care to their patients within the bounds of the clinical aspects of the patient's conditions, and with due consideration being given to the needs and desires of the patient."

In the past, orthodontics, like medicine, was to an extent paternalistic (ie, the doctor knows what is best, and the patient should not question his or her recommendations). Currently, however, orthodontics is practiced with the requirement of obtaining informed consent from patients who are autonomous and have a right to govern their health care as long as it "does no harm." This, coupled with a multitude of information and misinformation that is easily accessible by patients, challenges orthodontists to effectively communicate with their patients.

Clinical practice requires clinical experience and judgment in formulating treatment decisions. Because there are no universally accepted protocols in orthodontic practice, orthodontists may default to what they know best or what works in their hands. At the same time, they may be required to make a choice in using a particular treatment technique without having had appropriate training, such

as the use of orthodontic temporary skeletal anchorage devices. Orthodontic manufacturers are often in a position to provide this training, but their primary motivation may be to sell product and not to provide clinicians with objective education. Perhaps the lack of science may be not only a result of the lack of orthodontist demand for it but also related to the knowledge that errors in orthodontic treatment usually do not affect patients' lives to the same extent as potential harm from drugs or major surgery. How else might we account for the lack of universally accepted treatment modalities and yet a vast array of opinions and beliefs by orthodontists?

O'Brien and Sandler[20] argue that clinical decisions are largely governed by anecdotal evidence and the training and experience of the clinician. This may lead clinicians to remember their "good cases" that are often several standard deviations from the mean. The results of orthodontic trials are often refuted by the clinician because they may challenge long-held beliefs (cognitive biases). As pointed out by Hicks and Kluemper,[21] our brains generally use two modes of reasoning: heuristic or so-called right-brain (intuitive, automatic, implicit processing) and analytic or left-brain (deliberate, rule-based, explicit processing) reasoning. Cognitive biases and errors in clinical orthodontics arise under conditions of uncertainty, leading to greater reliance on heuristic thinking and possibly predictable errors in judgment.

Given the overwhelming volume of orthodontic literature published each year, how does the busy clinician have the time to read and make sense of the available evidence and then apply it to daily practice? The recent emphasis on systematic reviews and meta-analyses may allow the practicing orthodontist better access to the totality of evidence during clinical practice. On the other hand, because systematic reviews are relatively new in the field of orthodontics and there is a lack of high-quality studies, the results are often inconclusive and necessitate further high-quality research. However, the introduction of systematic reviews in conjunction with the refinement of clinical trial methodology and the standardization of publication guidelines is likely to increase the quality of orthodontic evidence in the long term. Already the American Dental Association (ADA) has developed an evidence-based website[22] with the objective of publishing critical summaries of systematic reviews from dental research that would present the available evidence, conclusions, and clinical recommendations to the practicing dentist.

With EBCP, there is more potential to be critical and questioning of new technologies, biased views, and unsubstantiated claims. For instance, in the past, even though the straight-wire or pre-adjusted edgewise appliances achieved universal acceptance, few had scrutinized whether they had any clinical advantages or disadvantages like we have done and currently do for self-ligating brackets. Do they shorten treatment time, reduce chair time, or lessen discomfort? Are they more hygienic, and do they achieve superior treatment results? Harradine pointed out that "no study ever demonstrated that pre-adjusted edgewise appliances were superior to plain edgewise, but the former are overwhelmingly preferred for reasons that are regarded by clinicians as being self-evident and in no need of the highest order of scientific proof."[23] For example, in a retrospective study comparing the treatment results of the Roth (straight-wire) appliance and standard edgewise appliance using two occlusal indices, no significant differences were found between the two appliances.[24] In fact, despite using the Roth appliance, experienced orthodontists still found it difficult to obtain all of Andrews's Six Keys to Normal Occlusion.[25]

In summary, orthodontics has been described as an art and a science, but the art in the practice of orthodontics seems to have eclipsed the science. This chapter presented the rationale for incorporating an EBCP model into clinical practice. Also, a cursory review of the current guidelines and standards for developing and reporting RCTs, systematic reviews, and meta-analyses were described. The purpose of this book is to provide the orthodontist with an evidence-based perspective on a variety of important orthodontic topics and to challenge the practicing orthodontist to reflect on his or her current treatment protocols from an evidence-based perspective. Dr Lysle Johnston, Jr, has questioned the value our profession has for academia and science, stating that "In effect, the specialty will have to decide if academia is anything more than a front for a calling that seems to have decided that science is irrelevant . . . and to survive, more is needed than fantastic hands and great results. Easier, quicker, better: in 2011, any two will do."[26] Perhaps this book will give the practitioner more appreciation of what academics and researchers do and how evidence impacts clinical orthodontic decision making and practice.

References

1. Rinchuse DJ, Rinchuse DJ, Kandasamy S. Evidence-based versus experienced-based views on occlusion and TMD. Am J Orthod Dentofacial Orthop 2005;127:249–254.
2. Ismail AI, Bader JD. Practical science: Evidence-based dentistry in clinical practice. J Am Dent Assoc 2004;135:78–83.
3. Harbour R, Miller J. A new system for grading recommendations in evidence based guidelines. BMJ 2001;323:334–336.
4. Santoro MA, Gorrie TM (eds). Ethics and the Pharmaceutical Industry. Cambridge: Cambridge University Press, 2005.
5. Equator Network. http://www.equator-network.org. Accessed 3 February 2012.
6. Moher D, Hopewell S, Schulz KF, et al. CONSORT 2010 explanation and elaboration: Updated guidelines for reporting parallel group randomised trials. Int J Surg 2012;10:28–55.
7. Liberati A, Altman DG, Tetzlaff J, et al. The PRISMA statement for reporting systematic reviews and meta-analyses of studies that evaluate health care interventions: Explanation and elaboration. J Clin Epidemiol 2009;62:c1–e34.
8. von Elm E, Altman DG, Egger M, et al. The Strengthening the Reporting of Observational Studies in Epidemiology (STROBE) statement: Guidelines for reporting observational studies [in Spanish]. Rev Esp Salud Publica 2008;82:251–259.
9. Stroup DF, Berlin JA, Morton SC, et al. Meta-analysis of observational studies in epidemiology: A proposal for reporting. Meta-analysis Of Observational Studies in Epidemiology (MOOSE) group. JAMA 2000;283:2008–2012.
10. Bossuyt PM, Reitsma JB, Bruns DE, et al. Towards complete and accurate reporting of studies of diagnostic accuracy: The STARD initiative. The Standards for Reporting of Diagnostic Accuracy Group. BMJ 2003;326:41–44.
11. Shea BJ, Grimshaw JM, Wells GA, et al. Development of AMSTAR: A measurement tool to assess the methodological quality of systematic reviews. BMC Med Res Methodol 2007;7:10.
12. Ebell MH, Siwek J, Weiss BD, et al. Strength of recommendation taxonomy (SORT): A patient-centered approach to grading evidence in the medical literature. Am Fam Physician 2004;69:548–556.
13. Higgins JPT, Green S (eds). Cochrane Handbook for Systematic Reviews of Interventions Version 5.1.0 [updated March 2011]. The Cochrane Collaboration 2011. Available from www.cochrane-handbook.org. Accessed 3 February 2012.
14. Borenstein M, Hedges LV, Higgins JPT, Rothstein HR. Introduction to Meta-Analysis. Chichester: Wiley, 2009.
15. GRADE Working Group website. http://www.gradeworkinggroup.org. Accessed 8 February 2012.
16. Guyatt G, Oxman AD, Akl EA, et al. GRADE guidelines: 1. Introduction—GRADE evidence profiles and summary of findings tables. J Clin Epidemiol 2011;64:383–94.
17. Forrest JL, Miller SA. Evidence-Based Decision Making: A Traditional Guide for Dental Professionals. Philadelphia: Lippincott, Williams & Wilkins, 2008.
18. Jerrold L. Litigation, legislation, and ethics. When patients lie to their doctors. Am J Orthod Dentofacial Orthop 2011;139:417–418.
19. The American Association of Orthodontists. Principles of Ethics and Code of Professional Conduct, adopted May 1994, amended 2005.
20. O'Brien K, Sandler J. In the land of no evidence, is the salesman king? Am J Orthod Dentofacial Orthop 2010;138:247–249.
21. Hicks EP, Kluemper GT. Heuristic reasoning and cognitive biases: Are they hindrances to judgments and decision making in orthodontics? Am J Orthod Dentofacial Orthop 2011;139:287–304.
22. ADA Center for Evidence-Based Dentistry. http://ebd.ada.org. Accessed 3 February 2012.
23. Harradine N. Northcroft Memorial Lecture self-ligation: Past, present and future. J Orthod 2009;36:260–271.
24. Kattner PF, Schneider BJ. Comparison of Roth appliance and standard edgewise appliances treatment results. Am J Orthod Dentofacial Orthop 1993;103:24–32.
25. Andrews LF. The six keys to normal occlusion. Am J Orthod 1972;62:296–309.
26. Bowman SJ. Educator profile: An interview with Dr J Lysle E. Johnston, Jr, DDS, MS, PhD: Part 1. Orthod Pract US 2011;2:6–9.

Daniel J. Rinchuse
DMD, MS, MDS, PhD

Peter G. Miles
BDSc, MDS

CHAPTER

2 | Early Intervention: The Evidence For and Against

In this chapter, various aspects of early intervention are evaluated, and some of the controversies surrounding early intervention are examined. Topics covered include the advantages and disadvantages of early treatment, early expansion, E-space preservation, and the efficacy of the mandibular lingual arch.

Class II Early Treatment

Because of the controversy regarding early treatment and particularly early treatment of Class II malocclusion, the arguments against and for early treatment are presented separately.

The evidence against early treatment

The early randomized controlled trial (RCT) studies showing no efficacy are primarily those regarding treatment of Class II malocclusions with functional appliances such as the bionator, Fränkel, twin block, headgear, or bite plate.[1–4] These studies show a temporary effect of functional appliances in early phase I or stage 1 treatment, but the effects are lost during the second phase, so there is no net effect. Dr Lysle Johnston calls this process a "mortgage on growth,"[5] meaning that you borrow a little growth prematurely during phase I treatment, but you pay it back later. Therefore, the overall effect of the second phase of treatment is the same as that obtained in patients who received late treatment only. In other words, you cannot grow mandibles, and there is limited advantage to two-stage treatment.

However, these RCTs are best for establishing causality, and because they are generally highly controlled with a narrow perspective, they might not be suitable for general-izations. Other limitations of RCTs, particularly in regard to efficacy of Class II treatment outcomes, include the following: They are expensive and time-consuming; clinical trials with orthodontic appliances are difficult because the appliance is one of several factors affecting the outcome; blinding is rarely possible; compliance is mostly self-reported; dropouts may be the ones not responding to treatment; and results show the average effect of treatment and disregard the many phenotypes of Class II, allowing the possibility that a more refined, stratified sample would produce different results.

The Cochrane Review has provided systematic reviews of literature based on primary research[6] with very low levels of bias with regard to early intervention with functional appliances for treatment of Class II malocclusions. For Class II, division 1 malocclusions, the evidence suggests that there is no advantage to providing two-stage orthodontic treatment for children with prominent maxillary anterior teeth over one-stage treatment during early adolescence.[7] Early orthodontic treatment seems to have no real effect on the overall outcome of treatment during adolescence. There appear to be minor improvements to the skeletal pattern when functional appliances are used in early adolescence, but these changes do not appear to be clinically significant.[7]

An RCT was designed to evaluate the efficacy of early orthodontic treatment of Class II malocclusion on the incidence of incisor trauma in the initial phase of treatment in headgear or bite plane, bionator, and observation (no treatment) groups followed by a second phase with fixed appliances.[8] In this investigation, early treatment was shown not to affect the incidence of incisor injury, and the majority of injuries that occurred before or during treatment were minor. Thus, the cost-benefit ratio of orthodontic treatment primarily to prevent incisor injury may not be justified. In this study, it was reported that a significant number of the children already had some incisor trauma before early orthodontic treatment commenced, and early orthodontic treatment would need to start at the time the permanent maxillary incisors erupted in order to evaluate the effectiveness of preventing dental injuries. Therefore, further research is needed to support the claim that certain Class II malocclusions with maxillary protrusion have accident-prone profiles and warrant early orthodontic treatment from a cost-benefit perspective.

Von Bremen and Pancherz[9] showed that for Class II, division 1 malocclusion, treatment in the permanent dentition was more efficient for both duration and outcome than treatment in early or late mixed dentition. In addition, treatment with fixed appliances such as the Herbst was more efficient than treatment with functional appliances with or without preceding expansion with maxillary plates or treatment with a combination of functional and fixed appliances.

In a systematic review, Millet et al[10] concluded that "there is no evidence to recommend or discourage any type of orthodontic treatment" for children with deep bite and retroclined maxillary anterior teeth (Class II, division 2 malocclusion),[10] although this information would be useful to the orthodontist. They propose two possible treatment options: a removable (functional) appliance that fits the maxillary and mandibular teeth followed by fixed braces, or extraction (usually two maxillary teeth) followed by fixed braces. However, they point out that currently "there is no evidence to show whether orthodontic treatment without taking out teeth in children with deep bite and retroclined upper front teeth is better or worse than orthodontic treatment involving taking out teeth or no orthodontic treatment."[10]

The evidence for early treatment

In a prospective RCT, Wheeler et al[11] demonstrated that both headgear and the bionator are effective in achieving phase I treatment goals, but the headgear group experienced more relapse between the end of treatment and the end of phase I. However, some would argue that the headgear should not have been completely stopped and a maintenance protocol should have been used.

Dugoni[12] compiled a list of limitations of the early-treatment studies:

1. These studies did not provide an individualized treatment protocol for subjects. Would an individualized comprehensive approach to phase I treatment have made a difference in their findings?
2. There were limited treatment goals for phase I treatment.
3. All subjects with overjets equal to or greater than 7 mm were included.
4. However, Class II subjects with < 7 mm of overjet were not included.
5. All treated subjects had 15 months of treatment.
6. All subjects were treated with phase II comprehensive treatment.

7. Evaluation of phase II records showed that many phase I subjects did not have resolution of tooth alignment, overbite, overjet, and crossbites.

According to Dugoni's protocol, after phase I, patients should have a supervised retention period until all permanent teeth have erupted (except third molars). A maxillary removable retainer and a mandibular lingual arch are continued if indicated. Also, headgear is sometimes continued to correct a Class II molar or to prevent relapse back toward the original Class II relationship.[13] One could argue that if headgear is continued during this retention phase, then it could be considered ongoing treatment and therefore less cost-effective. The clinical trials in the United Kingdom and at the University of North Carolina clearly indicated that early Class II correction had no long-term benefit, so it would then come down to being able to identify those cases that possibly could avoid a second phase of treatment. For example, patients with mesofacial and brachyfacial Class II relationships with a reasonable alignment once the overjet is corrected (assuming it is corrected in the first phase) may be happy to accept the resulting alignment and occlusion. However, this is conjecture and ideally would be the subject of future research. Figure 2-1 shows a patient who underwent a twin block for overjet correction and improvement of the deep bite followed by a Hawley retainer with a bite plane to allow posterior settling. The patient and family decided that the alignment, which had been improved by selective trimming and adjustment of the plates, was acceptable, and no further treatment was undertaken.

The efficacy of a comprehensive early treatment (CET) protocol was evaluated in a retrospective study of 305 Class I, Class II, and a small number of Class III patients who presented between the ages of 7½ and 9½ years randomly selected from the clinical practices of three experienced orthodontists who routinely employ this treatment philosophy (Oh HS and Dugoni SA, personal communication, 2012). The main treatment employed in 191 of the subjects was fixed mechanotherapy (maxillary 2 × 4 appliance) supplemented by extraoral forces (headgear) to restrain forward growth of the maxilla combined with treatment directed at preservation of E-space. The conclusion of the study was that CET is an effective modality for fully correcting certain kinds of malocclusions for many patients and making second phase treatment more reliable for other patients. However, because there was no control group, the authors of this study acknowledged some confounders in that growth and chance are not accounted for. Instead, this study compared its treatment outcomes with RCTs at the University of North Carolina and the University of Florida that evaluated the effectiveness of early treatment with functional appliances. This study is also prone to the common limitations of retrospective research such as incomplete or missing records for 31% of the sample, which can potentially bias the result. Phase I CET was an average of 21.5 months followed by active supervision over 2.9 years, which involved continued headgear wear, a maxillary retainer adjusted for guidance of eruption, and

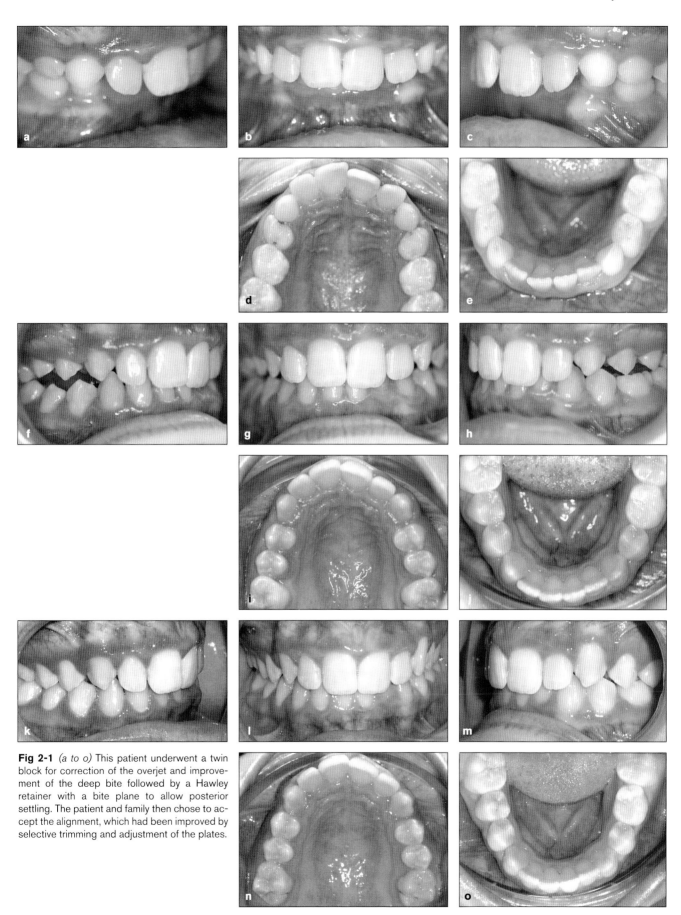

Fig 2-1 *(a to o)* This patient underwent a twin block for correction of the overjet and improvement of the deep bite followed by a Hawley retainer with a bite plane to allow posterior settling. The patient and family then chose to accept the alignment, which had been improved by selective trimming and adjustment of the plates.

a mandibular lingual arch. The authors found that 46% of the CET cohort did not undergo a fully bonded second phase of treatment. The remaining 54% had full fixed appliances with or without extractions. This second phase of treatment was an average of 1.9 years (± 0.7 years). When the sample was evaluated, the average overjet was 5.5 mm at the beginning of phase I CET, which is smaller than that of the patients included in the trials in the United Kingdom and at the University of North Carolina (overjet ≥ 7 mm). However, the goal was also different because it was aimed not only at correction of the overjet/Class II malocclusion but also at improving the alignment to limit or prevent a second phase of treatment. The overjet was reduced by 2.7 mm from an average of 5.5 mm, so at the end of CET it was 2.8 mm.

To apply this information to clinical practice, we need to consider the time and cost involved in an early phase of CET and the possible outcome of avoiding a second phase of treatment. A second phase was avoided in almost one-half of the subjects, most likely because they were happy with the outcome and did not wish to pursue further treatment. However, it is also possible that some subjects could not afford another phase of treatment or were worn out by the initial treatment and accepted the current condition.[14] Further studies of this type will hopefully help to identify subjects most likely to respond successfully to an early CET and those more successfully deferred to one-phase treatment. Another sample of this same study included deferred treatment, and the authors stated that this will be evaluated in the future. Based on these results, and until further studies are available to support or refute them, it would seem that almost one-half of mild Class II subjects who cooperate well with headgear and have mild to moderate crowding (5 mm maximum) that can be addressed with a maxillary 2 × 4 and a mandibular lingual arch but no other occlusal or eruption problems may seem suitable for such an approach. The success rate would also likely be lower than 46% because retrospective research tends to overestimate the response when compared with prospective clinical trials.

In another study evaluating early orthodontic treatment in the public health system in a Finnish population, 52% of the cohort received treatment between the ages of 8 and 15 years.[15] Subjects assessed to require treatment at age 8 years included patients with anterior or lateral crossbites, increased overjet (> 6 mm), deep overbite with palatal contact, and severe crowding. The early-treatment protocol (ages 8 to 12 years) included a quad-helix appliance for posterior crossbite, usually headgear if sagittal correction was required, and the use of palatal and lingual arches for space maintenance. During this time, the cases with a definite need for treatment as assessed by the Dental Health Component (DHC = 4 or 5) of the Index of Orthodontic Treatment Need decreased by about 20%, while those not indicated for treatment (DHC of 1 to 2) increased by about 20%. However, because there was no control group, it is unknown how many cases may have improved with no intervention. Conversely, 32% changed from the "no treatment need" category at age 8 years to the moderate or definite treatment need group by age 15 years.

Expansion

The indications and justification for maxillary expansion are the following: *(1)* restricted maxillary arch width, *(2)* mandibular functional shift, *(3)* increase in arch length in the absence of a posterior crossbite to enhance a nonextraction protocol, and *(4)* to improve a Class II relationship by provoking spontaneous mandibular growth or positioning response to maxillary expansion.[16] The latter two indications are advocated with a rapid palatal expander in the absence of a posterior crossbite. The belief is that the maxillary arch form governs the mandibular arch form so that if the maxillary arch form is changed, the mandibular arch form will also change, widening appropriately. The greatest gain in maxillary arch length is from proclination of the incisors followed by expansion of the intercanine width.[17] Therefore, reciprocal expansion of the mandibular intercanine width might result in the largest gain in arch length. If reciprocal expansion of the mandibular arch does not occur, then active expansion of the mandibular arch, possibly with a Schwarz appliance, has been recommended. Furthermore, advocates[18,19] of maxillary expansion in the absence of a crossbite believe that this may also result in correction of Class II malocclusion by "unlocking" the mandible, in the same way that having a larger shoe will free the foot to move forward. Subsequently, mandibular growth will make this initial postural change permanent.

There is no question that expansion of the arches can be achieved. However, regarding the issue of reciprocal expansion, even if it did occur in the mandibular intercanine width, stability would be a concern. Dr Hays Nance[20] was one of the first to advocate preservation of the patient's original mandibular intercanine width.[21] Gianelly[22] pointed out that any expansion of the mandibular intercanine width is not stable and that it should remain essentially unchanged during treatment.[23] A meta-analysis by Burke et al[24] of mandibular intercanine width in treatment and postretention found that mandibular intercanine width tends to expand during treatment by 0.8 to 2.0 mm and tends to constrict postretention by 1.2 to 1.9 mm, irrespective of pretreatment classification or whether treatment was extraction or nonextraction. In an evidence-based review, Gianelly[25] showed that reciprocal expansion of the mandibular intercanine width is an uncommon occurrence and that when it does occur, it is less than 1 mm.

Similarly, Bowman[26] argued that expansion in the absence of a posterior crossbite to resolve crowding is unscientific and predisposes patients to periodontal problems, pushes teeth out of the envelope of supporting alveolar bone, and is not stable. Furthermore, Bowman states that to avoid premolar extractions with 5 mm of crowding in each quadrant, 12 mm of stable expansion would be required. This amount of stable expansion has not been demonstrated in the known orthodontic literature.

Regarding the predictability and efficacy of maxillary expansion to correct a Class II malocclusion in the absence of a posterior crossbite, again Gianelly[25] argued that this

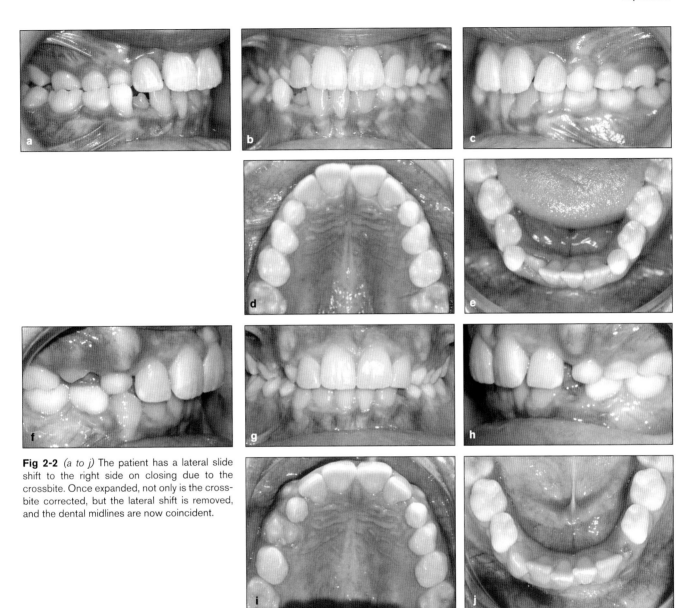

Fig 2-2 *(a to j)* The patient has a lateral slide shift to the right side on closing due to the crossbite. Once expanded, not only is the crossbite corrected, but the lateral shift is removed, and the dental midlines are now coincident.

expansion is no greater than what might occur from normal growth and development. Therefore, it is difficult to justify maxillary expansion in the absence of a posterior crossbite to correct maxillary and/or mandibular crowding or to correct a Class II malocclusion. In a small retrospective study of 13 Class II subjects who underwent expansion and then observation only, 7 of the 13 subjects underwent improvement in the Class II relationship, while this relationship actually worsened in 5 of the remaining subjects.[27] The authors concluded that their results do not support the "foot in the shoe" theory and that maxillary expansion does not predictably improve Class II dental relationships, although a larger sample size may increase the "power" and be more definitive/predictive.

In a systematic review of five papers on the long-term (more than 1 year) postretention stability of expansion,

Schiffman and Tuncay[28] demonstrated that only 2.4 mm of stable expansion remained. However, it can be argued that this amount may be no greater than what can be expected from normal growth. For example, Marshall et al[29] showed that maxillary molars upright lingually 3.3 degrees and maxillary intermolar width increased by 2.8 mm between 7.5 and 26.4 years of age. Similarly, the mandibular molars upright by 5.0 degrees, and mandibular intermolar width increases by 2.2 mm. Therefore, any maxillary expansion may not be stable beyond what might be expected from growth. This is not to say that maxillary expansion is not indicated or warranted. In the presence of a posterior crossbite with a lateral shift (Fig 2-2), the benefit of treatment appears to be obvious because if left untreated, it can possibly lead to asymmetric growth and uneven remodeling of the glenoid fossa,[30] although this does not appear

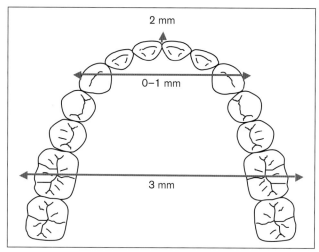

Fig 2-3 Arch expansion limits as suggested in Profitt et al.[40]

	Arch perimeter gain in the mandibular arch using various space-creation strategies for nonextraction treatment in the adult dentition*
Table 2-1	

Space-creation strategy	Arch perimeter gain
Intercanine width stable	0.0 mm
Intermolar width expansion of 3 mm	0.9 mm
Incisor advancement of 2 mm	2.2 mm
Interproximal reduction of 0.5 mm per contact from first premolar to first premolar	2.6 mm
Total	**5.7 mm**

*To keep within the potential boundaries of stability, only mild crowding of about 3 mm can be treated in the mandibular arch by expansion alone. The addition of interproximal reduction can add about 2.5 mm to this arch perimeter gain.

to make the subject any more or less prone to future temporomandibular joint disorder symptoms.[31] However, the timing of early expansion can still be debated. In their meta-analysis of the expansion literature, Schiffman and Tuncay[28] concluded that "early correction of a developing crossbite may or may not be beneficial." The Cochrane Library review of orthodontic treatment of posterior crossbites[32] stated that early treatment of posterior crossbites by removal of premature contacts appears to prevent them from being passed on to the adult dentition. When selective grinding alone is not effective, a removable or other expansion device to widen the maxillary arch will reduce the risk of a posterior crossbite being perpetuated. However, these conclusions were based on only two small studies by Thilander et al[33] and Lindner.[34]

The American Association of Orthodontists Council on Scientific Affairs (COSA) undertakes an evidence-based approach, often through systematic reviews, to provide answers to the numerous questions posed to it. Several questions in regard to expansion have been addressed. First, three questions with regard to self-ligating brackets were reviewed: (1) Does lateral expansion of the dental arch by self-ligating brackets "grow" buccal alveolar bone? (2) Is lateral expansion of the dental arch by self-ligating bracket systems comparable with lateral expansion gained by rapid maxillary expansion followed by conventional edgewise treatment? (3) Is lateral expansion of the dental arch gained by self-ligating bracket systems stable in the long term? COSA for all three questions concluded that there was a lack of peer-reviewed data available and weak and low-level evidence to support these claims.[35]

Another question posed to COSA was the efficacy of long-term (more than 1 year) stability of maxillary transverse expansion associated with fixed or removable appliances.[15] One study, a systematic review by Lagravere et al[36] that met their inclusion criteria, found that after 1 year

there remained 3.7 mm of expansion in adolescents and 4.8 mm in adults. However, this systematic review was associated with weak evidence, and there were limitations and confounders. So, again we may be back to our former premise that any stable expansion beyond normal growth may be suspect. Finally, an interesting hypothesis is that brachyfacial types might be amenable to greater expansion compared with dolichofacial types, who generally have weaker mandibular muscle forces.[37,38]

Now we can apply this information on expansion clinically. Because the mandibular arch tends to dictate the treatment protocol, and we feel we can conservatively apply a small amount of expansion and proclination to an individual case to avoid extractions, how much space can we expect to gain? (Proclining the mandibular incisors more than 95 degrees with decreased gingival thickness of less than 0.5 mm may enhance the severity and amount of recession.[39]) If we apply the limitations to arch development (Fig 2-3), as suggested by Profitt et al,[40] of 3 mm of intermolar expansion and 2 mm of mandibular incisor proclination and keep the intercanine width stable, we can then use data on perimeter gain[17] to calculate the space created (Table 2-1). Keeping the canines stable adds no space, while expanding the intermolar width adds only 0.9 mm of arch perimeter. The greatest increase to arch perimeter gain is the proclination or flaring of incisors with 2 mm of advancement, adding 2.2 mm of space. Altogether, this arch development has added 3.1 mm of arch perimeter. To improve the arch perimeter gain, we could consider adding interproximal reduction. By stripping 0.5 mm per contact from first premolar to first premolar (seven contacts), we would gain an additional 3.5 mm. However, it is unlikely that 100% of this space would be utilized because of some anchorage loss, so we will assume we would be able to use ¾ of this, leaving 2.6 mm of additional arch perimeter gain. In total then, we have now been able to treat

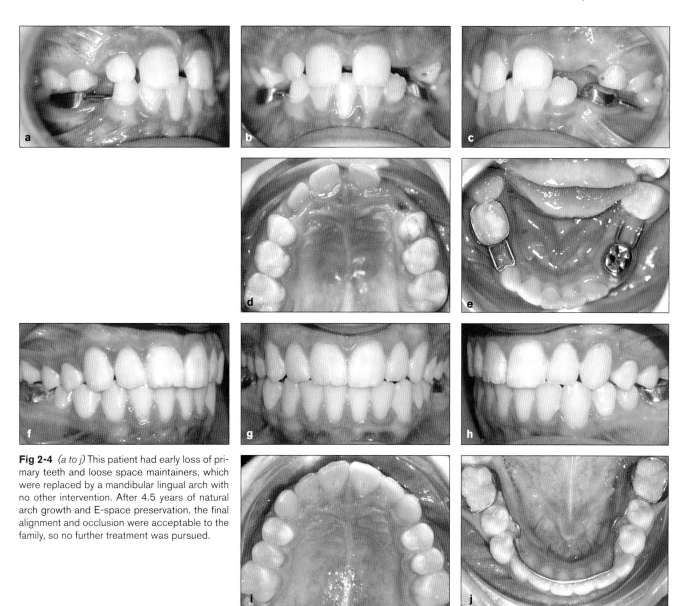

Fig 2-4 *(a to j)* This patient had early loss of primary teeth and loose space maintainers, which were replaced by a mandibular lingual arch with no other intervention. After 4.5 years of natural arch growth and E-space preservation. the final alignment and occlusion were acceptable to the family, so no further treatment was pursued.

5.7 mm of crowding in the mandibular arch with minimal potential impact on the equilibrium of the enveloping soft tissue forces and arch stability. These numbers can be modified to some extent with more or less interproximal reduction and/or the preservation of mandibular E-space, but the principal holds as to the limits achievable.

E-Space Preservation

A more conservative nonextraction approach for resolution of crowding is arch length preservation by the use of *leeway space*, or *E-space* (primary second molars) (Fig 2-4). *Leeway space* is the space available due to the differences in mesiodistal widths of the primary canine, first

molar, and second molar compared with the widths of the permanent successors (canine and first and second premolars). Therefore, if leeway space can be preserved, then about 4 to 5 mm of space/arch length in the maxillary and mandibular arches may be gained. The preservation of E-space is the best way to manage tooth size–arch length discrepancies. Therefore, with proper management of E-space in the late mixed dentition (at roughly 10½ years of age), approximately 76% of Class I and Class II malocclusions with good facial balance and 4 to 5 mm of crowding can be resolved without extractions. At that time, the orthodontist can decide whether nonextraction or extraction is preferred. The treatment can be completed in one phase within a reasonable time frame.[41,42] Currently, this protocol probably has the most evidence to support its utility.[43,44] According to Gianelly[42], approximately 10% of orthodon-

Table 2-2	Arch perimeter gain in the mandibular arch using various space-creation strategies for nonextraction treatment with E-space management during early treatment*
Space-creation strategy	**Arch perimeter gain**
Preservation of E-space	4.0 mm
Intercanine width stable	0.0 mm
Intermolar width expansion of 3 mm	0.9 mm
Incisor advancement of 1 mm	1.0 mm
Interproximal reduction of 0.5 mm per contact from first premolar to first premolar	2.6 mm
Total perimeter gain	**8.5 mm**

*By the addition of E-space management, a significantly greater amount of crowding can be potentially treated in the mandibular arch in a nonextraction manner. It is interesting to note in this scenario that E-space maintenance is the main factor in managing crowding, while arch expansion is the least effective strategy.

tic cases are truly phase I. Serial extractions and lingual arches are passive treatments and therefore not active mechanotherapy. For that reason, they are not included in the following phase I treatments:

- Incisor crossbites or crossbites complicated by a functional shift of the mandible
- Class III malocclusions, particularly those involving maxillary retrognathism
- Excessively protrusive and proclined maxillary incisors (accident-prone profile)
- Habits such as finger sucking

Efficacy of the Mandibular Lingual Arch

In orthodontics, the mandibular lingual arch (also known as *lower lingual arch* [LLA]) has been used for various reasons such as maintenance of arch perimeter/length, prevention of mesial tipping and drifting of permanent mandibular first molars, and as a space maintainer after premature loss of primary teeth. One possible iatrogenic effect of an LLA is proclination of the mandibular incisors by the tongue. In an RCT[45] evaluating the efficacy of an LLA to maintain arch length, comparisons were made among three groups: *(1)* control group, *(2)* LLA made of 0.9-mm stainless steel (SS), and *(3)* LLA made of 1.25-mm SS. The mandibular incisors proclined and moved forward, and there was space loss of the primary mandibular second molars in both treatment groups. Furthermore, the 0.9-mm SS group showed greater arch length preservation than the 1.25-mm SS group. On the other hand, a systematic review by Viglianisi[46] found the LLA to be effective for controlling mesial movement of molars and lingual tipping of incisors. However, only two studies[47,48] met the inclusion and exclusion criteria for this systematic review.

It also can be argued that E-space management may be more appropriate for brachyfacial patients than for doli-

chofacial patients, who may be more appropriately treated with extractions.[36] For instance, Vaden[49] is inclined toward extraction of premolars in most dolichofacial patients. This difference in response to an LLA in different facial types is supported by Fichera et al,[50] who found that arch length was preserved in dolichofacial types but with slight mandibular incisor advancement of 0.5 mm and mesial migration of the molars of 0.5 mm compared with meso- and brachyfacial types. Based on the limited evidence, the clinical significance of this difference is dubious.

We can then include this additional E-space into our calculation for resolving mandibular arch crowding (Table 2-2), but we need to consider that the LLA may have resulted in some incisor proclination already. Therefore, we will reduce the additional proclination during treatment in the adult dentition to only 1 mm, which adds only 1 mm of arch perimeter according to Germane et al.[17] We can now see that we can potentially resolve up to 8.5 mm of mandibular arch crowding, when deemed appropriate, in a nonextraction and theoretically stable manner by *(1)* preserving E-space, *(2)* expanding the intermolar width by 3 mm, *(3)* advancing the incisors by an additional 1 mm, and *(4)* performing 0.5 mm of interproximal reduction from first premolar to first premolar. Ideally, this approach would be the subject of future research.

Of all the space-gaining strategies discussed, the preservation of mandibular arch E-space is the most effective, but is it without risks? When the second primary molar is lost, there is some mesial drift of the mandibular permanent first molar, which potentially creates additional space for the second permanent molar to erupt. A study evaluating 200 patients treated with a nonextraction protocol including E-space maintenance with an LLA found that 8.5% of the mandibular second molars became impacted.[51] Because there was no control group, the authors of the study compared their results with literature-reported rates of impaction at 0.2% to 2.3%. The authors concluded that preservation of E-space results in a significant increase in the risk of an impacted mandibular second molar occurring. Potential risk factors for mesially impacted mandibular second molars could include genetic and racial predisposition as well as a lack of space between the first molar and the ascending ramus.[52] The risk of impaction must then be weighed against the potential space gain, and hopefully future research will give better guides in selecting those patients most suitable for space preservation. When impaction does occur, one retrospective study suggests that the exposure and uprighting of the second molar has a significantly higher chance of success (71%) versus extraction and allowing the third molar tooth to replace it (11%).[53]

Conclusion

In this chapter, we discussed the controversy regarding early intervention for the management of Class II malocclusions, expansion and the controversy of expansion in the absence of a posterior crossbite to gain arch length and provoke mandibular advancement in Class II patients, the efficacy of a mandibular lingual arch, and the rationale of E-space preservation as a strategy to resolve crowding and protrusion in mild to moderate Class I and Class II malocclusions.

With a sense of equipoise, balance between the arguments for and against early treatment, the early-treatment studies with regard to functional appliances are not at odds with the argument for early treatment as proposed by Dugoni and Oh et al (personal communication, 2012). Despite the arguments appearing as conflicting views, the differences are not real differences at all because they have approached the interest in early treatment from two varying frames of references. For instance, the early-treatment studies at the University of North Carolina and the University of Florida had specific treatment goals and research questions, which mainly addressed whether or not functional appliances could modify growth and whether or not their efficacy could result in shorter and more effective and efficient phase II outcomes. On the other hand, the primary goal of the University of the Pacific study by Oh et al was the evaluation of early correction of malocclusions using fixed mechanotherapy with extraoral forces to restrain forward growth of the maxilla, distalize the dentition, and if needed preserve the E-space (personal communication, 2012). Also, this protocol advocated individualized treatment and a supervised retention protocol between phases.

As clinicians, our experiences can be biased by our observations of what "works in our hands" regarding early orthodontic intervention for Class II malocclusions. High-quality evidence demonstrates that early treatment with functional appliances has little efficacy when compared with later treatment. However, fixed mechanotherapy with specific treatment goals may have merit for selected patients. The difficult part then becomes identifying those individuals that may benefit sufficiently from an initial early phase of treatment that can either eliminate or substantially simplify a second phase of treatment. As retrospective research tends to overestimate the actual efficacy of a treat-

ment, based on the 15% avoidance of phase II treatment in the early-treatment group in the UK study,[54] the 20% improvement in the Finnish study,[14] and the 46% avoidance in selected cases in the University of the Pacific study,[13] it may be possible that perhaps up to 10% to 20% of cases could benefit from an early phase of treatment involving a mandibular holding arch, limited alignment of the anterior dentition, and some headgear wear. These could include the mild to moderate crowded Class I and milder Class II cases, but the cost-effectiveness and predictability would need to be assessed in more detail in future research.

Summary points

- Functional appliances may have little utility in an initial phase I treatment protocol in most cases; however, fixed appliances with an individualized treatment protocol for selected patients, followed by a supervised retention period, may be justified but requires further research.
- It may be difficult to defend the concept of maxillary expansion in the absence of a posterior crossbite to alleviate moderate to severe crowding in both the maxilla and mandible and to correct Class II malocclusions.
- It may be difficult to justify maxillary expansion as an alternative to extraction treatment to resolve moderate to severe crowding considering that the stability of this expansion 1-year posttreatment is suspect, perhaps only 2 to 3 mm of interpremolar and intermolar expansion remains stable, and the space gain is modest.
- E-space preservation to eliminate extractions in approximately 76% of Class I and Class II patients with pleasing facial profiles with mild to moderate crowding appears to have merit. However, proper diagnosis and close observation should be done to prevent impaction of the mandibular permanent second molars.
- There is still controversy surrounding and weak evidence to support the concept that an LLA is effective for controlling mesial movement of molars and lingual tipping of incisors.

References

1. Keeling SD, Wheeler TT, King GJ, et al. Anteroposterior skeletal and dental changes after early Class II treatment with bionators and headgear. Am J Orthod Dentofacial Orthop 1998;113:40–50.
2. Ghafari J, Shofer FS, Jacobsson-Hunt U, Markowitz DI, Laster LL. Headgear versus functional regulator in the early treatment of Class II, division 1 malocclusion: A randomized clinical trial. Am J Orthod Dentofacial Orthop 1998;113:51–61.
3. Tulloch JF, Phillips C, Proffit WR. Benefits of early Class II treatment: Progress report of a two-phase randomized clinical trial. Am J Orthod Dentofacial Orthop 1998;113:62–72.
4. O'Brien K, Wright J, Conboy F, et al. Effectiveness of early orthodontic treatment with the Twin-block appliance: A multicenter, randomized, controlled trial. Part 1: Dental and skeletal effects. Am J Orthod Dentofacial Orthop 2003;124:234–243.
5. Johnston LE Jr. Functional appliances: A mortgage on mandibular position. Aust Orthod J 1996;14:154–157.

6. Niederman R, Clarkson J, Richards D. The Affordable Care Act and evidence-based care. J Am Dent Assoc 2011;142:364–367.

7. Harrison JE, O'Brien KD, Worthington HV. Orthodontic treatment of prominent upper front teeth in children. Cochrane Database Syst Rev 2007;(4):CD003452.

8. Chen DR, McGorray SP, Dolce C, Wheeler TT. Effect of early Class II treatment on the incidence of incisor trauma. Am J Orthod Dentofacial Orthop 2011;140:e155–e160.

9. Von Bremen J, Pancherz H. Efficiency of early and late Class II division 1 treatment. Am J Orthod Dentofacial Orthop 2002;121:31–37.

10. Millet DT, Cunninham SJ, O'Brien KD, Benson P, Williams A, de Oliveira CM. Orthodontic treatment of deep bite and retroclined upper front teeth in children. Cochrane Database Syst Rev 2006;(4):CD005972.

11. Wheeler TT, McGorray SP, Dolce C, Taylor MG, King GJ. Effectiveness of early treatment of Class II malocclusion. Am J Orthod Dentofacial Orthop 2002;121:9–17.

12. Dugoni SA. When to treat? A new perspective on early treatment. Lecture Summaries. http://www.cdabo.org/lectures.asp. Accessed 8 February 2012.

13. Dugoni S, Aubert M, Baumrind S. Differential diagnosis and treatment planning for early mixed dentition malocclusions. Am J Orthod Dentofacial Orthop 2006;129:580–581.

14. Hsieh T, Pinskaya Y, Roberts WE. Assessment of orthodontic treatment outcomes: Early treatment versus late treatment. Angle Orthod 2005;75:162–170.

15. Kerosuo H, Väkiparta M, Nyström M, Heikinheimo K. The seven-year outcome of an early orthodontic treatment strategy. J Dent Res 2008;87:584–588.

16. Marshall S, English JD Jr, Huang GJ, et al. Ask us. Long-term stability of maxillary expansion. Am J Orthod Dentofacial Orthop 2008;133:780–781.

17. Germane N, Lindauer SJ, Rubenstein LK, Revere JH Jr, Isaacson RJ. Increase in arch perimeter due orthodontic expansion. Am J Orthod Dentofacial Orthop 1991;100:421–427.

18. McNamara JA Jr. Early intervention in the transverse dimension: Is it worth the effort? Am J Orthod Dentofacial Orthop 2002;121:572–574.

19. McNamara JA Jr, Brudon WL. Orthodontics and dentofacial orthopedics. Ann Arbor, MI: Needham, 2001.

20. Nance HN. The limitations of orthodontic treatment: Mixed dentition diagnosis and treatment. Am J Orthod 1947;33:177–223.

21. Wahl N. Orthodontics in 3 millennia. Chapter 6: More early 20th-century appliances and the extraction controversy. Am J Orthod Dentofacial Orthop 2005;128:795–800.

22. Gianelly A. Bidimensional Technique: Theory and Practice. Islandia, NY: GAC International, 2000.

23. Gianelly A. Evidence-based therapy: An orthodontic dilemma. Am J Orthod Dentofacial Orthop 2006;129:596–598.

24. Burke SP, Silveira AM, Goldsmith LJ, Yancey JM, Stewart AV, Scarfe WC. A meta-analysis of mandibular intercanine width in treatment and postretention. Angle Orthod 1998;68:53–60.

25. Gianelly A. Rapid palatal expansion in the absence of crossbites: Added value? Am J Orthod Dentofacial Orthop 2003;124:362–365.

26. Bowman SJ. More than lip service: Facial esthetics in orthodontics. J Am Dent Assoc 1999;130:1173–1181.

27. Volk T, Sadowsky C, BeGole EA, Boice P. Rapid palatal expansion for spontaneous Class II correction. Am J Orthod Dentofacial Orthop 2010;137:310–315.

28. Schiffman PH, Tuncay OC. Maxillary expansion: A meta analysis. Clin Orthod Res 2001;4:86–96.

29. Marshall S, Dawson D, Southard KA, Lee AN, Casko JS, Southard TE. Transverse molar movements during growth. Am J Orthod Dentofacial Orthop 2003;124:615–624.

30. Pirttiniemi P, Kantomaa T, Lahtela P. Relationship between craniofacial and condyle path asymmetry in unilateral cross-bite patients. Eur J Orthod 1990;12:408–413.

31. Tullberg M, Tsarapatsani P, Huggare J, Kopp S. Long-term follow-up of early treatment of unilateral forced posterior crossbite with regard to temporomandibular disorders and associated symptoms. Acta Odontol Scand 2001;59:280–284.

32. Harrison JE, Ashby D. Orthodontic treatment for posterior cross-bites. Cochrane Database Syst Rev 2001;(1):CD000979.

33. Thilander B, Wahlund S, Lennartsson B. The effect of early interceptive treatment in children with posterior cross-bite. Eur J Orthod 1984;6:25–34.

34. Lindner A. Longitudinal study on the effect of early interceptive treatment in 4-year-old children with unilateral cross-bite. Scand J Dent Res 1989;97:432–438.

35. Marshall SD, Currier GF, Hatch NE, et al. Ask us. Self-ligating bracket claims. Am J Orthod Dentofacial Orthop 2010;138:128–131.

36. Lagravere MO, Major PW, Flores-Mir C. Long-term dental arch changes with rapid maxillary expansion: A systematic review. Angle Orthod 2005;75:155–161.

37. Zaher AR, Bishara SE, Jakobsen JR. Posttreatment changes in different facial types. Angle Orthod 1994;64:425–436.

38. Pepicelli A, Woods M, Briggs C. The mandibular muscles and their importance in orthodontics: A contemporary review. Am J Orthod Dentofacial Orthop 2005;128:774–780.

39. Burrow SJ. To extract or not to extract: A diagnostic decision, not a marketing decision. Am J Orthod Dentofacial Orthop 2008;133:341–342.

40. Profitt W, Fields Jr HW, Sarver DM. Contemporary Orthodontics. St Louis: Mosby, 2006:282.

41. Gianelly AA. Leeway space and the resolution of crowding in the mixed dentition. Semin Orthod 1995;1:188–194.

42. Gianelly A. Timing of treatment. Pract Rev Orthod 1996;8(3).

43. Little RM. Stability and relapse: Early treatment of arch length deficiency. Am J Orthod Dentofacial Orthop 2002;121:578–581.

44. Dugoni S, Lee J, Varela J, Dugoni AA. Early mixed dentition treatment: Postretention evaluation of stability and relapse. Angle Orthod 1995;65:311–320.

45. Owais AI, Rousan ME, Badran SA, Abu Alhaija ES. Effectiveness of a lower lingual arch as a space holding device. Eur J Orthod 2011;33:37–42.

46. Viglianisi A. Effects of lingual arch used as space maintainer on mandibular arch dimension: A systematic review. Am J Orthod Dentofacial Orthop 2010;138:382.e1–382.e4.

47. Villalobos FJ, Sinha PK, Nanda RS. Longitudinal assessment of vertical and sagittal control in the mandibular arch by the mandibular fixed lingual arch. Am J Orthod Dentofacial Orthop 2000;118:366–370.

48. Rebellato J, Lindauer SJ, Rubenstein LK, Isaacson RJ, Davidovitch M, Vroom K. Lower arch perimeter preservation using the lingual arch. Am J Orthod Dentofacial Orthop 1997;112:449–456.

49. Vaden JL. Nonsurgical treatment of the patient with vertical discrepancy. Am J Orthod Dentofacial Orthop 1998;113:567–582.

50. Fichera G, Greco M, Leonardi R. Effectiveness of the passive lingual arch for E space maintenance in subjects with anterior or posterior rotation of the mandible: A retrospective study. Med Princ Pract 2011;20:165–170.

51. Sonis A, Ackerman M. E-space preservation: Is there a relationship to mandibular second molar impaction? Angle Orthod 2011;81:1045–1049.

52. Shapira Y, Finkelstein T, Shpack N, Lai YH, Kuftinec MM, Vardimon A. Mandibular second molar impaction. Part I: Genetic traits and characteristics. Am J Orthod Dentofacial Orthop 2011;140:32–37.

53. Magnusson C, Kjellberg H. Impaction and retention of second molars: Diagnosis, treatment and outcome. A retrospective follow-up study. Angle Orthod 2009;79:422–427.

54. O'Brien K, Wright J, Conboy F, et al. Early treatment for Class II Division 1 malocclusion with the Twin-block appliance: A multicenter, randomized, controlled trial. Am J Orthod Dentofacial Orthop 2009;135:573–579.

Peter G. Miles
BDSc, MDS

Theodore Eliades
DDS, MS, Dr Med, PhD

Nikolaos Pandis
DDS, MS, Dr med dent, MSc

CHAPTER

3 | Bonding and Adhesives in Orthodontics

Introduction

Treatment efficiency in orthodontics relies on several factors, including accurate bracket positioning and effective bonding of brackets to the enamel. The advent of direct bonding of orthodontic attachments to the etched enamel surface as first described by Newman[1] was a major advance in orthodontic treatment. He described a technique using 40% phosphoric acid for 60 seconds, and this technique remained basically unchanged for another 25 years. Shorter etch times were later examined in clinical trials, and no significant difference in bond failure rates were found between 60-second and 15-second etch times.[2,3] Hence, over time we have seen a reduction in practitioner acid etch times from 60 seconds in 1986 to an average of 30 seconds by 1996, which has remained the same up to 2008.[4] Despite this reduction in etch times, the reported average bond failure in orthodontic offices has remained at 5%; however, this data comes from a survey,[4] so it may well underestimate the true breakage rate. Bracket debonding during treatment is inconvenient and costly to both the orthodontist and the patient. In our own practices, our goal is to have as low a bond failure risk as possible, so it is preferable to be 5% or lower. As demonstrated in Table 3-1, a practice with an average of 250 case starts per year and an average treatment time of 24 months can save 4 repairs per day (or 776 per year) if the bond failure risk can be reduced from 10% to 2%.

So what steps should we take and what information can we gather from the literature to help us in such a basic skill as the bonding of orthodontic brackets? Some may choose to base their choice of adhesive or primer on the myriad of laboratory studies that have been published over the years. However, there are a number of problems with this approach. The American Dental Association Council on Dental Materials reported that most laboratory bonding studies cannot predict the clinical behavior of the adhesives tested.[5] Some of the limitations of in vitro studies include that most in vitro studies are conducted within a short time after bonding (often within 24 hours), so the potential influence of the oral environment on the bonding material cannot be taken into account. Thermocycling cannot replicate the effects of bond degradation by saliva, and the loading rates are slow compared with chewing. Bond strength can also be affected clinically by pH and microbial degradation.[6,7] In a systematic review of bond studies, many factors were found to play a significant role in the final bond strength measured in laboratory studies.[8] For example, water storage can decrease bond strength by an average 10.7 MPa, each second of curing time with a halogen light can increase bond strength by 0.077 MPa, and each millimeter per minute of greater crosshead speed of the Instron machine increases bond strength by 1.3 MPa. The authors of the review concluded that many in vitro studies fail to report test conditions that could significantly affect the outcome.[8]

Some clinicians will judge or select an adhesive from a laboratory study based on its mean or median bond strength without also considering the variation. For example, Fig 3-1 shows two curves representing bond strengths in MPa for two adhesives, both having the same mean bond strength of 13 MPa, which is considered adequate for the orthodontic bonding of brackets. However, if we pick an arbitrary bond strength of about 8 MPa, as suggested by Reynolds[9] as the minimum (6 to 8 MPa) required bond strength to survive clinically, we can see that the adhesive represented by the blue curve has substantially fewer brackets that could potentially fail compared with the adhesive represented by the pink curve. For these reasons, even a well-controlled, statistically valid laboratory study of bond strength should merely serve as a precursor to a controlled clinical investigation. It is important for the clinician to realize that most bond strength tests are

Table 3-1	Failure rates and their respective number of repairs per day and year*	
Failure rate (%)	Repairs per day	Repairs per year
10	5.3	970
5	2.6	485
2	1.1	194

*For a practice with 250 new case starts per year bonded back to the first molars (with 15% involving extraction of four teeth), with an average treatment time of 24 months, and assuming a 4-day work week for 46 weeks of the year.

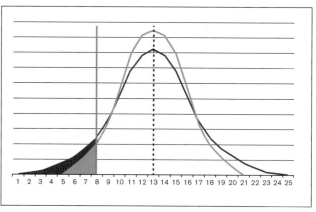

Fig 3-1 These two curves represent two adhesives with an identical mean bond strength of 13 MPa, so both would appear clinically suitable. However, the pink adhesive curve has a greater range, resulting in more brackets with lower bond strengths (< 8 MPa) and a greater potential for more brackets to debond clinically.

performed in vitro and that intraoral bond strengths may not be as high as those recorded in the laboratory setting.[10] For example, in a study comparing in vitro bond strength with in vivo bond strength, the mean bond strength values of the in vivo groups were approximately 40% lower than those for the in vitro groups.[11] For all of these reasons, this chapter emphasizes the importance of clinical studies and draws support from laboratory studies.

Pumice Prophylaxis

Many procedures in medicine and dentistry are performed in a certain way because that is how they were initially described. As already mentioned, for many years acid etching was performed for 60 seconds because that is how it was first used to bond attachments, but later it was discovered that etching for as little as 15 seconds is just as effective, although etching for 20 seconds may be more prudent to allow for variation in enamel type and operator error. Similarly, it has been accepted that pumice prophylaxis is required prior to the acid etching of enamel, but is this a necessary step?

In a clinical investigation of 614 directly bonded brackets randomly assigned to pumice or no pumice prophylaxis, no significant difference was found in the failure of attachments.[12] In a split-mouth study involving 85 patients, no significant difference was found in the rate of bond failure when pumicing was omitted.[13] Another clinical trial in 60 patients over an 18-month observation period also found no difference in bond failure (P = 0.67).[14] However, when similar studies were performed using self-etching primers (SEPs), increased bond failure probabilities ranging from 2.6 to 4.75 times higher were recorded if pumice prophy-

laxis was omitted.[15,16] Pandis and Eliades[17] suggested that a clean surface was more important for SEPs because the chalky appearance of enamel that results from traditional etching, signaling that the surface is well prepared, is not visible clinically when using an SEP.

Self-Etching Primers

SEPs have been increasing in popularity since their introduction. According to a 2008 survey,[4] approximately 30% of orthodontists in the United States use SEPs. There are many different versions of SEPs available, and several laboratory studies suggest that they are suitable for clinical use; however, the best available clinical evidence is discussed here.

A split-mouth clinical trial in 37 patients using Transbond Plus SEP (3M Unitek) versus the two-step conventional etch and prime (CEP) technique and Transbond XT Primer (3M Unitek) found identical risks of failure (0.6%) over 6 months.[18] In contrast, another clinical trial of two different SEPs used with Transbond XT Adhesive (3M Unitek) found a marked difference between the Transbond Plus SEP, exhibiting about a 1% failure risk, and the One-Step SEP (Reliance), which demonstrated an 8.1% failure risk.[17] Because the same adhesive had been used with both primers, the authors concluded that clinicians should be careful not to mix different brands of primers and adhesives. In support of this conclusion, another prospective randomized controlled trial (RCT) comparing Transbond Plus SEP and Clearfil Protect Bond (Kuraray) when bonding brackets with Transbond XT found 4.4 times as many failures with the Clearfil (P = 0.002).[19] Therefore, it seems that, at least when used with the Transbond XT Adhesive, the Transbond Plus SEP is a suitable alternative to the conventional acid etching with Transbond XT primer. More clinical trials are necessary to ensure that this applies to other primers and their matched adhesives.

SEPs may save some clinical time compared with the CEP technique. One study found that an SEP took 25 seconds less per bracket than the CEP technique; in a patient requiring 20 brackets to be bonded, that means an average reduction in clinical chairside time of about 8.5 minutes.[20] In this study, the times were averaged per quadrant, and the acid etch times were not recorded (eg, 20 seconds versus 60 seconds). In addition, the time to pumice the teeth prior to bonding, which is not routinely required for conventional etching, was not included in this study. The reported 8.5 minutes of saved time seems disproportionally large when compared with a paper describing indirect bonding in which a total of 8 minutes was required to conventionally etch, prime, place the indirect bonding trays, and light cure all brackets in both arches.[21] Considering that each tooth with an SEP must be pumiced and then rubbed with the conditioner for approximately 3 seconds prior to bonding, this 8.5 minutes of saved time seems to be not much less than the time required to etch, rinse, and bond when using a conventional primer. However, when bonding an individual tooth, particularly in a fidgety patient or in a moisture-prone area, the time saving may be advantageous. Efficiency in terms of time may then come down to personal preference, what procedures staff can perform, and how this staff is utilized in an individual office.

Saliva Contamination

When bonding orthodontic attachments, clinicians make every effort to avoid saliva contamination to protect the etched enamel surface. It may be useful to consider the use of an antisialogogue such as atropine sulfate prior to bracket placement. In an RCT, atropine sulfate was found to be an acceptable premedication by most patients (76%), and it had no effect on the bracket survival rate over 12 months.[22] A more recent systematic review on the effect of antisialogogues in dentistry found that there is evidence that antisialogogues work and inconclusive evidence that they reduce bond failure; the authors concluded that the use of antisialogogues for dental procedures in general is questionable.[23] The use of atropine sulfate on a routine basis therefore seems unwarranted.

In vitro laboratory research has suggested that after conventional etching, adequate mean shear bond strengths may still be maintained with saliva contamination after application of a hydrophobic or hydrophilic primer.[24,25] However, bond strengths improved if the surface was dried and a second coat of primer was applied. When using the CEP technique, it may be suitable to dry and reapply primer if only minimal saliva contamination has occurred, but

unfortunately no clinical research exists to validate these laboratory studies.

However, a clinical study evaluating the effect of saliva contamination on the failure of brackets etched with Transbond Plus SEP concluded that saliva contamination results in a higher bond failure risk, especially when it occurs prior to the application of an SEP. The study involved 46 patients in three groups—deliberate saliva contamination prior to application of an SEP, deliberate saliva contamination after application of an SEP, and a control group with no saliva contamination—with a total of 531 brackets being placed and observed over a minimum 6-month observation period.[26] Although there was no statistically significant difference in bond failure risk ($P = 0.11$) between the groups, the brackets of the teeth that underwent saliva contamination before SEP application had a higher failure risk (10.5%) compared with both the control group (6.1%) and the group who underwent saliva contamination after SEP application (4.4%). The risk of bond failure was almost twice that of the contamination after group, so this could have been a Type II error in that an inadequate sample size resulted in a lack of power and that a larger sample may have found a statistically significant difference.

The results of laboratory studies with SEPs vary. One found no difference in bond failure with saliva contamination,[27] others found a reduction in bond strength when the saliva was contaminated before SEP application,[28,29] while others found a reduction when the saliva was contaminated after SEP application.[29,30] It is of interest to note that when teeth were contaminated with blood, a significant reduction in shear bond strength was observed, independent of when the contamination occurred during the bonding process.[31]

The results of these laboratory studies indicate that following blood contamination, it is advisable to reinitiate the procedure rather than apply a new coat of the primer or SEP. Small amounts of saliva contamination may be tolerated, but it is prudent to reinitiate the bonding sequence if there is excessive saliva contamination before or after the application of an SEP.[10]

Bonding to Bleached Enamel

The vital bleaching of enamel is now a relatively common procedure and readily available in many forms. But does recent bleaching of teeth affect bond strength? Laboratory studies have varied in their findings, but this variance seems to be related to the amount of time between bleaching and bonding. When brackets were bonded immediately after at-home bleaching, most laboratory studies found that bond strength was reduced, but when there was a delay of 24 hours or more, the bond strength was not significantly affected.[32–36] However, another in vitro study using a 35% hydrogen bleaching agent found no significant difference in shear bond strength.[37]

In a split-mouth clinical trial evaluating the bracket survival rate of brackets bonded to bleached and unbleached teeth, a significantly higher rate of bond failure was found with bleached teeth (16.6%) compared with unbleached teeth (1.8%) over 6 months. Brackets bonded within 24 hours of bleaching resulted in a significantly higher clinical failure rate (14.5%) compared with those bonded after 3 weeks (2.1%). This study used Transbond Plus SEP, so the results may not be transferable to the CEP technique.[38]

Based on the limited clinical evidence, it currently seems prudent for patients to cease dental bleaching 3 weeks prior to the bonding of orthodontic attachments when using an SEP. There is no clinical data for using conventional etching and primers, but the laboratory data suggests that a delay of 24 hours may be adequate; however, further clinical research is required to confirm this.

Microetching/Air Abrasion

Bond failure risks vary between studies and between different regions of the mouth, with most failures usually reported on the mandibular posterior teeth.[4] Bond failure occurs more frequently on the second premolars than on the anterior teeth, and an even higher number of failures has been reported on the molars.[2,39] A total failure risk of 14.8% has been reported for posterior teeth, with first and second molars failing 9.7% and 20% of the time, respectively.[40] This study also reported that mandibular molars had more bond failures (21%) than maxillary molars (7.5%). Similar bond failure risks, with more failures occurring on the mandibular molars than on the maxillary molars, have been reported by others.[41,42]

Apart from pumice prophylaxis, enamel can also be prepared for bonding by air abrasion or microetching of the surface. Laboratory research demonstrates that acid-etched enamel surfaces have higher bond strengths than air-abraded surfaces that were not acid etched.[43–45] Therefore, microetching of enamel without acid etching is not recommended clinically. Microetching alone is unsuitable for routine enamel conditioning, but, if used prior to acid etching, it may result in higher bond strengths.

Two clinical trials by the same group reported an overall bond failure risk of 14.8% on the posterior mandibular teeth when an SEP was used and a lower failure risk of 8% when all of the teeth were air abraded prior to etching.[40,46] However, the observation period was shorter in the latter study (15 months versus 26 months), so it is difficult to say whether the microetching or the length of the observation period was more influential on the outcome. The possibility that time was more influential is supported by another clinical trial, which reported an increasing bond failure risk over time: 3.0%, 5.3%, and 14.8% at 1, 6, and 12 months, respectively.[47]

To evaluate the effect of microetching prior to acid etching, a split-mouth clinical trial recorded the bond failure of 384 mandibular premolars and first molars in a sample of 64 patients.[48] No pumice prophylaxis was used. One side was microetched prior to acid etching while the other side was conventionally acid etched only. During the 6-month observation period, two brackets (1%) came loose on the microetched/acid-etched enamel side, and four bonds (2.1%) failed on the conventionally acid-etched side. This difference was not clinically or statistically significant ($P = 0.41$). The study therefore concluded that the addition of microetching prior to acid etching does not result in fewer bond failures during the first 6 months of treatment. This result is supported by another split-mouth clinical trial in which orthodontic attachments were bonded to severely fluorosed enamel, which reported that there was no advantage in microetching fluorosed enamel when using an adhesion promoter.[49]

Bonding to Porcelain/Ceramic

With many adults now seeking orthodontic treatment, there is sometimes the requirement of bonding an attachment to a ceramic restoration. There are several options available for the preparation of the ceramic surface, but, unfortunately, there are no prospective clinical trials to guide us as to the most successful method while minimizing the risk of damage to the ceramic restoration. Clinical trials can be designed to evaluate not only the rate of bond failure but also the relative risk of damage to the restoration during treatment as well as when the bracket is removed at the completion of treatment. In the laboratory setting, the rate of debonding of the bracket is significantly slower when compared with a patient biting down and suddenly debonding a bracket. At the completion of treatment, the clinician can take more care during bracket removal to reduce the risk of ceramic fracture. In this section, we examine the laboratory data on the various preparation techniques, namely conventional acid etching, air abrasion/microetching, hydrofluoric acid (HFA) etching, the application of silane, and combinations of these.

When bonding to air-abraded ceramic surfaces, Zachrisson et al[50] found that air abrasion alone or in combination with conventional acid etching did not provide sufficient bond strength for clinical use (2.8 to 3.4 MPa). However, when air abrasion (Fig 3-2) was used in combination with silane application or 2 minutes of HFA etching, the bond strengths were significantly improved and were considered clinically suitable (11.5 to 11.6 MPa). Alhaija[51] also found that the addition of HFA significantly improved the bond strength over air abrasion alone.

However, Bourke and Rock[52] concluded that the removal of the porcelain glaze or use of HFA prior to bonding was unnecessary to secure a target bond strength of 6 to 8 MPa. The use of HFA did increase the bond strength, but it was also associated with increased porcelain surface damage. Overall, the best bond strengths were achieved when silane was involved. Based on their results, they suggested the best regimen for orthodontic bonding to feldspathic porcelain was to apply conventional phosphoric acid for 60 seconds and prime with silane prior to bonding. Kocadereli et al[53] also found that air abrasion alone did not achieve acceptable bond strength (24 N), but any procedure involving silane did (80 to 96 N). The use of HFA combined with silane produced the most retentive surface.

Schmage et al[54] also found suitable bond strengths with either HFA alone or any combination involving silane application (12 to 16 MPa). This study also evaluated a silicatization (silica coating) technique, which involved air abrading with a silicon dioxide (silica) material for 13 seconds followed by silane application. The conventional air abrasive is usually aluminum trioxide. This technique achieved satisfactory bond strengths (15 MPa), but cohesive failures were observed in the ceramic during removal of the brackets. For this reason, adhesive failures are preferred to avoid ceramic fractures during debonding.[55] Thurmond et al[56] have suggested that if bond strengths between the ceramic and the composite resin are higher than 13 MPa, the fracture will be cohesive, so the goal is to obtain a high enough bond strength for clinical success but not so high as to substantially increase the risk of ceramic fracture. Nebbe and Stein[57] found a significant number of porcelain fractures in both glazed (36%) and deglazed (71%) porcelain when silane had been applied. Therefore, it appears that there is a risk of damage to the ceramic with all of these techniques (silane, silicatization, air abrasion, and HFA), and patients need to be well informed of this risk. In many cases of mild abrasion, the porcelain surface can be polished to an acceptable result, but a significant fracture may result in a costly repair or even replacement of the restoration.

Another problem for the clinician is identifying what type of ceramic has been used. The constituents, crystalline structure, particle size, and microtopography by etching can vary between different ceramics and result in a variation in the bond strength achieved with the same surface treatment.[58] In a study evaluating the bonding properties of three different types of ceramic, again air abrasion alone did not provide an adequate bond strength.[59] The silica-coating technique and HFA plus silicatization produced the highest bond strengths. However, the higher bond strengths in the silica-coated HFA group and the air abrasion with silane group resulted in cohesive fractures in the ceramic, so debonding must be done carefully. In this study, the authors also presented estimated survival plots based on their bond strength data.[59] It is interesting to note that despite the adequate mean bond strengths achieved by all methods (other than air abrasion alone), the estimated bond failure (using Reynolds's 6 to 8 MPa as a guide[9]) could range from 5% to almost 40%. Although this failure rate varied with the type of porcelain, the most successful results, based on these plot estimations, were achieved when using either the silica-coating technique with silane or air abrasion with HFA.

Based on the bond strengths from the laboratory findings, it seems that either the use of silicatization or silanation (silane application) is suitable clinically. However,

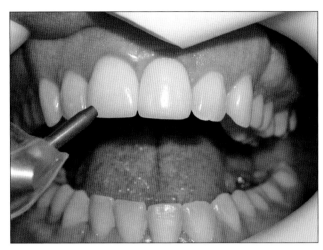

Fig 3-2 Light microetching has been demonstrated in laboratory research to improve bond strength to porcelain crowns or veneers when used in conjunction with HFA etching and/or silane application but offers no additional benefit when bonding to enamel.

when retrospectively evaluating failed brackets bonded to ceramic restorations, Zachrisson[60] stated that excellent clinical bonds to porcelain crowns were routinely achieved with the HFA and that the silane application alone was highly unreliable and the technique should be abandoned. Of the 183 attachments bonded to porcelain crowns or laminate veneers in 95 patients, 17 brackets came loose during the course of therapy (9.3%). The application of silane after HFA did not improve the clinical success and so was considered optional. However, care should be taken because HFA is corrosive and capable of causing severe tissue irritation. Because of this potential risk, a clinician may choose an alternative conditioning technique such as the silica-coating method. However, laboratory data may not represent the true clinical effectiveness of the silica-coating technique, so clinical research is required to elucidate the most effective and safest technique(s) when bonding to ceramic restorations.

Decalcification

Fixed orthodontic appliances make it difficult for young patients to maintain adequate oral hygiene during treatment. The bacteria in plaque produce organic acids, which cause dissolution of calcium and phosphate ions from the enamel surface. This can result in the formation of white spots (Fig 3-3) or early caries lesions in as little as 4 weeks.[61,62]

There are several materials and techniques available for etching and priming the enamel when bonding. The enamel can be conventionally acid etched with the application of a primer, or an SEP can be used. While many conventional hydrophobic primers are filled, many hy-

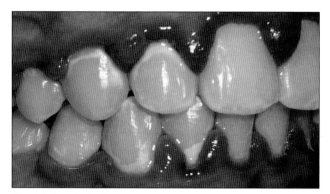

Fig 3-3 Decalcification is an undesirable outcome for all concerned and can result in the early termination of treatment.

drophilic primers and SEP formulations are unfilled. The advantage of a filled primer is that it may protect the enamel and reduce the risk of decalcification. This is supported by in vitro research.[63] An in vitro trial comparing Transbond Plus SEP with conventional acid etching followed by the application of Light Bond (Reliance), a fluoride-releasing sealant, demonstrated a 50% reduction in decalcification in the Light Bond compared with the SEP and the untreated control.[64] In a follow-up clinical trial comparing Transbond SEP and Light Bond, again a 50% reduction in the decalcification scores was demonstrated (27.5% versus 13.9%).[65] No significant difference was found in those patients with excellent oral hygiene, but patients with fair or poor oral hygiene compliance had higher decalcification scores in the SEP group than in the conventionally treated group. The authors concluded that using an SEP might save chair time but also provides less resistance to enamel decalcification, especially in patients with poor oral hygiene. Another study evaluating a fluoride-containing, filled sealant (ProSeal, Reliance) versus a non–fluoride-containing, unfilled primer (Transbond MIP, 3M Unitek) found no statistically or clinically significant difference between the two.[66] This contradiction with the previous study could possibly be due to differences in the treatment times (18 to 24 months in the former study versus 12 to 18 months in the latter). The longer treatment time would potentially increase the risk of decalcification, making any difference more apparent. Another possibility is that the hygiene may have been better maintained in the latter study, whereas in the former, the difference was only noted in those with poor oral hygiene. Finally, the disparity could be explained by the difference in the CEP method versus the SEP method. With an SEP, an acidic complex remains in the resin network when the primer polymerizes, lowering the pH at the enamel surface and maintaining a continuous acidic challenge.[65] With conventional etching, on the other hand, the acid is immediately removed by the rinsing step.

Apart from using filled sealers or fluoride-releasing sealants, another approach to protect the enamel from decalcification uses antibacterial components added to the primers. A clinical trial compared two SEPs, Transbond Plus SEP and Clearfil Protect Bond, which contains an antibacterial monomer.[19] The 24 patients in the trial were observed over 12 months, and no difference was found in the Plaque Index or decalcification scores between the two SEPs. However, as previously discussed, the odds of bond failure were found to be 4.2 times higher in the Clearfil Protect Bond group. Currently there are no antibacterial primers that are recommended.

Based on the limited clinical evidence, it appears that there is a potential increased risk of decalcification with the use of an SEP, although more research is required to confirm this. Therefore, it may be prudent to use a conventional acid etch and seal technique and consider a filled, fluoride-releasing sealant, particularly in patients with poor oral hygiene. There is the potential for a filled sealant to discolor during treatment, which the patient may find disappointing, but this discoloration is transient, whereas white spot lesions are not.

Another method to apply fluoride is to incorporate it into the adhesive. In a systematic review of the literature regarding fluoride-containing adhesives, the authors concluded that there is weak evidence that glass-ionomer cement (GIC) is more effective than composite resin in preventing white spot formation.[67] However, another systematic review of orthodontic adhesives supports the use of a composite resin adhesive over a conventional GIC adhesive because of the higher bond failures recorded using GIC.[68] No recommendation for clinical practice could be made based on these results, but the authors felt that some materials could be worthy of further investigation. Therefore, more standardized research is required before a clear answer as to the potential efficiency of fluoride-containing adhesives can be given.[67]

Gingivally Offset Brackets

As previously discussed, the highest bond failure risk occurs on the mandibular posterior teeth. It is therefore clinically useful to know what procedures can reduce this. In an RCT comparing conventional premolar brackets with gingivally offset premolar brackets from the same manufacturer, 10 times as many conventional brackets (8.3%) failed compared with the gingivally offset brackets (0.8%).[69] The clinical recommendation based on this result is therefore to use gingivally offset bases on mandibular premolar brackets. Ideally, this study would be repeated to confirm this finding. Another consideration is the use of bite protection wedges in reducing mandibular posterior bond failure, but this has not been investigated.

Indirect Bonding

Although indirect bonding is less accepted than direct bonding, it has been steadily increasing in popularity since 1996, when about 8% of survey respondents used indirect bonding versus 13% in 2008.[4] Bond failure rates for indirect bonding (13.9%) were initially higher when compared with direct bonding (2.5%).[70] Over time, however, modifications and improvements to the technique have resulted in similar bond strengths and failure rates.[71–73]

Again, limited clinical research exists for indirect bonding, and the results of laboratory studies can give misleading results for clinical practice. For example, in a laboratory trial of one direct bonding adhesive and two indirect bonding adhesives, no significant difference was found between the mean bond strengths (16.3, 13.8, and 14.8 MPa).[74] Therefore, it appears that all three adhesives are suitable for clinical use. The authors also conducted a Weibull survival analysis, which helps in the assessment of possible clinical failures at the lower range of bond strengths, and found a bracket survival rate of over 90% for all three adhesives. However, if the 6 to 8 MPa range, as suggested by Reynolds,[9] is used as a minimal bond strength for clinical practice, the Sondhi Rapid Set indirect adhesive (3M Unitek) exhibited approximately twice the bond failure risk (about 4% to 9%) when compared with the other indirect and direct adhesives tested (about 2% to 5%). This is supported by a prospective clinical trial that compared two chemical-cured indirect bonding adhesives.[75] The Sondhi Rapid Set adhesive was found to have a clinical bond failure risk (9.9%) seven times higher than that of the Maximum Cure adhesive (Reliance) (1.4%). Although all these adhesives yield clinically suitable mean bond strengths in the laboratory setting, it is clinically more efficient to use the adhesive with the significantly lower bond failure risk.

The above-mentioned indirect bonding adhesives were all chemically set because this allowed short curing times of approximately 2½ to 3 minutes. However, once the tray is placed in the mouth, it must be kept very still during this curing period. The advances in curing light technology, from halogen lights with longer curing times to plasma and now light-emitting diode (LED) lights with short curing times, has made the use of light-cured materials more feasible for indirect bonding (Fig 3-4). Curing times of 3 to 5 seconds through a porcelain or plastic bracket or from two sides of a metal bracket have made curing times comparable between light- and chemical-cured adhesives. In another prospective clinical trial comparing the flowable light-cured adhesive Filtek Flow (now known as *Transbond Supreme LV* [3M Unitek]) with the chemical-cured Maximum Cure, no significant difference was found in the bond failure risk over 6 months (2.4% versus 2.9%).[76] Therefore, both of these adhesives are considered clinically suitable for the indirect bonding of brackets.

The modern technique of indirect bonding most commonly involves the use of a custom base, where the brack-

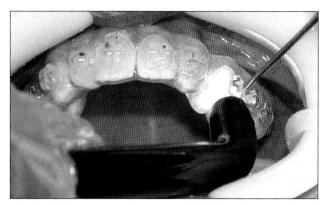

Fig 3-4 The advent of plasma and LED curing lights has allowed for the use of light-cured adhesives in indirect bonding. After the tray is seated, there is no need to rush as with chemical-cured adhesives. The tray and bracket can be visually checked and then held in place to ensure correct seating of the tray prior to light curing the adhesive.

et is placed on a cast of the patient's teeth using composite resin. This composite is then chemically cured, thermally/ heat cured, or light cured. One clinical trial[77] and another laboratory study[78] comparing heat-cured custom bases with light-cured custom bases found the light-cured bases to be superior, so light-cured composite is recommended in clinical practice. The custom base is then prepared for bonding, usually with very light microetching (1 second or less); some authors recommend the use of plastic conditioners to improve adhesion to the bonding adhesive. One laboratory study found that microetching significantly improved the shear bond strength of the custom base, while the additional use of the unfilled resin Ortho Solo (Ormco) as a plastic conditioner prior to bonding was not necessary.[79] In a prospective clinical trial using denture monomer (methyl methacrylate) as a custom base conditioner, no significant difference in bond failure was observed,[80] so it seems that apart from microetching, no other custom base conditioning is required prior to clinical indirect bonding.

Polymerization Lamps and Photocuring*

Light intensity variation in the material

Penetration of a light beam into the relatively thin layer of orthodontic adhesive depends on a number of factors related to the light beam itself, the application mode, and the material characteristics. It is well known that the distance of the source from the surface and the path that the

*Sections reprinted from Eliades[81] with permission.

incident beam will have to travel to reach the adhesive have a large effect on the intensity of incident light.[82] The applicable equation in this field is Lambert's law, which describes the variation of intensity with distance as

$$I = I_0 e^{-\gamma d}$$

where I is the light intensity at distance d, I_0 is the intensity departing from the source, and γ is the absorption coefficient of the medium (e is a constant).

In general, the translucency of a composite increases with an increasing match of the refractive indices of the matrix and fillers. The matrix relates to the comonomer system of bisphenol A glycidyl methacrylate (bis-GMA)/triethylene glycol dimethacrylate (TEGDMA) mixture, which is used to combine the favorable features of both monomers: the increased molecular weight of bis-GMA, which offers stability and a thicker consistency, and the decreased molecular weight and higher mobility of TEGDMA, which contributes to the larger degree of cure. Varying the proportion of these constituents, as well as other materials such as amines, accelerators, inhibitors, and initiators, may slightly affect the refractive index of the matrix (about 1.5 in methacrylate resins).[83]

Fillers are contained in the adhesive in a ratio of 0.6 to 0.7 (% wt) in the form of silica particles and barium glasses. These possess a refractive index of 1.55 at the wavelength of the photoinitiator.[84] The maximum light scattering appears to occur at a particle size equivalent to one-half the wavelength of the photoinitiator of the polymerization, which for camphoroquinone systems is 468 nm; therefore, the favorable filler size is set to about 230 nm. However, most adhesives include a large size variation of the filler particles, and in orthodontic adhesives, most filler systems are placed arbitrarily.

Light and polymerization initiation

Most light-cured adhesives employ camphoroquinone as the photoinitiator of polymerization. This molecule is contained in a concentration of 0.2% to 1% of the matrix and shows a peak absorbance wavelength of 468 nm, which implies that increased light intensity in other frequencies may not be effective to agitate the molecule into the excited state, which lasts for 0.05 ms.[83] This is important when choosing a light source based on the peak intensity reported by the manufacturer; it is critical that this peak should correspond to the absorbance wavelength of the photoinitiator, namely 468 nm.

Lamps and degree of cure of adhesives

Light-cured orthodontic adhesives require a light curing source of a defined wavelength and with sufficient intensity to initiate the polymerization reaction. Increased light

intensity and curing time have been advocated for fast polymerization and a high degree of cure.[85]

Since the introduction of the halogen lamp, the choice of light curing sources has expanded to include plasma arc, laser, and LED lights, which were introduced to the profession to facilitate shorter irradiation times.

Plasma lamps have a very high intensity compared with halogen lights (1,600 to 2,100 mW/cm²), an effective spectrum of 450 to 500 nm, and a significantly higher cost, which nevertheless is counterweighed by their reported increased life span of 5,000 hours relative to 40 to 100 hours for halogen lamps. The fiber-optic cable on these units can be fragile and costly to replace if broken. Orthodontic bonding with these light sources can be achieved with only 6 seconds of irradiation for stainless steel brackets or 3 seconds for ceramic brackets.[86,87]

Laser lights show an intensity of 700 to 1,000 mW/cm², with a basically monochromatic spectrum of variable wavelength (454, 458, 466, 472, 477, 488, and 497 nm). They are costly but have an almost infinite life span. Application of these light sources to orthodontic bonding has shown that 5 seconds of irradiation provided bond strength values comparable to those found for halogen.[88,89]

LED light curing units yield a maximum intensity of 1,100 mW/cm² at a spectrum of 420 to 600 nm, with more recent units reportedly reaching 1,600 mW/cm². LED lights are cost comparable to conventional halogen lights and possess a nearly infinite life span. The results of bond strength studies show contradicting evidence on the performance of these lights, with most investigations demonstrating comparable bond strength to halogen lights with the same irradiation duration and reduced strength when shorter time frames are applied.[90,91]

As analyzed above, two important parameters of light curing units are the amount of light energy emitted and the appropriate wavelength to efficiently excite the photoinitiator. However, others suggest that within the 490 to 450–nm wavelength range, light intensity and exposure time are more significant than light wavelength in determining degree of cure[83] because camphoroquinone exhibits a broad absorption spectrum at this range. Curing time has been directly associated with increased conversion in a study comparing high- and low-intensity halogen lights.[92] Nevertheless, an LED light with a lower intensity than a halogen light has been shown to produce a greater depth of cure,[90] implying a rather complicated interaction pattern of light intensity, emitted wavelength, curing time, and extent of absorption by the material.

The variation of percent degree of cure (%DC) as a function of bond strength has not been examined, and it is possible that bond strength is unaffected after a certain %DC is reached. Bond strength is a poor indicator of %DC because of the interference of bracket design, variation in load application, loading rate, teeth storage and preparation, and testing conditions, among other factors. However, the %DC has been shown to modulate the mechanical properties of the material[93,94] as well as the resistance to degradation and dissolution,[95] a key property, which cannot be explored using bond strength tests.

Lamps and bond strength

There are various steps that, if adopted, can result in an increase in the reliability of future research. These include the preference of reporting force (N) as opposed to pressure (MPa) values. Work in this area has shown that the stress distribution in the bracket base is not homogenous, and thus the report of force per surface is mistaken. Also, it is difficult to estimate the effective surface area of bracket bases because of the differences in the mesh gauge, even among brackets with identical dimensions. An additional measure entails the inclusion of a Weibull analysis, which can be used to predict the bond survival at specific stress increments.[96]

Lamps and bond failures

To avoid the assumption of bond strength protocols, bond failure studies have been designed to test the variable of retention of bonds throughout a set time, which ranges from 6 months to the entire treatment duration (18+ months). This process provides direct clinical evidence and is therefore preferred over the conventional bond strength tests whenever possible.

Although this type of study presents a major advantage related to its profound clinical relevance, it does not provide an insight into the cause or pattern of failure.[40] Moreover, failure rate protocols are very demanding from a setup perspective because they are laborious, require extended monitoring, and are difficult to apply in an ordinary practice setup. On the other hand, large clinical environments, such as those found in educational institutions, carry some unfavorable features, such as the intervention of multiple operators, the socioeconomic and dental status of patients seeking treatment in institutions, and variations in malocclusion classification and resultant mechanotherapy (ie, use of interarch elastics, variety of archwires, etc). These factors may introduce cross effects from various participant-related parameters, such as habits, masticatory forces (which vary with facial type), and diet.

The results of the limited evidence available from bond failure studies on this topic, including the handful of long-term trials on the clinical performance of high-intensity LED lamps, demonstrate that these lamps are incapable of reaching the success rates observed for plasma lamps, implying that an increase in irradiation should be implemented.

Data on bond failure report that, for the halogen lamp, it may be around 3% to 5%, depending on the study, with some authors reporting higher rates[97] and others showing rates as low as 3.4%.[98] This discrepancy may be attributed to different irradiation times. The overall risk of failure recorded with the halogen unit was not significantly different from the failure rate for the LED lamp. A higher risk of bond failure was most often found in the mandibular dental arch compared with the maxillary arch and in the posterior segments (premolars) compared with the anterior segments. There are no clinical studies in the literature evaluating the efficiency of LED lamps in orthodontic bonding. Previous in vitro studies found that LED and halogen lamps provided comparable shear bond strengths when bonding orthodontic brackets with an equivalent polymerization time.[98]

The distribution of failures between the two dental arches has shown considerable variation. Previous studies reported more failures in the mandibular dental arch, while others found no statistically significant difference between failures in the mandibular and maxillary arches.[99–102] Others noted more failures in the mandibular arch than in the maxillary arch and attributed them to occlusal interferences between the brackets of the two dental arches during the first phase of orthodontic therapy, the gravity of the bolus of food, and the presence of more initial crowding in the mandibular dental arch—especially in the anterior segment—in most of the patients of this sample.[103] Regarding association between the risk of failure and dental arch side (left or right), previous studies have reported contradictory results.[102] The variability observed between these studies could be assigned to differences in mastication habits between patients, pressure during tooth brushing between right- or left-handed patients, as well as moisture control and handling of materials and bonding procedure between right- and left-handed operators.

The finding reported by some studies on the higher failure rates in premolars than in anterior teeth has been attributed to higher masticatory forces exerted on posterior teeth,[104–106] access difficulties during bonding,[107] and differences in the morphology and structure of the superficial enamel layer between posterior and anterior teeth. Because some studies report more failures in boys than in girls, it seems that individual preferences, which are gender specific and related to the character of the participants and the attention to diet and care of appliances, may have an effect on the outcome.

Lamps and the biologic action of blue light

Various reports have focused on the potentially biologically hazardous effects of light sources on several tissues. Blue light (wavelength of 380 to 500 nm) is commonly used to initiate polymerization of dental resin composites for a variety of applications. Although initially blue light was characterized as relatively harmless, more recent studies have shown that it affects several aspects of cell physiology. Particularly, it has been reported that it disturbs mitochondrial function,[108–113] thus causing an oxidative stress that leads to activation of the stress-responsive pathways,[114] oxidative DNA damage,[115] or even the inhibition of mitosis.[116] The group of investigations cited above has suggested that blue light affects DNA integrity, cellular mitosis, and mitochondrial status in various cell types through the generation of reactive oxygen species. These investigations employed a variety of mouse and human, normal and transformed cell types, as well as a vast array of assays, which extended from assessment of cell vitality to markers of cells' metabolism and oxidative status. This multiplicity of testing protocols has resulted in a variety of effects described.

The result of the sole investigation adopting the time exposures seen in an orthodontic routine bond up has shown that blue light did not affect the viability of these cells in that no signs of cytotoxicity were observed.[117] In addition, there was no immediate effect on the regulation of proliferation; until 24 hours after irradiation, there was no inhibition of DNA synthesis, a prerequisite for cell proliferation. To evaluate the long-term effect, absolute cell counting was performed, as opposed to indirect assays such as, for example, the MTT assay, because the former provides information not only on the culture's cell number but also on the mitochondrial status of cells while the latter is known to be disturbed by blue light irradiation. One week after treatment, all types of irradiation induced a significant inhibition of cell proliferation compared with untreated cultures.

Several studies have shown that the exposure to blue light leads to the generation of reactive oxygen species, proposing that these are responsible for the adverse biologic effects of blue light. However, in the study by Taoufik et al,[117] the use of the potent antioxidant N-acetyl-cysteine was unable to annul the inhibitory effect of irradiation on cell proliferation. One possible explanation for this may relate to the extracellular environment used in various studies. Irradiation of cells in this study was performed in phosphate-buffered saline (PBS) and in the absence of culture medium.

It has been recently shown that blue light suppresses mitochondrial activity in normal human epidermal keratinocytes and mouse BALB fibroblasts only when cells are maintained in culture medium during exposure and not in PBS.[118] Accordingly, the effect of blue light in mitochondrial status and reactive oxygen species production in different environments requires further investigation. An immediate cellular response to irradiation involves alteration of proliferation in order to provide time for repair of the DNA damage before entering into mitosis, thereby avoiding mutations and aneuploidy. Moreover, the results of a DNA assay did not suggest intense DNA damage that would activate intracellular pathways in order to inhibit proliferation (no DNA breaks were identified).

In summary, the evidence on the biologic effects of blue light are indicative of an action that is probably not an immediate reaction, is confined to long-term effects, and is not mediated by an oxidation mechanism or DNA damage. The array of effects described suggests that high-energy sources such as plasma lamps should be used with caution, especially when bonding mandibular tubes where a close contact between the tissue and the lamp tip occurs.

Conclusion

Although the bonding of orthodontic attachments has been commonplace for some time, there are a limited number of clinical trials available for many of our clinical questions. One difficulty in comparing in vivo bonding studies is the lack of uniformity in the observation period. Therefore, it would be useful if investigators used the same time frame or related bond failures to the length of treatment.

Summary points

- In the absence of obvious plaque, prophylaxis is not required before conventional acid etching of enamel. However, it must be done when using an SEP.
- Conventional acid etching can be done for less than 60 seconds, with a minimum of 15 seconds.
- Microetching the mandibular posterior teeth prior to acid etching does not significantly improve bond failure risk in the first 6 months of treatment.
- SEPs may save some clinical time but also may offer less protection against decalcification compared with a filled, fluoride-releasing sealant in patients with poor oral hygiene.
- There is little evidence that gingivally offset mandibular premolar brackets have a lower clinical failure rate compared with standard brackets, but further studies are required.
- Current evidence supports the use of alternative curing lights (to halogen) because of either more efficient handling (LED) or reduced irradiation time (plasma). However, the overall degree of cure seems to be unaffected because this is dictated by the energy (intensity $\times$ duration) provided to the adhesive, which in principle remains the same.

References

1. Newman GV. Epoxy adhesives for orthodontic attachments: A progress report. Am J Orthod 1965;51:901–912.
2. Kinch AP, Taylor H, Warltier R, Oliver RG, Newcombe RG. A clinical trial comparing the failure rates of directly bonded brackets using etch times of 15 or 60 seconds. Am J Orthod Dentofacial Orthop 1988;94:476–483.
3. Sadowsky PL, Retief DH, Cox PR, Hernández-Orsini R, Rape WG, Bradley EL. Effects of etchant concentration and duration on the retention of orthodontic brackets: An in vivo study. Am J Orthod Dentofacial Orthop 1990;98:417–421.
4. Keim RG, Gottlieb EL, Nelson AH, Vogels DS 3rd. 2008 JCO Study of Orthodontic Diagnosis and Treatment Procedures, Part 1: Results and trends. J Clin Orthod 2008;42:625–640.
5. Swartz M. Limitations of in vitro orthodontic bond strength testing. J Clin Orthod 2007;41:207–210.
6. Kandil SH, Kamar AA, Shaabam SA, Taymour NM, Morsi SE. Effect of temperature and aging on the mechanical properties of dental polymeric composite materials. Biomaterials 1989;8:540–545.
7. Matasa CG. Microbial attack of orthodontic adhesives. Am J Orthod Dentofacial Orthop 1995;108:132–141.

8. Finnema KJ, Ozcan M, Post WJ, Ren Y, Dijkstra PU. In-vitro orthodontic bond strength testing: A systematic review and meta-analysis. Am J Orthod Dentofacial Orthop 2010;137:615–622.

9. Reynolds IR. A review of direct orthodontic bonding. Br J Orthod 1975;2:143–146.

10. Bishara SE, Ostby AW. Bonding and debonding from metal to ceramic: Research and its clinical application. Semin Orthod 2010; 16:24–36.

11. Hajrassie MK, Khier SE. In-vivo and in-vitro comparison of bond strengths of orthodontic brackets bonded to enamel and debonded at various times. Am J Orthod Dentofacial Orthop 2007;131: 384–390.

12. Barry GR. A clinical investigation of the effects of omission of pumice prophylaxis on band and bond failure. Br J Orthod 1995; 22:245–248.

13. Lindauer SJ, Browning H, Shroff B, Marshall F, Anderson RH, Moon PC. Effect of pumice prophylaxis on the bond strength of orthodontic brackets. Am J Orthod Dentofacial Orthop 1997;111:599–605.

14. Ireland AJ, Sherriff M. The effect of pumicing on the in vivo use of a resin modified glass poly(alkenoate) cement and a conventional no-mix composite for bonding orthodontic brackets. J Orthod 2002;29:217–220.

15. Burgess AM, Sherriff M, Ireland AJ. Self-etching primers: Is prophylactic pumicing necessary? A randomized clinical trial. Angle Orthod 2006;76:114–118.

16. Lill DJ, Lindauer SJ, Tüfekçi E, Shroff B. Importance of pumice prophylaxis for bonding with self-etch primer. Am J Orthod Dentofacial Orthop 2008;133:423–426.

17. Pandis N, Eliades T. A comparative in vivo assessment of the long-term failure rate of 2 self-etching primers. Am J Orthod Dentofacial Orthop 2005;128:96–98.

18. Elekdag-Turk S, Isci D, Turk T, Cakmak F. Six-month bracket failure rate evaluation of a self-etching primer. Eur J Orthod 2008;30:211–216.

19. Paschos E, Kurochkina N, Huth KC, Hansson CS, Rudzki-Janson I. Failure rate of brackets bonded with antimicrobial and fluoride-releasing, self-etching primer and the effect on prevention of enamel demineralization. Am J Orthod Dentofacial Orthop 2009;135:613–620.

20. Aljubouri YD, Millett DT, Gilmour WH. Six and 12 months' evaluation of a self-etching primer versus two-stage etch and prime for orthodontic bonding: A randomized clinical trial. Eur J Orthod 2004;26:565–571.

21. Miles PG. Indirect bonding with a flowable light-cured adhesive. J Clin Orthod 2002;36:646–647.

22. Ponduri S, Turnbull N, Birnie D, Ireland AJ, Sandy JR. Does atropine sulphate improve orthodontic bond survival? A randomized clinical trial. Am J Orthod Dentofacial Orthop 2007;132:663–670.

23. Kuijpers MA, Vissink A, Ren Y, Kuijpers-Jagtman AM. The effect of antisialogogues in dentistry: A systematic review with a focus on bond failure in orthodontics. J Am Dent Assoc 2010;141:954–965.

24. Webster MJ, Nanda RS, Duncanson MG, Khajotia SS, Sinha PK. The effect of saliva on shear bond strengths of hydrophilic bonding systems. Am J Orthod Dentofacial Orthop 2001;119:54–58.

25. Schaneveldt S, Foley TF. Bond strength comparison of moisture insensitive primers. Am J Orthod Dentofacial Orthop 2002;122: 267–273.

26. Campoy MD, Plasencia E, Vicente A, Bravo LA, Cibria R. Effect of saliva contamination on bracket failure with a self-etching primer: A prospective controlled clinical trial. Am J Orthod Dentofacial Orthop 2010;137:679–683.

27. Zeppieri IL, Chung CH, Mante FK. Effect of saliva on shear bond strength of an orthodontic adhesive used with moisture-insensitive and self-etching primers. Am J Orthod Dentofacial Orthop 2003; 124:414–419.

28. Larmour CJ, Stirrups DR. An ex vivo assessment of a bonding technique using a self-etching primer. J Orthod 2003;30:225–228.

29. Townsend RD, Dunn WJ. The effect of saliva contamination on enamel and dentin using a self-etching adhesive. J Am Dent Assoc 2004;135:895–901.

30. Cacciafesta V, Sfondrini MF, De Angelis M, Scribante A, Klersy C. Effect of water and saliva contamination on shear bond strength of brackets bonded with conventional, hydrophilic, and self-etching primers. Am J Orthod Dentofacial Orthop 2003;123:633–640.

31. Oonsombat C, Bishara SE, Ajlouni R. The effect of blood contamination on the shear bond strength of orthodontic brackets with the use of a new self-etch primer. Am J Orthod Dentofacial Orthop 2003;123:547–550.

32. Miles PG, Pontier JP, Bahiraei D, Close J. The effect of carbamide peroxide bleach on the tensile bond strength of ceramic brackets: An in vitro study. Am J Orthod Dentofacial Orthop 1994;106;371–375.

33. Bishara SE, Sulieman A, Olson M. Effect of enamel bleaching on the bonding strength of orthodontic brackets. Am J Orthod Dentofacial Orthop 1993;104;444–447.

34. Homewood C, Tyas M, Woods M. Bonding to previously bleached teeth. Aust Orthod J 2001;17:27–34.

35. Patusco VC, Montenegro G, Lenza MA, de Carvalho AA. Bond strength of metallic brackets after dental bleaching. Angle Orthod 2009;79:122–126.

36. Bishara SE, Oonsombat C, Soliman MM, Ajlouni R, Laffoone JF. The effect of tooth bleaching on the shear bond strength of orthodontic brackets. Am J Orthod Dentofacial Orthop 2005;128:755–760.

37. Uysal T, Basciftci FA, Uşümez S, Sari Z, Buyukerkmen A. Can previously bleached teeth be bonded safely? Am J Orthod Dentofacial Orthop 2003;123:628–632.

38. Mullins JM, Kao EC, Martin CA, Gunel E, Ngan P. Tooth whitening effects on bracket bond strength in vivo. Angle Orthod 2009;79: 777–783.

39. Sonis AL, Snell W. An evaluation of a fluoride-releasing, visible light-activated bonding system for orthodontic bracket placement. Am J Orthod Dentofacial Orthop 1989;95:306–311.

40. Pandis N, Christensen L, Eliades T. Long-term clinical failure rate of molar tubes bonded with a self-etching primer. Angle Orthod 2005;75:1000–1002.

41. Millett DT, Hallgren A, Fornell AC, Robertson M. Bonded molar tubes: A retrospective evaluation of clinical performance. Am J Orthod Dentofacial Orthop 1999;115:667–674.

42. Zachrisson BJ. A posttreatment evaluation of direct bonding in orthodontics. Am J Orthod 1977;71:173–189.

43. Gray GB, Carey GP, Jagger DC. An in vitro investigation of a comparison of bond strengths of composite to etched and air-abraded human enamel surfaces. J Prosthodont 2006;15:2–8.

44. Olsen ME, Bishara SE, Damon P, Jakobsen JR. Comparison of shear bond strength and surface structure between conventional acid etching and air-abrasion of human enamel. Am J Orthod Dentofacial Orthop 1997;112:502–506.

45. Abu Alhaija ES, Al-Wahadni AM. Evaluation of shear bond strength with different enamel pre-treatments. Eur J Orthod 2004;26:179–184.

46. Pandis N, Polychronopoulou A, Eliades T. A comparative assessment of the failure rate of molar tubes bonded with a self-etching primer and conventional acid-etching. World J Orthod 2006;7:41–44.

47. House K, Ireland AJ, Sherriff M. An investigation into the use of a single component self-etching primer adhesive system for orthodontic bonding: A randomized controlled clinical trial. J Orthod 2006;33:38–44.

48. Miles PG. Does microetching enamel reduce bracket failure when indirect bonding mandibular posterior teeth? Aust Orthod J 2008; 24:1–4.

49. Noble J, Karaiskos NE, Wiltshire WA. In vivo bonding of orthodontic brackets to fluorosed enamel using an adhesion promotor. Angle Orthod 2008;78:357–360.

50. Zachrisson YO, Zachrisson BU, Büyükyilmaz T. Surface preparation for orthodontic bonding to porcelain. Am J Orthod Dentofacial Orthop 1996;109:420–430.

51. Abu Alhaija ES, Abu AlReesh IA, AlWahadni AM. Factors affecting the shear bond strength of metal and ceramic brackets bonded to different ceramic surfaces. Eur J Orthod 2010;32:274–280.

52. Bourke BM, Rock WP. Factors affecting the shear bond strength of orthodontic brackets to porcelain. Br J Orthod 1999;26:285–290.

53. Kocadereli I, Canay S, Akça K. Tensile bond strength of ceramic orthodontic brackets bonded to porcelain surfaces. Am J Orthod Dentofacial Orthop 2001;119:617–620.

54. Schmage P, Nergiz I, Herrmann W, Ozcan M. Influence of various surface-conditioning methods on the bond strength of metal brackets to ceramic surfaces. Am J Orthod Dentofacial Orthop 2003; 123:540–546.

55. Smith GA, McInnes-Ledoux P, Ledoux WR, Weinberg R. Orthodontic bonding to porcelain—Bond strength and refinishing. Am J Orthod Dentofacial Orthop 1988;94:245–252.

56. Thurmond JW, Barkmeier WW, Wilwerding TM. Effect of porcelain surface treatments on bond strengths of composite resin bonded to porcelain. J Prosthet Dent 1994;72:355–359.

57. Nebbe B, Stein E. Orthodontic brackets bonded to glazed and deglazed porcelain surfaces. Am J Orthod Dentofacial Orthop 1996; 109:431–436.

58. Sorensen JA, Engelman MJ, Torres TJ, Avera SP. Shear bond strength of composite resin to porcelain. Int J Prosthodont 1991; 4:17–23.

59. Karan S, Büyükyilmaz T, Toroğlu MS. Orthodontic bonding to several ceramic surfaces: Are there acceptable alternatives to conventional methods? Am J Orthod Dentofacial Orthop 2007;132: 144.e7–144.e14.

60. Zachrisson BU. Orthodontic bonding to artificial tooth surfaces: Clinical versus laboratory findings. Am J Orthod Dentofacial Orthop 2000;117:592–594.

61. O'Reilly MM, Featherstone JD. Demineralization and remineralization around orthodontic appliances: An in vivo study. Am J Orthod Dentofacial Orthop 1987;92:33–40.

62. Gorton J, Featherstone JD. In vivo inhibition of demineralization around orthodontic brackets. Am J Orthod Dentofacial Orthop 2003;123:10–14.

63. Hu W, Featherstone JD. Prevention of enamel demineralization: An in-vitro study using light-cured filled sealant. Am J Orthod Dentofacial Orthop 2005;128:592–600.

64. Tanna N, Kao E, Gladwin M, Ngan PW. Effects of sealant and self-etching primer on enamel decalcification. Part I: An in-vitro study. Am J Orthod Dentofacial Orthop 2009;135:199–205.

65. Ghiz MA, Ngan P, Kao E, Martin C, Gunel E. Effects of sealant and self-etching primer on enamel decalcification. Part II: An in-vivo study. Am J Orthod Dentofacial Orthop 2009;135:206–213.

66. Leizer C, Weinstein M, Borislow AJ, Braitman LE. Efficacy of a filled-resin sealant in preventing decalcification during orthodontic treatment. Am J Orthod Dentofacial Orthop 2010;137:796–800.

67. Rogers S, Chadwick B, Treasure E. Fluoride-containing orthodontic adhesives and decalcification in patients with fixed appliances: A systematic review. Am J Orthod Dentofacial Orthop 2010;138: 390.e1–390.e8.

68. Mandall NA, Millett DT, Mattick CR, Hickman J, Worthington HV, Macfarlane TV. Orthodontic adhesives: A systematic review. J Orthod 2002;29:205–210.

69. Thind BS, Stirrups DR, Hewage S. Bond failure of gingivally offset mandibular premolar brackets: A randomized controlled clinical trial. Am J Orthod Dentofacial Orthop 2009;135:49–53.

70. Zachrisson BU, Brobakken BO. Clinical comparison of direct versus indirect bonding with different bracket types and adhesives. Am J Orthod 1978;74:62–78.

71. Read MJ, O'Brien KD. A clinical trial of an indirect bonding technique with a visible light-cured adhesive. Am J Orthod Dentofacial Orthop 1990;98:259–262.

72. Aguirre MJ, King GJ, Waldron JM. Assessment of bracket placement and bond strength when comparing direct bonding to indirect bonding techniques. Am J Orthod Dentofacial Orthop 1982;82: 269–276.

73. Hocevar RA, Vincent HF. Indirect versus direct bonding: Bond strength and failure location. Am J Orthod Dentofacial Orthop 1988;94:367–371.

74. Linn BJ, Berzins DW, Dhuru VB, Bradley TG. A comparison of bond strength between direct- and indirect-bonding methods. Angle Orthod 2006;76:289–294.

75. Miles PG, Weyant RJ. A clinical comparison of two chemically-cured adhesives used for indirect bonding. J Orthod 2003;30:331–336.

76. Miles PG, Weyant RJ. A comparison of two indirect bonding adhesives. Angle Orthod 2005;75:1019–1023.

77. Miles PG. A comparison of retention rates of brackets with thermally-cured and light-cured custom bases in indirect bonding procedures. Aust Orthod J 2000;16:115–117.

78. Klocke A, Shi J, Kahl-Nieke B, Bismayer U. Bond strength with custom base indirect bonding techniques. Angle Orthod 2002;73: 176–180.

79. Thompson MA, Drummond JL, BeGole EA. Bond strength analysis of custom base variables in indirect bonding techniques. Am J Orthod Dentofacial Orthop 2008;133:9.e15–9.e20.

80. Miles P. Indirect bonding—Do custom bases need a plastic conditioner? A randomised clinical trial. Aust Orthod J 2010;26:109–112.

81. Eliades T. Polymerization lamps and photocuring in orthodontics. Semin Orthod 2010;16:83–90.

82. Watts DC, Amer O, Combe E. Characteristics of visible light-cured composite systems. Br Dent J 1984;156:209–215.

83. Watts C, Silikas N. In situ photopolymerization and polymerization shrinkage phenomena. In: Eliades G, Watts DC, Eliades T (eds). Dental Hard Tissues and Bonding: Interfacial Phenomena and Related Properties. Heidelberg: Springer, 2005:123–154.

84. Suzuki H, Taira M, Wakasa K, Yamaki M. Refractive-index-adjustable fillers for visible-light-cured dental resin composites: Preparation of TiO_2-SiO_2 glass powder by the sol-gel process. J Dent Res 1991;70:883–888.

85. Niepraschk M, Rahiotis C, Bradley TG, Eliades T, Eliades G. Effect of various curing lights on the degree of cure of orthodontic adhesives. Am J Orthod Dentofacial Orthop 2007;132:382–384.

86. Yoon TH, Lee YK, Lim BS, Kim CW. Degree of polymerization of resin composites by different light sources. J Oral Rehabil 2002; 29:1165–1173.

87. Signorelli MD, Kao E, Ngan PW, Gladwin MA. Comparison of bond strength between orthodontic brackets bonded with halogen and plasma arc curing lights: An in-vitro and in-vivo study. Am J Orthod Dentofacial Orthop 2006;129:277–282.

88. Talbot TQ, Blankenau RJ, Zobitz ME, Weaver AL, Lohse CM, Rebellato J. Effect of argon laser irradiation on shear bond strength of orthodontic brackets: An in vitro study. Am J Orthod Dentofacial Orthop 2000;118:274–279.

89. Lalani N, Foley TF, Voth R, Banting D, Mamandras A. Polymerization with the argon laser: Curing time and shear bond strength. Angle Orthod 2000;70:28–33.

90. Mills RW, Jandt KD, Ashworth SH. Dental composite depth of cure with halogen and blue light emitting diode technology. Br Dent J 1999;186:388–391.

91. Kauppi MR, Combe EC. Polymerization of orthodontic adhesives using modern high-intensity visible curing lights. Am J Orthod Dentofacial Orthop 2003;124:316–322.

92. Nomoto R. Effect of light wavelength on polymerization of light-cured resins. Dent Mater J 1997;16:60–73.

93. Asmussen E. Restorative resins: Hardness and strength vs. quantity of remaining double bonds. Scand J Dent Res 1982;90:484–489.

94. Ferracane JL, Greener EH. The effect of resin formulation on the degree of conversion and mechanical properties of dental restorative resins. J Biomed Mater Res 1986;20:121–131.

95. Söderholm K-JM, Zigan M, Ragan M, Fischlschweiger W, Bergman M. Hydropytic degradation of dental composites. J Dent Res 1984;63:1248–1254.

96. Scougall-Vilchis RJ, Ohashi S, Yamamoto K. Effects of 6 self-etching primers on shear bond strength of orthodontic brackets. Am J Orthod Dentofacial Orthop 2009;135:424.e1–424.e7.

97. Flaut I, Wehrbein H. The effects of argon laser curing of a resin adhesive on bracket retention and enamel decalcification: A prospective clinical trial. Eur J Orthod 2004;26:553–560.

98. Pettemerides AP, Sherriff M, Ireland AJ. An in vivo study to compare a plasma arc light and a conventional quartz halogen curing light in orthodontic bonding. Eur J Orthod 2004;26:573–577.

99. Lovius BB, Pender N, Hewage S, O'Dowling I, Tomkins A. A clinical trial of a light activated material over an 18 month period. Br J Orthod 1987;14:11–20.

100. Trimpeneers LM, Dermaut LR. A clinical trial comparing the failure rates of two orthodontic bonding systems. Am J Orthod Dentofacial Orthop 1996;110:547–550.

101. Sunna S, Rock WP. Clinical performance of orthodontic brackets and adhesive systems: A randomized clinical trial. Br J Orthod 1998;25:283–287.

102. Shammaa I, Ngan P, Kim H, et al. Comparison of bracket debonding force between two conventional resin adhesives and a resin-reinforced glass ionomer cement: An in vitro and in vivo study. Angle Orthod 1999;69:463–469.

103. Koupis NS, Eliades T, Athanasiou AE. Clinical evaluation of bracket bonding using two different polymerization sources. Angle Orthod 2008;78:922–925.

104. Armas Galindo HR, Sadowsky PL, Vlachos C, Jacobson A, Wallace D. An in vivo comparison between a visible light-cured bonding system and a chemically cured bonding system. Am J Orthod Dentofacial Orthop 1998;113:271–275.

105. Chung CH, Piatti A. Clinical comparison of the bond failure rates between fluoride-releasing and non-fluoride-releasing composite resins. J Clin Orthod 2000;34:409–412.

106. Cacciafesta V, Sfondrini MF, Scribante A. Plasma arc versus halogen light-curing of adhesive-precoated orthodontic brackets: A 12-month clinical study of bond failures. Am J Orthod Dentofacial Orthop 2004;126:194–199.

107. Millett DT, Hallgren A, Cattanach D, et al. A 5-year clinical review of bond failure with a light-cured resin adhesive. Angle Orthod 1998;68:351–356.

108. Aggarwal BB, Quintanilha AT, Cammack R, Packer L. Damage to mitochondrial electron transport and energy coupling by visible light. Biochim Biophys Acta 1978;502:367–382.

109. Lockwood DB, Wataha JC, Lewis JB, Tseng WY, Messer RL, Hsu SD. Blue light generates reactive oxygen species (ROS) differentially in tumor vs. normal epithelial cells. Dent Mater 2005;21:683–688.

110. Omata Y, Lewis JB, Rotenberg S, et al. Intra- and extracellular reactive oxygen species generated by blue light. J Biomed Mater Res A 2006;77:470–477.

111. Krishnamoorthy RR, Crawford MJ, Chaturvedi MM, et al. Photo-oxidative stress down-modulates the activity of nuclear factor-κB involvement of caspase-1, leading to apoptosis of photoreceptor cells. J Biol Chem 1999;274:3734–3743.

112. Pflaum M, Kielbassa C, Garmyn M, Epe B. Oxidative DNA damage induced by visible light in mammalian cells: Extent, inhibition by antioxidants and genotoxic effects. Mutat Res 1998;408:137–146.

113. Gorgidze LA, Oshemkova SA, Vorobjev IA. Blue light inhibits mitosis in tissue culture cells. Biosci Rep 1998;18:215–224.

114. Wataha JC, Lewis JB, Lockwood PE, et al. Blue light differentially modulates cell survival and growth. J Dent Res 2004;83:104–108.

115. Wataha JC, Lockwood PE, Lewis JB, Rueggeberg FA, Messer RL. Biological effects of blue light from dental curing units. Dent Mater 2004;20:150–157.

116. Rogakou EP, Boon C, Redon C, Bonner WM. Megabase chromatin domains involved in DNA double-strand breaks in vivo. J Cell Biol 1999;146:905–915.

117. Taoufik K, Mavrogonatou E, Eliades T, Papagiannoulis L, Eliades G, Kletsas D. Effect of blue light on the proliferation of human gingival fibroblasts. Dent Mater 2008;24:895–900.

118. Sodowska AM, Manuel-Y-Keenoy B, De Backer WA. Antioxidant and anti-inflammatory efficacy of NAC in the treatment of COPD: Discordant in vitro and in vivo dose-effects: A review. Pulm Pharmacol Ther 2007;20:9–22.

William A. Brantley
PhD

CHAPTER

4 | Wires Used in Orthodontic Practice

Introduction

Orthodontists have many choices for clinical selection of wires to be used during patient treatment. Four major types—stainless steel (SS), cobalt-chromium (Co-Cr), beta-titanium (β-Ti), and nickel-titanium (Ni-Ti)—are currently in widespread use, and these wires can be either single-strand or multistrand. This chapter presents information about the compositions and properties of these different wires and then discusses clinical studies that have examined their efficacy. Additional information about orthodontic wires can be found in two review articles[1,2] and two book chapters.[3,4]

This chapter begins with a description of the desirable characteristics of orthodontic wires, followed by summaries of the manufacturing process, important mechanical properties, and relevant mechanics concepts. After this foundation information is presented, each of the major wire types is discussed, with greater emphasis on Ni-Ti and β-Ti wires. The chapter concludes with a critical review of reports on clinical performance.

Desirable Characteristics of Orthodontic Wires

Orthodontic wires should (1) produce clinically acceptable levels of biomechanical forces when activated in the oral environment, (2) be biocompatible, (3) have adequate ability for clinical manipulation, and (4) not be expensive.

Biocompatibility requires that the wires not undergo significant corrosion under clinical conditions and release ions that will be toxic for patients. For some clinical applications, the ability of wires to be joined by soldering or welding to form more complex appliances is desirable. None of the four wire types meet all of these desirable characteristics, so the clinical selection should depend on the particular patient case and the different combinations of properties offered by each wire.

Manufacturing Process for Orthodontic Wires

Round orthodontic wires are manufactured by a drawing process, in which an original cast ingot of the alloy is subjected to several stages with intermediate heat treatments.[3,4] Rectangular and square orthodontic wires are manufactured from round wires with the use of a Turks Head machine, which employs two pairs of rollers, with one pair arranged vertically and the other pair arranged horizontally. As a result, rectangular and square wires inevitably have rounded corners (beveled edges), which affects the torque delivery with orthodontic brackets.[5] Details of the wire manufacturing process are proprietary with the manufacturers, but it is well known that variations in processing parameters have significant effects on wire properties. Scanning electron microscope (SEM) images found in publications cited later in this chapter show evidence of the wire manufacturing process.

Important Mechanical Properties of Orthodontic Wires and Mechanical Testing

The major mechanical property of importance for orthodontic wire alloys is the *elastic modulus*, which is directly proportional to the biomechanical force produced when the archwire is activated clinically.[6] For metallic materials used in engineering, the elastic modulus is normally measured with the tension test (Young's modulus, *E*) and is the ratio between stress and strain over the elastic range where the specimen elongation disappears when the applied force is removed. Because it is difficult to determine the precise onset of permanent deformation, the stress for a designated small amount of permanent tensile strain (sometimes termed *offset*), such as 0.1% or 0.2%, is instead reported as the yield strength (*YS*). Another important mechanical property for orthodontic wires is *resilience*, or, equivalently, the *modulus of resilience*, which is the area under the elastic portion of the stress-strain curve in tension. Resilience (*R*) is often expressed as

$$R = \frac{(YS)^2}{2E}$$

and represents the approximate elastic biomechanical energy available.

However, tension testing of orthodontic wires is not straightforward.[7] Special grips must be employed because of their small cross-sectional dimensions, and special precautions are needed to avoid premature fracture within the grips if an accurate measurement of permanent elongation in the central gauge portion of the wire specimen after fracture (ductility) is to be obtained. Consequently, orthodontic wires have generally been tested in some mode of bending, which is much easier to perform than tension testing and is relevant for clinical conditions. The original American Dental Association (ADA) Specification No. 32 for orthodontic wires, which was developed by a committee made up of members from universities, orthodontic companies, and private practice, stipulated a cantilever bending test to evaluate the mechanical properties,[8] and other investigators have used three-point and four-point bending tests.[9]

Mechanical property evaluation of orthodontic wires should follow the current International Organization for Standardization (ISO) standard,[10] which has been adopted by the ADA. The ISO standard subdivides orthodontic wires into Type 1 and Type 2, depending on whether they display linear elastic or nonlinear elastic behavior, respectively, during unloading at temperatures up to 50°C. SS, Co-Cr, and β-Ti wires display linear elastic behavior. Some Ni-Ti wires appear to display linear elastic behavior, while other Ni-Ti wires clearly display nonlinear elastic behavior. The elastic behavior of Ni-Ti wires is discussed in more detail in the later section devoted specifically to these wires.

Type 1 wires may be tested in tension or three-point bending, and the standard stipulates the testing conditions and specimen dimensions.[10] If a tension test is performed, the elastic modulus in GPa, 0.2% proof strength (yield strength) in MPa, and percentage elongation after fracture are determined. When a three-point bending test is performed (10 mm test span length between supports), the *bending stiffness* (the slope of the initial linear elastic portion of the force-deflection curve) in N/mm and the *0.1-mm offset bending force* in N, which causes a permanent offset of 0.1 mm in the specimen, are determined. Type 1 wires may be tested at room temperature (23°C ± 2°C) because their mechanical properties have little temperature dependence. Although not included in the ISO standard, the elastic modulus (Young's modulus) in three-point bending can be determined from the linear portion of the force-deflection plot using the appropriate relationship from solid mechanics.[9]

For Type 2 wires, the ISO standard only indicates use of a three-point bending test, which must be performed at 36°C ± 1°C.[10] The specimens (10-mm test span length) are loaded to a bending deflection of 3.1 mm, and the bending force during unloading is determined at successively decreasing deflections of 3.0, 2.0, 1.0, and 0.5 mm.

Classic Terminology for Orthodontic Wire Properties and Solid Mechanics Terms

Classic terminology of *stiffness*, *strength*, and *range* for orthodontic wires has been employed.[11] For bending tests, *stiffness* refers to the linear slope for the initial elastic range, *strength* refers to the maximum force or moment at the end of the elastic range where yielding (permanent deformation) of the wire begins, and *range* refers to the maximum deflection at which the wire behaves elastically. Burstone and Goldberg[12] introduced the property of *springback*, which is equal to the maximum elastic deflection or activation that can be achieved and subsequently recovered with a wire. From a practical viewpoint, *springback* (*SB*) can be defined from the results of a tension test as the quotient of yield strength (*YS*) and elastic modulus (*E*) or

$$SB = \frac{YS}{E}$$

for the wire being tested because it is very difficult to determine the precise onset of permanent deformation. A desirable high springback can be achieved with an appropriate combination of high yield strength and low elastic modulus. When lighter forces are desired for orthodontic tooth movement, a lower value of elastic modulus for the wire is needed. In the following sections, these mechanical properties are compared for the major wire types. From the definitions of the classic terms, *stiffness* is the quotient of strength and range.[9] Kusy[11] has developed nomograms showing relationships among these three elastic properties for bending and torsion of SS, Ni-Ti, and β-Ti wires with a wide variety of cross-sectional dimensions.

The elastic bending stiffness for a straight orthodontic wire is a more complex property than the elastic stiffness (elastic modulus) measured in a tension test, which is the quotient of tensile stress and tensile strain, as previously noted. The elastic bending stiffness, or *flexural rigidity*, is the product of contributions from the wire alloy and the geometry of the wire.[9] The alloy contribution is the elastic modulus (*E*), and the geometry contribution is the *moment of inertia* (*I*). The elastic bending stiffness also varies inversely with the length of the wire.

The moment of inertia (*I*) is a solid mechanics parameter that emerges from a derivation of the elastic flexure formula for a beam, relating the applied bending moment and the resulting stress distribution.[9] For the elastic bending of a symmetric beam (such as a round, rectangular, or square orthodontic wire), the stress varies from a maximum in tension at the outer curvature to a maximum in compression at the inner curvature. At the mid-plane of the elastically bent wire, called the *neutral surface*, there is zero stress and strain. When viewed in cross section, this mid-plane of zero stress and strain is called the *neutral axis*.

If a series of single-strand orthodontic wires of the same length manufactured from the same alloy with identical values of elastic modulus are compared, the relative values of moment of inertia provide a comparison of the elastic bending stiffness.[9] For a round wire,

$$I = \frac{\pi d^4}{64}$$

where *d* is the diameter. For a rectangular wire,

$$I = \frac{wt^3}{12}$$

where *w* is the width and *t* is the thickness (the cross-sectional dimension in the plane of bending). For rectangular wires, the two different bending directions can be termed *edgewise* and *flatwise*, following the terminology used by Kusy.[11] When the wide variation in cross-sectional dimensions is considered, it can be seen that the moment of inertia (and thus the elastic bending stiffness) varies enormously for the clinically used orthodontic wires.[9] The stiffness of an orthodontic wire can be considerably reduced if several small-diameter wires are twisted together to form a multistrand wire. Rucker and Kusy[13–15] have discussed the theoretical aspects and performed bending and tension test measurements for multistrand wires in a series of articles that focused on the elastic properties of SS and Ni-Ti leveling wires.

Stainless Steel Wires

The SS (iron-chromium alloy) wire was the principal orthodontic wire by the 1950s,[2] and orthodontic companies currently offer a variety of these wires. Verstrynge et al[16] have reported the general compositions of 10 SS orthodontic wires from nine companies, determined by x-ray energy-dispersive spectrometric analysis (EDS) with an SEM. Mechanical properties were determined with tension tests (Table 4-1) and three-point bending tests, and Vickers hardness was also measured; only 0.017 × 0.025–inch wires were evaluated. All 10 wires were austenitic SS alloys. Nine wires were AISI (American Iron and Steel Institute) Type 304, containing approximately 18% chromium, 8% nickel, and small amounts of other elements (balance iron), traditionally termed *18-8 stainless steels*. The tenth was a nickel-free wire of the type covered by ASTM (American Society for Testing and Materials) standard F2229 for nitrogen-strengthened, manganese-chromium-molybdenum (Mn-Cr-Mo), low-nickel SS wires used in surgical implants. Mean values of elastic modulus measured with the tension test varied from 166 to 184 GPa, and there was good agreement with values obtained with the three-point bending test. Mean 0.2% offset yield strength varied from 1,540 to 1,970 MPa, and springback varied from 0.009 to 0.011. Mean Vickers hardness for the 10 SS wires varied from approximately 240 to 290 kg/mm[2]. Surfaces of the SS wire products were examined with an SEM, and Fig 4-1 shows an example with parallel linear features that resulted from the manufacturing process.

The mean values of elastic modulus and yield strength reported by Verstrynge et al[16] are comparable with tension test results in an earlier study[7] for several sizes of as-received SS wires, principally from one company. In that study, heat treatment caused increases in yield strength and resilience for all wires and in elastic modulus for some wires; this treatment has been recommended for SS wires to provide stress relief and prevent fracture during clinical manipulation.[3,7]

The austenitic structure provides formability, and other advantages of these wires include low cost, excellent corrosion resistance arising from a chromium oxide surface film, and the ability to be joined by soldering and welding.[3,4] SS wires have low surface roughness[19] and generally exhibited the lowest coefficients of friction for different combinations of SS and alumina brackets and the dry and wet (saliva) states.[20,21] Some orthodontists have concerns about the high elastic modulus for SS wires, along with their potential for nickel release into the oral environment. However, nickel sensitization of orthodontic patients with intraoral devices is considered to be highly improbable, although sensitization of patients with extraoral devices containing nickel cannot be excluded.[22] Austenitic SS wires are susceptible to intergranular corrosion when heated in the temperature range of 400°C to 900°C, and caution is needed during joining or stress-relief heat treatments for orthodontic appliances.[3,4]

Table 4-1	Recently reported values of mechanical properties for as-received orthodontic wires		
Alloy type	**Elastic modulus (GPa)**	**Yield strength (MPa)**	**Springback**
SS*	166–184	1,540–1,970	0.009–0.011
SS†	176–186	—	—
Co-Cr‡	175–192	1,040–1,160	0.006
Co-Cr†	189–206	—	—
Ni-Ti§			
0.016-inch	33 and 37	440	0.013
0.018-inch	32 and 37	490	0.014
0.017 × 0.025–inch	58–60	310	0.005
β-Ti*	64–72	770–1,010	0.011–0.014
Titanium alloy* (Ti-6Al-4V)	93	1,250	0.013

*From Verstrynge et al[16] and tension tests on 0.017 × 0.025–inch wires, reporting 0.2% offset yield strength.

†From Tian and Darvell[17] using very accurate cantilever bending tests on different sizes of one SS wire and four tempers of Elgiloy (Rocky Mountain Orthodontics). Yield strength and springback were not reported.

‡From Kusy et al[18] using tension tests to measure 0.1% offset yield strength (YS) and three-point and four-point bending tests to measure elastic modulus (E). Values of springback are calculated from these values of E and YS.

§From Rucker and Kusy[15] using tension tests to measure 0.1% offset yield strength and three-point bending tests to measure elastic modulus. Values of springback are again calculated and averaged for these wire sizes.

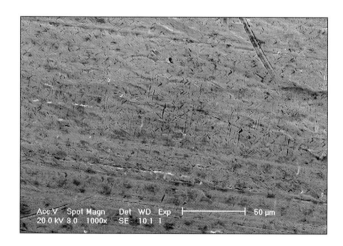

Fig 4-1 SEM image at ×1,000 original magnification of SS wire (Ortho Organizers). (Reprinted from Verstrynge et al[16] with permission.)

Another recent article[23] has presented information about three types of the popular Australian austenitic SS wires, manufactured by A.J. Wilcock in diameters ranging from 0.012 to 0.024 inch and in several grades of varying resilience. Mean values of elastic modulus for the 0.016-inch- and 0.018-inch-diameter Australian wires obtained with tension tests ranged from 173 to 177 GPa, but values of springback were not determined. The carbon content of these wires was much higher than that for standard 18-8 wire alloys, and mean values of Vickers hardness (approximately 640 to 660 kg/mm²) were also much higher than the values reported by Verstrynge et al[16] for other SS wires. This much higher hardness was attributed to the increased carbon content and differences in the manufacturing processes. SEM images revealed surface striations from the manufacturing process, along with irregularities and porosity, which varied for the three types of Australian wire that were evaluated. The authors concluded that the increased hardness of Australian wire, compared with other SS wires, might increase brittleness, cause difficulty for the clinician in placing bends, and account for the tendency of higher grades to fracture during bending, as well as negatively affect sliding mechanics during therapy, particularly if titanium brackets are used. They noted that the hardness of conventional SS wires and SS brackets are similar.

Cobalt-Chromium Wires

A Co-Cr alloy was developed for a watch spring by the Elgin Watch Company in the 1950s,[2] and a popular orthodontic wire alloy has been marketed as Elgiloy (Rocky Mountain Orthodontics). The composition is 40% cobalt, 20% chromium, 15.81% iron, 15% nickel, 7% molybdenum, 2% manganese, 0.15% carbon, and 0.04% beryllium. These wires are available in four color-coded tempers. Three tempers can be manipulated in the as-received condition and then heat treated to produce improved yield strength and resilience; heat treatment is not recommended for the most resilient temper, which already has very high spring qualities in the as-received condition. In an earlier study, as-received Elgiloy wires of the four tempers and a wide variety of sizes had values of elastic modulus (E) measured in tension ranging from about 150 to 180 GPa and 0.1% offset yield strength (YS) ranging from about 830 to 1,240 MPa.[7] Kusy et al[18] subsequently performed an extensive study of the mechanical properties of the four tempers of Elgiloy wires, using bending tests to determine E and tension tests to determine the 0.1% offset YS. Overall mean values ranged from about 170 to 190 GPa for E and from about 1,040 to 1,160 MPa for YS; substantial variations in these properties were found for different wire sizes and tempers. Recently, using a very accurate cantilever bending test with long spans, low loads, and a laser displacement sensor, Tian and Darvell[17] found that mean elastic modulus values for as-received Elgiloy wires of the four tempers ranged from 190 to 206 GPa, and higher values were found for WIPTAM wires (Elephant Dental), another Co-Cr alloy. Values of mechanical properties for as-received Co-Cr alloys from the studies by Kusy et al[18] and Tian and Darvell[17] are provided in Table 4-1. Elgiloy wires have excellent formability (other than the most resilient temper) and excellent corrosion resistance from a chromium oxide surface film; however, they are more expensive than SS wires.[3,4] Older measurements also found lower springback compared with SS wires.[3,7] The surface roughness of Elgiloy wire is higher than that of SS wire but lower than that of Ni-Ti and β-Ti wires,[19] and Elgiloy wire generally exhibited lower frictional coefficients with brackets compared with both of these wires.[20,21] Other companies also market Co-Cr orthodontic wires, but studies of their mechanical properties have not appeared in the orthodontic literature. Although recent articles indicate that Elgiloy orthodontic wires can be cytotoxic under some laboratory conditions,[24,25] no clinical evidence exists of biocompatibility problems for patients.

Nickel-Titanium Wires

Ni-Ti wires for orthodontics date from the pioneering work by Andreasen et al[26,27] reported in the early 1970s. Their studies followed the seminal research by Buehler and his colleagues[28,29] on Ni-Ti *shape memory alloys*, which was published in the previous decade. These alloys were named *Nitinol* after their *ni*ckel and *ti*tanium compositions and the *N*aval *O*rdnance *L*aboratory where the studies were performed. The first commercial Ni-Ti orthodontic wire was introduced by the Unitek company (now 3M Unitek) as Nitinol (now Nitinol Classic) and had the unique advantages of a very low elastic modulus and very wide working range compared with SS and Co-Cr wires.[30] Nitinol Classic is now classified as *nonsuperelastic*.[3] However, in the years following the introduction of Nitinol, two new Ni-Ti orthodontic wires having *superelastic* (termed *pseudoelastic* in the materials science literature) behavior were introduced: Chinese Ni-Ti,[31] marketed as Sentalloy by GAC International (now Dentsply GAC International), and Japanese Ni-Ti,[32] marketed as Ni-Ti by Ormco. The first wire (Neo Sentalloy) possessing true shape memory in the oral environment was introduced by GAC International in the early 1990s.[33] Ni-Ti wires of this type are now available from many companies.

Ni-Ti orthodontic wires have nearly equiatomic nickel and titanium compositions, with other secondary elements intentionally added by manufacturers, hence the term *NiTi wires*. There are two principal NiTi phases, with different mechanical properties[2] and atomic arrangements,[3] and their proportions and characteristics determine the properties of the given NiTi wire.[3] Transformations between these phases can occur with changes in temperature or stress and take place by a twinning process on the atomic scale, which provides the mechanism for the shape memory effect.[2–4] Austenitic NiTi (*austenite*) is the high-temperature, low-stress phase, while martensitic NiTi (*martensite*) is the structure that exists for conditions of low-temperature and high-stress. R-phase is an intermediate structure that can form during the forward (heating) and reverse (cooling) transformations between martensite and austenite.[3] Because of their different crystal structures, the NiTi phases in orthodontic wires can be identified by x-ray diffraction.[3,34–36] The most convenient analytic technique to provide information about transformations between the NiTi phases with changes in wire temperature is differential scanning calorimetry (DSC).[3,37–39]

Four phase transformation temperatures are typically specified for Ni-Ti orthodontic wires. The temperatures for the start and finish of the transformation from martensite to austenite, when the wire is heated, are designated as A_s and A_f, respectively. The temperatures for the start and finish of the transformation from austenite to martensite, when the wire is cooled, are designated as M_s and M_f, respectively. In the ISO standard for orthodontic wires, the A_f temperature for Type 2 wires, determined by DSC, must be specified to the nearest 1°C.[10]

Figure 4-2 shows the considerable differences in mechanical properties for the original Nitinol (termed *work-hardened Ni-Ti*) and Japanese Ni-Ti alloys compared with SS and Co-Cr alloys for 0.016-inch-diameter wires.[32] The slopes (elastic modulus) of the initial tensile stress-strain plots (elastic range) are similar for the latter two wires,

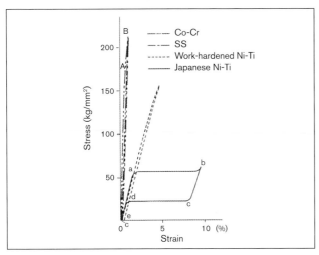

Fig 4-2 Comparison of stress-strain curves obtained with the tension test for SS, Co-Cr, Nitinol, and Japanese Ni-Ti orthodontic wires. (Reprinted from Miura et al[32] with permission.)

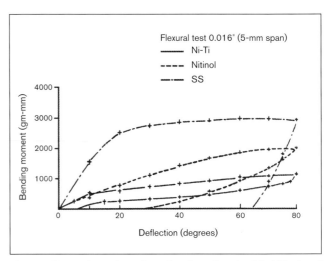

Fig 4-3 Comparison of cantilever bending plots for SS, Nitinol, and Chinese Ni-Ti orthodontic wires. (Reprinted from Burstone et al[31] with permission.)

and these are much greater than the slopes of the initial plots for the two Ni-Ti wires, which are also similar. The work-hardened Ni-Ti wire experienced a small amount of permanent strain (region from *0* to *e* on the horizontal axis) after removal of the stress. For Japanese Ni-Ti wire, there are two horizontal superelastic regions following the initial elastic range (*0* to *a*). The region from *a* to *b* is termed the *upper superelastic plateau* for loading, and the region from *c* to *d* is termed the *lower superelastic plateau* for unloading. The region from *a* to *b* corresponds to the stress-induced transformation of the wire from austenite to martensite during loading, and the region from *c* to *d* corresponds to the reverse transformation of martensite to austenite during the first stage of unloading. The final unloading of the wire corresponds to the region from *d* to *0*, and all of the elastic strain in austenite will disappear. If the Japanese Ni-Ti wire is subjected to stress exceeding that for the upper superelastic plateau, the stress-strain curve will continue beyond *b* in a manner similar to the work-hardened Ni-Ti wire, and there will be some permanent deformation after removal of the stress and recovery of the superelastic and elastic strains.

In Fig 4-2, the nonsuperelastic Nitinol wire appears to have linear elastic behavior, but careful tension tests have shown that this wire actually displays nonlinear elastic behavior.[14] The nonlinear elastic behavior for the superelastic Japanese Ni-Ti wire[32] is evident in this figure because the range of elastic strain extends to the end of the horizontal line for the upper superelastic plateau stress. The stress levels for the superelastic plateaus can be modified conveniently with the use of elevated temperature[32] or electrical resistance[40] heat treatment, and this has been exploited commercially to produce a Ni-Ti archwire with variable force delivery (BioForce, Dentsply GAC International).

In bending, the elastic stress varies linearly from zero at the center of the wire to maximum tensile and compres-

sive values at opposite surfaces,[9] and the superelastic plateaus are not sharply defined.[3,41] This can be seen in Fig 4-3, which compares the cantilever bending test results for the original Chinese Ni-Ti and Nitinol wires with SS orthodontic wires, using 5-mm test spans appropriate for interbracket distances.[31] In this study, the wire specimens were bent to an angular deflection of 80 degrees, which resulted in permanent deformation, and then unloaded. Springback (the difference between 80 degrees and the final angular deflection after unloading) is much greater for Chinese Ni-Ti wire compared to Nitinol. Superelastic and nonsuperelastic Ni-Ti wires are readily identified by differences in springback.[41]

Transformations in the superelastic wire Nitinol SE (3M Unitek) and the shape memory wire Neo Sentalloy during heating are shown in Figs 4-4 and 4-5, respectively. The temperature-modulated DSC[39] plots present much more detail about the wire transformations than is possible with conventional DSC[38] because use of a small sinusoidal temperature variation superimposed on the linear heating or cooling ramp enables the presentation of nonreversing heat flow processes, which can be seen in these two figures. Transformations involving austenite (A), martensite (M), and R-phase (R) have been labeled in these figures. M′ is a low-temperature form of martensite that results from twinning.[42] (For these experiments, the wire specimens were first cooled from room temperature to approximately –150°C to assure complete transformation to martensite and then heated to 100°C to assure complete transformation to austenite. Then the specimens were cooled again to –150°C; the cooling plots are also provided by Brantley et al.[39]) Using the procedure in the ISO standard[10] of placing a tangent line to the right side of the peak corresponding to the transformation to austenite and locating the intersection with an extrapolation of the adjacent baseline, it is found that the A_f temperature for Nitinol SE is greater than

Fig 4-4 Heating curve for Nitinol SE orthodontic wire obtained with temperature-modulated DSC. Rev, reversing. (Reprinted from Brantley et al[39] with permission.)

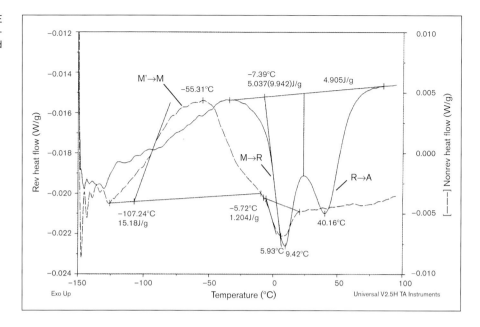

Fig 4-5 Heating curve for Neo Sentalloy orthodontic wire obtained with temperature-modulated DSC. Rev, reversing. (Reprinted from Brantley et al[39] with permission.)

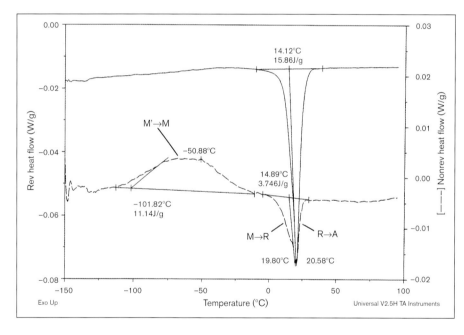

50°C and the A_f temperature for Neo Sentalloy is below body temperature (37°C). Heating curves obtained by conventional DSC[38] are adequate to determine the A_f temperature for orthodontic wires but present considerably less information than those obtained by temperature-modulated DSC.[39] Transformation peaks for Nitinol Classic are very weak because the work-hardened martensitic structure does not undergo much transformation to austenite.[37,38,43]

Popular Copper Ni-Ti orthodontic wires are marketed by Ormco with A_f temperatures of 27°C, 35°C, and 40°C. The relative force delivered by the Copper Ni-Ti wire decreases with increasing A_f temperature, and the clinician is thus provided with options for selecting the wire size and force for individual patients. Figure 4-6 presents the heating temperature-modulated DSC plot for 35°C Copper Ni-Ti,[39] and the A_f temperature determined from this curve is close to the value reported by the manufacturer. Kusy[2] reported that Copper Ni-Ti wires contain very small percentages of chromium to compensate for the effect of the copper addition on raising the Ni-Ti transformation temperature above that of the oral environment.

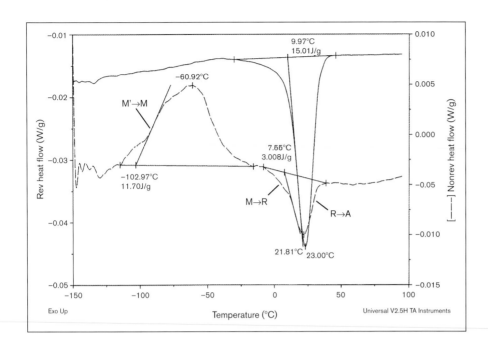

Fig 4-6 Heating curve for 35°C Copper Ni-Ti orthodontic wire obtained with temperature-modulated DSC. Rev, reversing. (Reprinted from Brantley et al[39] with permission.)

Another classification for Ni-Ti orthodontic wires was introduced by Kusy[44]: *martensitic-stabilized* (eg, Nitinol Classic), *martensitic-active* (eg, Sentalloy), and *austenitic-active* (eg, Ni-Ti). Martensitic-stabilized wires are subjected to sufficient mechanical deformation during drawing and other processing steps that the shape memory effect (SME) is suppressed; these are nonsuperelastic wires. Martensitic-active wires change to the austenitic structure when placed in the mouth by a *thermoelastic effect*; this effect can be observed when a deformed archwire segment is warmed in the hands and returns to its original shape. These wires exhibit shape memory in the oral environment. (Brantley et al[43] studied the transformations that occur when Sentalloy is heated.) Austenitic-active wires undergo a stress-induced pseudoelastic transformation to martensite when subjected to sufficient mechanical deformation in the oral environment and then return to austenite upon deactivation; these are superelastic wires. Kusy[2] noted that precise composition control by manufacturers of the starting Ni-Ti alloy ingots can be achieved to obtain the desired transformation temperatures for orthodontic wires used in the oral environment.

Rucker and Kusy[15] evaluated three sizes of Ni-Ti leveling archwires from one manufacturer (Dentaurum) and found that mean values of elastic modulus obtained with three-point bending tests ranged from 32 to 37 GPa for 0.016-inch- and 0.018-inch-diameter wires and from 58 to 60 GPa for 0.017 × 0.025–inch rectangular wires. Mean values of 0.1% offset yield strength obtained from tension tests ranged from 310 MPa for the 0.017 × 0.025–inch rectangular wire to 490 MPa for the 0.018-inch-diameter wire. These values of elastic modulus and yield strength are summarized in Table 4-1. Recently, Iijima et al[45] determined the elastic modulus of Nitinol Classic and 35°C

Copper Ni-Ti using three-point bending and tension tests and found approximate mean values of 40 GPa for Nitinol Classic and 50 GPa and 22 GPa, respectively, for austenitic and martensitic 35°C Copper Ni-Ti. Table 4-1 shows that values of elastic modulus and yield strength for Ni-Ti wires are much lower than those for SS wires, and springback is usually greater. In an older study in which tension tests were performed on many sizes of Nitinol Classic, substantial variations in mean values of elastic modulus and 0.1% offset yield strength were also found.[7]

While the low elastic modulus and generally wide elastic range are advantages of Ni-Ti wires, there are concerns about difficulty for manipulation, surface roughness, corrosion and release of nickel ions into the oral environment, and degradation of mechanical properties by fluoride ions. Ni-Ti wires are also more expensive than SS and Co-Cr wires.

Measurements of surface roughness by Bourauel et al[46] for 11 Ni-Ti wires using atomic force microscopy, laser specular reflectance, and profilometry revealed that some products had much rougher surfaces compared with the SS wire product used for comparison. These authors pointed out the importance of surface roughness for wire friction with brackets, esthetics, corrosion behavior, and biocompatibility. In vitro electrochemical corrosion experiments by this research group,[47] using a modified Fusayama electrolyte (an artificial saliva) and including numerous bending cycles to simulate mastication, revealed substantial variations in corrosion tendency; breakdown potential of the surface oxide film, which provides corrosion resistance; surface roughness; and nickel ion release for four Ni-Ti wire products. They concluded that variations in surface topography and microstructural phases resulting from differences in wire processing by manufacturers might be sources for differences in corrosion tendency. The role of phase transformations on the corrosion of Ni-Ti wires has also been suggested from the results of another in vitro study.[48]

Fluoride attacks the protective oxide surface film on Ni-Ti orthodontic wires, causing corrosion and nickel release; this has been an active area of research because of concern about effects of fluoride ions found in toothpastes, mouthrinses, and topical fluoride applications. The in vitro electrochemical corrosion behavior was compared recently for four Ni-Ti wire products in an acidic artificial saliva containing several fluoride concentrations.[49] Corrosion resistance varied among these products and decreased with increasing fluoride concentration. There was no evident correspondence with differences in surface topography for the four products, and all products experienced severe corrosion when exposed to the 0.5% fluoride concentration. Another recent in vitro study found that the release of nickel from two products into an artificial saliva solution was greater when the wires were subjected to continuous three-point bending, which was attributed to buckling or cracking of the protective surface oxide film.[50] However, examination of topographic changes and measurement of nickel release from lingual archwires immersed up to 30 days in Hank's Balanced Salt Solution showed that amounts of nickel release from Ni-Ti and Copper Ni-Ti were below the levels known to cause cell damage, although changes in surface roughness of Copper Ni-Ti seemed to have clinical significance.[51] A third in vitro electrochemical study has shown that Ni-Ti orthodontic wires are susceptible to pitting corrosion in chloride ion solutions and to general corrosion attack in fluoride solutions.[52] A fourth in vitro study using extracts from Ni-Ti and SS wires, which were collected by an electrochemical procedure in an artificial saliva containing chloride ions and acidulated sodium fluoride and analyzed by atomic absorption spectroscopy, found that the released ions from both wires were cytotoxic but noted that the laboratory environment did not simulate in vivo conditions.[53]

Principles of in vitro electrochemical corrosion testing performed in the aforementioned studies are summarized by Brantley.[6] While such tests, in which corrosion is forced to occur by applying increasing electrical potential, provide useful information, they should be considered primarily for screening purposes to compare relative corrosion behavior of similar alloys. Commonly employed electrolytes, such as saline solutions or artificial salivas, cannot fully simulate the complex chemical conditions of the oral environment, as emphasized by Kao et al.[53]

Other recent studies have investigated the effects of fluoride ions and the oral environment on the mechanical properties of Ni-Ti wires. Superelastic Ni-Ti wires that were immersed in an acidulated phosphate fluoride solution and subjected to a tension test experienced hydrogen embrittlement.[54] However, in another study, examination of Ni-Ti archwires that had fractured intraorally suggests that the observed brittle fracture was not caused by hydrogen embrittlement because an increase in alloy hardness at the exposed surface was absent.[55] Fracture sites for the retrieved archwires were preferentially located at the mid-span between premolar and molar, and failure was attributed to the complex stress distribution from masticatory forces and engagement in the bracket. These authors made the important comment that laboratory tension tests substantially underestimate the loading experienced by archwires in vivo.

Walker et al[56] compared unloading behavior in three-point bending, using a methodology based on the ISO standard,[10] for a conventional superelastic Ni-Ti wire (Ormco) and Copper Ni-Ti wire (specific A_f temperature not provided) following exposure to an acidulated fluoride agent, a neutral fluoride agent, or distilled water (control) for 1½ hours at 37°C. This time period simulated 3 months of daily one-minute topical applications. Mechanical testing was performed in distilled water at 37°C. While the unloading elastic modulus and yield strength of the conventional superelastic wire were significantly decreased by exposure to both fluoride agents, no significant effect was found for Copper Ni-Ti with either agent. Changes in surface topography due to corrosion were observed after exposure to the fluoride agents, with more severe attack on the Copper Ni-Ti wire surfaces.

A recent clinical study[57] closely followed the ISO standard methodology[10] to compare the unloading three-point bending properties at 37°C for two groups of 0.016 × 0.022–inch superelastic Ni-Ti wire products (G&H Wire Company) after exposure in the oral environment and a third group serving as a control that was not exposed intraorally. During the 6-week period of study, the first group of patients used a fluoride-containing toothpaste and fluoride mouthrinse combination, and the second group used a nonfluoridated toothpaste. Both groups of exposed wires experienced degradation in unloading force compared with the unexposed control wires. The wire group exposed to the fluoride regimen experienced slightly more force degradation than the group exposed to the nonfluoridated toothpaste for the 3.1-mm and 3.0-mm deflections but less degradation for deflections of 1.0 mm and 0.5 mm.

Further laboratory and clinical research is required to appreciate the full implications of the different unloading behaviors observed by Walker et al[56] and Vo et al.[57] Additional insight into the fundamental materials science mechanisms is needed, and it is highly important to obtain information about responses of other superelastic wire products to commercial fluoride regimens and unfluoridated toothpastes under conditions relevant to tooth movement in vivo.

Surface modification of Ni-Ti wires has also been an active area of research. From in vitro electrochemical study of the corrosion of ion-implanted Ni-Ti wire (IonGuard Neo Sentalloy, GAC International) in artificial saliva and fluoride mouthrinse solutions, Iijima et al[58] concluded that the modified surface may improve corrosion properties compared to Neo Sentalloy wire that was not ion implanted. Recent laboratory studies have shown that a diamondlike carbon coating reduces friction,[59] and esthetic metallic and

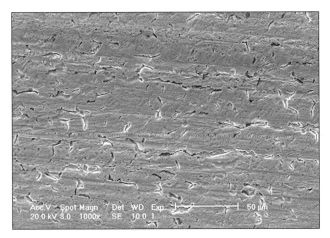

Fig 4-7 SEM image at ×1,000 original magnification of β-Ti wire (TMA). (Reprinted from Verstrynge et al[16] with permission.)

polymer coatings influence the unloading force in bending while increasing surface roughness.[60] Other studies have shown that for unloading, epoxy-coated esthetic wires produce lower force than uncoated Ni-Ti- wires,[61] and the retrieved coated archwires produced lower force than the as-received coated archwires.[62] Moreover, profilometry and microscopic examination of the retrieved 0.016-inch-diameter, epoxy-coated Ni-Ti archwires that had been used in vivo for a mean period of 33 days revealed increased surface roughness, discoloration, ditching, and delamination.[62] An average of 25% of the original coatings was lost, which greatly reduced the esthetics of the retrieved archwires. Further clinical research is needed to evaluate whether coated Ni-Ti wires can yield improved performance for orthodontic therapy because the oral environment is a much more stringent medium for survival and function of these wires than the laboratory.

Beta-Titanium Wires

β-Ti was the last of the four major metallic wire alloys to be introduced to the profession. The potential of β-Ti for orthodontics was originally realized by Burstone and Goldberg,[63,64] and an orthodontic wire named *TMA* (*titanium-molybdenum alloy*) was marketed by Ormco around 1980. The nominal composition of the original alloy evaluated by Burstone and Goldberg was approximately 11% molybdenum, 6% zirconium, and 4% tin, with the balance titanium; this alloy was well known in engineering materials as *β-III titanium*.[64,65] Molybdenum stabilizes the high-temperature β-Ti crystal structure, and zirconium and tin improve mechanical properties[66] and suppress formation of an embrittling omega phase during annealing heat treatment for processing by the manufacturer.[67] The β-Ti crystal structure has higher ductility than the room-temperature α-titanium structure, resulting in high formability, which

enables the manipulation of β-Ti wires to form complex orthodontic appliances.[64]

β-Ti wires are more expensive than SS and Co-Cr wires, but they are popular because of several favorable properties. β-Ti wires have an elastic modulus intermediate between that of SS and Co-Cr wires, along with high springback.[63,64] β-Ti is the only orthodontic alloy with true weldability,[63] which is useful for the fabrication of more complex appliances, and detailed information about welding these wires has been published.[68,69] Iijima et al[70–73] have recently examined β-Ti wires joined by infrared brazing/soldering, laser welding, and electrical resistance welding and concluded that the joined wires would be suitable for clinical use.

β-Ti wires are expected to be more biocompatible than the other three major wire alloys because nickel is absent from their compositions; corrosion resistance is provided by the thin titanium oxide surface film. A review article has indicated that there are no concerns about cytotoxicity for molybdenum, zirconium, and tin.[74] However, there has been concern for β-Ti orthodontic wires from several laboratory studies investigating the breakdown of the titanium oxide surface film by fluoride ions in topical fluoride prophylactic agents, resulting in hydrogen absorption that might cause degradation of mechanical properties and even delayed fracture due to hydrogen embrittlement.[75–78] Recent studies have evaluated thin films of titanium aluminum nitride (TiAlN) placed by cathodic arc physical vapor deposition and tungsten carbide/carbon (WC/C) placed by magnetron sputtering on the surface of β-Ti wires.[79,80] While the TiAlN coating was superior in reducing property changes caused by prolonged immersion in a mouthrinse solution with high fluoride ion concentration,[79] the WC/C coating was more effective in reducing frictional properties.[80]

In the original study by Kusy et al[19] using laser specular reflectance, β-Ti wire (TMA) had a rougher surface than one SS wire product and wires of two Elgiloy tempers, although not as rough as the surfaces of two Ni-Ti wires (Nitinol and Titanal [Lancer Orthodontics]). Figure 4-7 shows a recent SEM image of the surface of the TMA β-Ti from the Verstrynge et al[16] publication, and parallel linear features from the manufacturing process can be seen.

Subsequently, using a model laboratory system that employed SS flats to simulate brackets, a wide range of sliding velocities for archwire specimens, and prevailing atmospheric conditions at 34°C, Kusy and Whitley[81] found that β-Ti (TMA) consistently had the highest coefficients of friction compared with representative SS, Elgiloy, and Ni-Ti wires. From additional in vitro experiments, they concluded that the high friction of β-Ti wires under laboratory conditions originated from cold welding to SS brackets and adherence to alumina brackets caused by mechanical abrasion.[20,82]

Kusy and Whitley collaborated with colleagues at Spire Corporation on an innovative nitrogen ion implantation process for β-Ti wire (TMA).[83] Polycrystalline alumina flats (simulating ceramic brackets) were also implanted with titanium ions. Static and kinetic frictional coefficients for sliding of ion-implanted β-Ti wires against the ion-implanted alumina flats were similar to coefficients for control (not implanted) couples of SS, Co-Cr, and Ni-Ti wires against control (not implanted) polycrystalline alumina flats. Subsequently, ion implantation was commercially employed for β-Ti wires (Low-Friction TMA, Ormco); a clinical study that evaluated these ion-implanted wires is discussed in a later section of this chapter. Ion implantation has also been utilized commercially for Ni-Ti wires (IonGuard Neo Sentalloy, GAC International), and this surface treatment was found to reduce the nickel ion release.[84]

After expiration of the patent for the original TMA wire, new β-Ti orthodontic wires were introduced by Dentsply GAC International (Resolve) and 3M Unitek (Beta III Titanium). Both manufacturers claim that their β-Ti wires are carefully processed and microfinished (Resolve) or polished (Beta III Titanium) to yield a smoother surface for reduced friction with brackets during sliding mechanics. Subsequently, β-Ti wires were marketed by many other companies.

In the previously discussed article by Verstrynge et al,[16] compositions, mechanical properties (Table 4-1), and surface roughness were also reported for twelve 0.017 × 0.025–inch titanium alloy wires from ten companies. From their EDS/SEM analyses, the wires could be classified into four groups: *(1)* nine wires were β-III titanium with general composition of Ti-11.5Mo-6Zr-4.5Sn, including one with nitrogen ion implantation, *(2)* one wire was Beta C Titanium (Highland Metals) with general composition of Ti-3Al-8V-6Cr-4Mo-4Zr,[65] *(3)* one wire had an approximate Ti-6Al-4V composition and was an α-β titanium alloy with a two-phase microstructure (TiMolium, TP Orthodontics), and *(4)* one wire was a different type of β-Ti with an approximate Ti-45Nb composition (Titanium Niobium FA, Ormco). The β-stabilizing element niobium is beneficial for reducing stress corrosion cracking of the β-Ti alloys.[65]

Mean values of elastic modulus measured with the tension test ranged from 64 to 72 GPa for seven β-III titanium wires, but a much higher mean value (93 GPa) was found for the eighth wire (TiMolium Ti-6Al-4V alloy) that was reported.[16] In comparison, mean values measured with the three-point bending test for 11 wires ranged from 65 to 88 GPa, and the mean value for TiMolium was 100 GPa. Mean values of elastic modulus measured with the three-point bending test were substantially higher than those measured with the tension test for four β-III titanium wires and the Ti-6Al-4V wire. Mean values of 0.2% offset yield strength for the seven β-III titanium wires measured with the tension test ranged from 770 to 1,100 GPa, and the mean value for the Ti-6Al-4V wire was 1,250 MPa. Mean Vickers hardness for the 12 wires ranged from approximately 100 kg/mm² for Titanium Niobium FA to 190 kg/mm² for TiMolium, with similar values for the other β-Ti wires. Springback ranged from 0.012 to 0.014 for the eight titanium alloy wires whose mechanical properties were determined with the tension test. Surface roughness was measured by a profilometer with a 3-μm diamond tip that contacted the wire specimen. The average distance from the mean line traversed by the tip (R_a) ranged from 0.07 to 0.17 μm for the 12 titanium wire products, while the maximum peak-to-valley distance of the profile (R_t) had much greater values ranging from 1.15 to 2.78 μm.

In another article, Kusy et al[85] reported a study of six of these titanium alloy wires, comparing the compositions determined by EDS/SEM analyses, surface roughness obtained by laser reflectance spectroscopy, and sliding resistances measured with a custom laboratory apparatus simulating a three-bracket system. More precise elemental compositions were presented for the five β-III titanium alloys and the α-β titanium alloy compared with the general compositions provided by Verstrynge et al.[16] The six titanium alloy wire products could be classified into two groups, based on specular reflectance and optical surface roughness: *(1)* Beta III Titanium, Resolve, and CAN (Ortho Organizers) wires had a lower overall value (0.148 μm) of mean root-mean-squared (RMS) optical roughness; *(2)* TMA, Low-Friction TMA, and TiMolium had a higher overall value (0.195 μm) of mean RMS optical roughness. Differences in values of surface roughness for these six wire products measured in the studies by Kusy et al[85] and Verstrynge et al[16] arise because of the optical and profilometry techniques that were employed, respectively. Most importantly, for six different values of angulation covering the passive and active regions of sliding, the coefficients of friction found by Kusy et al[85] for these six wire products using the simulated three-bracket system varied only from 0.17 to 0.27 and was independent of surface roughness.

Archwire Selection and Clinical Studies

The preceding sections have shown that there are many choices for clinical wire selection, depending on the particular orthodontic patient and the decision about an optimum treatment plan. As one example of the general principles for archwire selection, the 3M Unitek Catalog[86] presents an archwire analysis for the initial phase (leveling, tipping, and rotating), the intermediate phase (space closure, arch form correction, and occlusal plane leveling), and the finishing phase (vertical detailing, individual rotations, refinement of interdigitation, and retention). Three approaches for the archwire sequence are suggested, using 3M Unitek products, when the wire criteria for each phase are considered: *(1)* The first choice for the three phases is Nitinol HA (heat-activated), followed by Nitinol Classic, followed by Beta III Titanium. *(2)* The second choice for the three phases is Nitinol SE, followed by Beta III Titanium, followed by Permachrome (SS). *(3)* The third choice for the three phases is Nitinol Classic, followed by Permachrome, followed by Flexiloy (Co-Cr-Ni alloy). A second presentation about archwire selection is found in the Ormco Orthodontic Products Catalog,[87] which presents a detailed wire stiffness guide showing the different arch-wire alloys and wire sizes offered by the company, with suggestions for selection that depend on whether the malocclusion is considered mild, moderate, or severe. A third presentation about archwire selection is provided in the Dentaurum Wire Manual,[88] which provides detailed information about the properties of wires offered by the company, along with suggestions for their use during the initial, intermediate, and final phases of treatment. Each major orthodontic company that markets archwires has recommendations about selection for different phases of patient therapy.

Because many different archwires are available for the four major alloys, it is instructive to examine important publications that have reported the efficacy of various products. Discussions of seven randomized controlled trials totaling 517 patients, in which initial archwires were employed for tooth alignment, are found in a recent Cochrane Collaboration review.[89] These seven clinical studies are summarized in order of publication in the following paragraphs.

Cobb et al[90] compared use of 0.016-inch-diameter ion-implanted Ni-Ti wire (Sentalloy), 0.016-inch-diameter Sentalloy that was not ion implanted, and 0.00175-inch-diameter triple-strand steel wire (Wildcat, GAC International) for initial alignment. For this study, there were 123 patients and 155 dental arches. Patients were randomly assigned to the archwire types, and both 0.018-inch- and 0.022-inch-slot edgewise appliances were employed. At the end of the 12-month study, no significant difference in the rate of tooth movement was found among the three archwires, despite the superelastic character of Sentalloy and the lower friction claimed by the manufacturer for ion-implanted Sentalloy. The rate of alignment was significantly faster in the mandibular arch for patients having the 0.022-inch-slot appliances.

Evans et al[91] compared three aligning archwires: 0.016-inch- and 0.022-inch-diameter medium-force martensitic-active Ni-Ti (Titanium Heat Memory Wire, American Orthodontics); 0.0155-inch-diameter multistrand SS (Dentaflex, Dentarium); and 0.016-inch- and 0.022-inch-diameter graded-force, martensite-active Ni-Ti (BioForce Sentalloy, GAC International). This 8-week study had 56 patients who needed maxillary and mandibular fixed appliances, and they were randomly assigned two of the three archwires. The two Ni-Ti archwire products did not show superior performance in the rate of tooth alignment compared with the less expensive SS archwire. The authors noted that variations in the metabolic responses of patients might obscure differences in the efficacy of the three wires and commented that the two Ni-Ti wires might not be sufficiently deformed during the initial alignment phase to fully utilize their superelastic property. This point was also emphasized by Rucker and Kusy[15] in discussing their laboratory evaluation of numerous leveling archwires.

O'Brien et al[92] reported the results of a study with a mean duration of 35 days in which a superelastic Ni-Ti wire (Titanol, Forestadent) and the nonsuperelastic wire Nitinol were compared. A total of 40 patients participated, with 20 randomly assigned to each archwire, which was placed in edgewise appliances. No significant difference in the amount of tooth movement was found between the two Ni-Ti wires, although there was a clinical impression that the superelastic wire was superior because it could be more readily engaged when the teeth were severely malpositioned.

Rather than investigating the efficacy of tooth alignment, Jones and Chan[93] compared the pain experienced by patients with two different aligning archwires: 0.014-inch-diameter heavy superelastic Japanese Ni-Ti and 0.015-inch-diameter multistrand SS (Twist Flex, 3M Unitek). After an initial archwire was randomly placed in 43 patients, 22 patients subsequently received a randomly allocated second archwire in the opposing arch. These investigators found that the pain score peaked in the morning after placement of the archwire, endured for 5 to 6 days, and was similar after insertion of the second archwire. (The Cochrane Collaboration review[89] notes that several other clinical studies have reported the return of pain levels to normal after 6 to 7 days following placement of the initial wires.) Over a 2-week period, no significant difference was found in the pain response between the patients with superelastic and multistrand SS archwires.

West et al[94] compared 0.0155-inch-diameter multistrand SS wire (Dentaflex) and 0.014-inch-diameter superelastic Ni-Ti wire (Ni-Ti) for initial tooth alignment in a 6-week study. A total of 62 patients participated, and the 74 dental arches were randomly assigned to the two archwire groups. Following a detailed statistical analysis, the degree of initial alignment achieved overall for patients with the two wires was judged to be similar. The superelastic Ni-Ti wire provided better alignment in the mandibular labial segment, where the interbracket distance was usually less. The authors commented that a longer clinical evaluation period might be indicated for the superelastic wire.

Fernandes et al[95] reported the outcome of another pain study for patients in the initial alignment phase who received either 0.014-inch-diameter superelastic Sentalloy Light (GAC International) or 0.014-inch-diameter non-superelastic Nitinol wires. The 128 patients were randomly assigned to one of these archwires, and assessments of pain/discomfort were made over the initial 7-day period. The discomfort increased continuously after insertion of either archwire, peaking in the first night, remaining high for the second night, and returning to a normal level after 7 days. During the first 10 hours, the pain/discomfort was less after placement of the Sentalloy archwire compared with the Nitinol archwire, although significant differences were only found for the first 4 hours. The pain experienced in the mandibular arch was significantly higher than that in the maxillary arch during the first 11 hours after placement of either archwire. The differences in initial pain/discomfort responses to the superelastic and nonsuperelastic Ni-Ti archwires is consistent, with lower force delivery of the former when strain reaches the level for the upper superelastic plateau (see Fig 4-2).

Pandis et al[96] employed a double-blind, randomized clinical trial comparing 0.016-inch-diameter 35°C Copper Ni-Ti and 0.016-inch-diameter Ni-Ti wire not containing copper (Modern Arch; specific product not identified). Sixty patients were randomly divided into two equal groups, and the archwire selected was not disclosed to the orthodontist or the patient. Self-ligating brackets (GAC International) with 0.022-inch slots were used, and the amount of crowding of the mandibular anterior teeth was assessed over a maximum period of 6 months; a strong statistical methodology was employed to analyze the clinical results. There was no significant difference in the efficacy of either archwire for alleviating the duration of crowding. The investigators made the important conclusion that differences in loading patterns for archwires under clinical and laboratory conditions might eliminate the advantage of Copper Ni-Ti that has been inferred from laboratory studies.

An additional clinical study that is not included in the Cochrane collaboration review[89] has been performed by Ong et al,[97] who compared alignment efficiency of orthodontic archwire sequences, rather than single archwire types, from three manufacturers. The 132 patients were randomly assigned to the one of the following wire sequences for the mandibular arch: *(1)* 3M Unitek: 0.014-inch-diameter Nitinol Classic and 0.017 × 0.017–inch Nitinol HA; *(2)* Dentsply GAC International: 0.014-inch-diameter Sentalloy and 0.016 × 0.022–inch BioForce; or *(3)* Ormco: 0.014-inch-diameter Damon Copper Ni-Ti and 0.014 × 0.025–inch Damon Copper Ni-Ti. (Information about the A_f temperature for Damon Copper Ni-Ti is not available.) All patients received 0.018 × 0.025–inch slot brackets (3M Unitek), and all three groups finished with the same working archwire, 0.016 × 0.022–inch SS (3M Unitek), for a common endpoint. Patients were blinded for group allocation throughout treatment, but this was not possible for the clinician providing treatment. Discomfort information was obtained over a 7-day period after insertion of each archwire, and alignment efficiency was measured by the time required to reach the working archwire. All three archwire sequences produced acceptable clinical results, with similar results for both alignment efficiency (approximate mean time of 4 months to reach working archwire) and patient discomfort. The 3M Unitek archwire sequence caused significantly less discomfort compared with the GAC International and Ormco sequences 24 hours after insertion of the working archwire. This was attributed to differences in progression of archwire material and the arch forms.

It is evident that many more clinical studies should be performed to evaluate currently marketed wires for use in orthodontics. The advantages of superelastic Ni-Ti wires (conventional and ion-implanted) and Copper Ni-Ti archwires, advocated by manufacturers and found in laboratory studies, over nonsuperelastic Ni-Ti and multistrand SS archwires have not been observed in clinical studies. Pandis and Bourauel[98] have recently assessed the clinical significance of superelasticity for Ni-Ti wires and concluded that their lack of effectiveness for alleviating the crowd-ing of teeth in vivo can be attributed to free play of the wire within the bracket walls as well as potential aging effects of the brackets and wires. They advocate additional clinical trials to gain insight into the complex processes occurring in vivo. Manufacturers are constantly improving the properties of wire products, such as the surface roughness of current β-Ti wires compared with the original TMA, and clinical evaluations of the new products are continually needed. Considerable care is needed for the design of clinical studies: Attention must be directed to having a sufficient number of patients, using a double-blind protocol whenever possible to avoid bias (often difficult in orthodontics), always employing appropriate manipulation for all materials, having sufficient duration of the investigation, and employing correct methods for statistical analyses of the results.[89]

Summary Points

There are several very important closing points that clinicians should remember after reading this chapter:

- The general compositions, advantages, and potential concerns for each of the four major wire types should be thoroughly understood. Each major type has a unique set of general properties, which should be considered carefully for rational selection in a given patient case. Moreover, wire products of the same alloy type can vary substantially in properties among manufacturers because of differences in metallurgic quality and care with processing.
- Websites for the major orthodontic companies provide valuable details about the general compositions and properties of their wire products. Worthwhile information is concisely presented about major clinically relevant features of the archwire products, along with excellent advice about selection for the various phases of orthodontic treatment.
- It is important to understand the terminology used to describe the structures and properties of orthodontic wires, as well as the general principles underlying the laboratory techniques that are employed to obtain this information. The mechanics terminology used to describe the force delivery of archwires, as well as the major factors involved, should also be understood.
- The science of orthodontics and current technology are continuously evolving. New metallic archwires are emerging from the research laboratory, and there is substantial interest in esthetic polymeric archwires (not discussed in this chapter), which may eventually replace the metallic archwires. It is essential to remain abreast of current literature, and the PubMed search engine (http://www.ncbi.nlm.nih.gov/pubmed/) is a valuable resource.
- One should be an informed skeptic about the claims from manufacturers or published laboratory studies

about the exceptional properties of any new archwire products. Clinical studies have shown that such claims often do not withstand comparison to existing products that are frequently less expensive. It is highly important to appreciate the guiding principles for properly conducted clinical studies and to recognize that the complex oral environment and loading conditions experienced by archwires are not readily mimicked in the research laboratory.

References

1. Kapila S, Sachdeva R. Mechanical properties and clinical applications of orthodontics wires. Am J Orthod Dentofacial Orthop 1989; 96:100–109.
2. Kusy RP. A review of contemporary archwires: Their properties and characteristics. Angle Orthod 1997;63:197–207.
3. Brantley WA. Orthodontic wires. In: Brantley WA, Eliades T (eds). Orthodontic Materials: Scientific and Clinical Aspects. Stuttgart: Thieme, 2001:77–103.
4. Brantley WA. Orthodontic wires. In: O'Brien WJ (ed). Dental Materials and Their Selection, ed 4. Chicago: Quintessence, 2008:276–292.
5. Sebanc J, Brantley WA, Pincsak JJ, Conover JP. Variability of effective root torque as a function of edge bevel on orthodontic arch wires. Am J Orthod 1984;86:43–51.
6. Brantley WA. Structures and properties of orthodontic materials. In: Brantley WA, Eliades T (eds). Orthodontic Materials: Scientific and Clinical Aspects. Stuttgart: Thieme, 2001:1–25.
7. Asgharnia MK, Brantley WA. Comparison of bending and tension tests for orthodontic wires. Am J Orthod 1986;89:228–236.
8. American Dental Association Council on Dental Materials and Devices. New American Dental Association specification no. 32 for orthodontic wires not containing precious metals. J Am Dent Assoc 1977;5;1169–1171.
9. Brantley WA, Eliades T, Litsky AS. Mechanics and mechanical testing of orthodontic materials. In: Brantley WA, Eliades T (eds). Orthodontic Materials: Scientific and Clinical Aspects. Stuttgart: Thieme, 2001:27–47.
10. ISO Standard 15841. Dentistry—Wires for use in orthodontics. Geneva: International Organization for Standardization, 2006. ANSI/ADA Specification No. 32—Orthodontic Wires: 2006 is an identical adoption of this ISO standard.
11. Kusy RP. On the use of nomograms to determine the elastic property ratios of orthodontic arch wires. Am J Orthod 1983;83:374–381.
12. Burstone CJ, Goldberg AJ. Maximum forces and deflections from orthodontic appliances. Am J Orthod 1983;84:95–103.
13. Rucker BK, Kusy RP. Theoretical investigation of elastic flexural properties for multistranded orthodontic archwires. J Biomed Mater Res 2002;62:338–349.
14. Rucker BK, Kusy RP. Elastic flexural properties of multistranded stainless steel versus conventional nickel titanium archwires. Angle Orthod 2002;72:302–309.
15. Rucker BK, Kusy RP. Elastic properties of alternative versus single-stranded leveling archwires. Am J Orthod Dentofacial Orthop 2002;122:528–541.
16. Verstrynge A, Van Humbeeck J, Willems G. In-vitro evaluation of the material characteristics of stainless steel and beta-titanium orthodontic wires. Am J Orthod Dentofacial Orthop 2006;130:460–470.
17. Tian K, Darvell BW. Determination of the flexural modulus of elasticity of orthodontic archwires. Dent Mater 2010;26:821–829.
18. Kusy RP, Mims L, Whitley JQ. Mechanical characteristics of various tempers of as-received cobalt-chromium archwires. Am J Orthod Dentofacial Orthop 2001;119:274–291.
19. Kusy RP, Whitley JQ, Mayhew MJ, Buckthal JE. Surface roughness of orthodontic archwires via laser spectroscopy. Angle Orthod 1988;58:33–45.
20. Kusy RP, Whitley JQ. Coefficients of friction for arch wires in stainless steel and polycrystalline alumina bracket slots. I. The dry state. Am J Orthod Dentofacial Orthop 1990;98:300–312.
21. Kusy RP, Whitley JQ, Prewitt MJ. Comparison of the frictional coefficients for selected archwire-bracket slot combinations in the dry and wet states. Angle Orthod 1991;61:293–302.
22. Hensten-Pettersen A, Jacobsen N, Grimsdóttir MR. Allergic reactions and safety concerns. In: Brantley WA, Eliades T (eds). Orthodontic Materials: Scientific and Clinical Aspects. Stuttgart: Thieme, 2001:287–299.
23. Pelsue BM, Zinelis S, Bradley TG, Berzins DW, Eliades T, Eliades G. Structure, composition, and mechanical properties of Australian orthodontic wires. Angle Orthod 2009;79:97–101.
24. Es-Souni M, Fischer-Brandies H, Es-Souni M. On the in vitro biocompatibility of Elgiloy, a Co-based alloy, compared to two titanium alloys. J Orofac Orthop 2003;64:16–26.
25. David A, Lobner D. In vivo cytotoxicity of orthodontic archwires in cortical cell cultures. Eur J Orthod 2004;26:421–426.
26. Andreasen GF, Brady PR. A use hypothesis for 55 Nitinol wire for orthodontics. Angle Orthod 1972;42:172–177.
27. Andreasen GF, Hilleman TB. An evaluation of 55 cobalt substituted Nitinol wire for use in orthodontics. J Am Dent Assoc 1971;82:1373–1375.
28. Buehler WJ, Gilfrich JV, Riley RC. Effect of low-temperature phase changes on the mechanical properties of alloys near the composition of TiNi. J Appl Phys 1963;34:1475–1477.
29. Buehler WJ, Wang FE. A summary of recent research on the nitinol alloys and their potential application in ocean engineering. Ocean Eng 1968;1:105–120.
30. Andreasen GF, Morrow RE. Laboratory and clinical analyses of nitinol wire. Am J Orthod 1978;73:142–151.
31. Burstone CJ, Qin B, Morton JY. Chinese NiTi wire—A new orthodontic alloy. Am J Orthod 1985;87:445–452.
32. Miura F, Mogi M, Ohura Y, Hamanaka H. The super-elastic property of the Japanese NiTi alloy wire for use in orthodontics. Am J Orthod Dentofacial Orthop 1986;90:1–10.
33. Fletcher ML, Miyake S, Brantley WA, Culbertson BM. DSC and bending studies of a new shape-memory orthodontic wire. J Dent Res 1992;71(AADR abstracts):169.
34. Thayer TA, Bagby MD, Moore RN, De Angelis RJ. X-ray diffraction of nitinol orthodontic arch wires. Am J Orthod Dentofacial Orthop 1995;107:604–612.
35. Iijima M, Brantley WA, Kawashima I, et al. Micro-X-ray diffraction observation of nickel-titanium orthodontic wires in simulated oral environment. Biomaterials 2004;25:171–176.
36. Iijima M, Brantley WA, Guo WH, Clark WAT, Yuasa T, Mizoguchi I. X-ray diffraction study of low-temperature phase transformations in nickel-titanium orthodontic wires. Dent Mater 2008;24:1454–1460.
37. Yoneyama T, Doi H, Hamanaka H, Okamoto Y, Mogi M, Miura F. Super-elasticity and thermal behavior of Ni-Ti alloy orthodontic arch wires. Dent Mater J 1992;11:1–10.
38. Bradley TG, Brantley WA, Culbertson BM. Differential scanning calorimetry (DSC) analyses of superelastic and nonsuperelastic nickel-titanium orthodontic wires. Am J Orthod Dentofacial Orthop 1996;109:589–597.
39. Brantley WA, Iijima M, Grentzer TH. Temperature-modulated DSC provides new insight about nickel-titanium wire transformations. Am J Orthod Dentofacial Orthop 2003;124:387–394.
40. Miura F, Mogi M, Ohura Y. Japanese NiTi alloy wire: Use of the direct electric resistance heat treatment method. Eur J Orthod 1988; 10:187–191.
41. Khier SE, Brantley WA, Fournelle RA. Bending properties of superelastic and nonsuperelastic nickel-titanium orthodontic wires. Am J Orthod Dentofacial Orthop 1991;99:310–318.
42. Brantley WA, Guo W, Clark WAT, Iijima M. Microstructural studies of 35°C Copper Ni-Ti orthodontic wire and TEM confirmation of low-temperature martensite transformation. Dent Mater 2008;24:204–210.

43. Brantley WA, Iijima M, Grentzer TH. Temperature-modulated DSC study of phase transformations in nickel-titanium orthodontic wires. Thermochim Acta 2002;392–393:329–337.

44. Kusy RP. Nitinol alloys: So, who's on first? [letter] Am J Orthod Dentofacial Orthop 1991;100:25A–26A.

45. Iijima M, Muguruma T, Brantley WA, Mizoguchi I. Comparison of nanoindentation, 3-point bending, and tension tests for orthodontic wires. Am J Orthod Dentofacial Orthop 2011;140:65–71.

46. Bourauel C, Fries T, Drescher D, Plietsch R. Surface roughness of orthodontic wires via atomic force microscopy, laser specular reflectance, and profilometry. Eur J Orthod 1998;20:79–92.

47. Widu F, Drescher D, Junker R, Bourauel C. Corrosion and biocompatibility of orthodontic wires. J Mater Sci Mater Med 1999;10:275–281.

48. Segal N, Hell J, Berzins DW. Influence of stress and phase on corrosion of a superelastic nickel-titanium orthodontic wire. Am J Orthod Dentofacial Orthop 2009;135:764–770.

49. Lee TH, Huang TK, Lin SY, Chen LK, Chou MY, Huang HH. Corrosion resistance of different nickel-titanium archwires in acidic fluoride-containing artificial saliva. Angle Orthod 2010;80:547–553.

50. Liu JK, Lee TM, Liu IH. Effect of loading force on the dissolution behavior and surface properties of nickel-titanium orthodontic archwires in artificial saliva. Am J Orthod Dentofacial Orthop 2011;140:166–176.

51. Suárez C, Vilar T, Gil J, Sevilla P. In vitro evaluation of surface topographic changes and nickel release of lingual orthodontic archwires. J Mater Sci Mater Med 2010;21:675–683.

52. Li X, Wang J, Han EH, Ke W. Influence of fluoride and chloride on corrosion behavior of NiTi orthodontic wires. Acta Biomater 2007;3:807–815.

53. Kao CT, Ding SJ, He H, Chou MY, Huang TH. Cytotoxicity of orthodontic wire corroded in fluoride solution in vitro. Angle Orthod 2007;77:349–354.

54. Yokoyama K, Kaneko K, Moriyama K, Asaoka K, Sakai J, Nagumo M. Hydrogen embrittlement of Ni-Ti superelastic alloy in fluoride solution. J Biomed Mater Res A 2003;65:182–187.

55. Zinelis S, Eliades T, Pandis N, Eliades G, Bourauel C. Why do nickel-titanium archwires fracture intraorally? Fractographic analysis and failure mechanism of in-vivo fractured wires. Am J Orthod Dentofacial Orthop 2007;132:84–89.

56. Walker MP, White RJ, Kula KS. Effect of fluoride prophylactic agents on the mechanical properties of nickel-titanium-based orthodontic wires. Am J Orthod Dentofacial Orthop 2005;127:662–669.

57. Vo J, Chudasama DN, Rinchuse DJ, Day R. A clinical trial to evaluate the effects of prophylactic fluoride agents on the superelastic properties of nickel-titanium wires. World J Orthod 2010;11:135–141.

58. Iijima M, Yuasa T, Endo K, Muguruma T, Ohno H, Mizoguchi I. Corrosion behavior of ion implanted nickel-titanium orthodontic wire in fluoride mouth rinse solutions. Dent Mater J 2010;29:53–58.

59. Muguruma T, Iijima M, Brantley WA, Mizoguchi I. Effects of a diamond-like carbon coating on the frictional properties of orthodontic wires. Angle Orthod 2011;81:141–148.

60. Iijima M, Muguruma T, Brantley W, et al. Effect of coating on properties of esthetic orthodontic nickel-titanium wires. Angle Orthod 2012;82:319–325.

61. Elayyan F, Silikas N, Bearn D. Mechanical properties of coated superelastic archwires in conventional and self-ligating orthodontic brackets. Am J Orthod Dentofacial Orthop 2010;137:213–217.

62. Elayyan F, Silikas N, Bearn D. Ex vivo surface and mechanical properties of coated orthodontic archwires. Eur J Orthod 2008;30:661–667.

63. Burstone CJ, Goldberg AJ. Beta titanium: A new orthodontic alloy. Am J Orthod 1980;77:121–132.

64. Goldberg J, Burstone CJ. An evaluation of beta titanium alloys for use in orthodontic appliances. J Dent Res 1979:58;593–599.

65. Donachie MJ Jr. Titanium: A Technical Guide, ed 2. Materials Park, OH: ASM International, 2000:1–3,13–24,101–103,128–130, 240–247.

66. Brick RM, Pense AW, Gordon RB. Structure and Properties of Engineering Materials, ed 4. New York: McGraw-Hill, 1977:234–245.

67. Wilson DF, Goldberg AJ. Alternative beta-titanium alloys for orthodontic wires. Dent Mater 1987:3:337–341.

68. Donovan MT, Lin JJ, Brantley WA, Conover JP. Weldability of beta titanium arch wires. Am J Orthod 1984;85:207–216.

69. Nelson KR, Burstone CJ, Goldberg AJ. Optimal welding of beta titanium orthodontic wires. Am J Orthod Dentofacial Orthop 1987; 92:213–219.

70. Iijima M, Brantley WA, Kawashima I, et al. Microstructures of beta-titanium orthodontic wires joined by infrared brazing. J Biomed Mater Res B Appl Biomater 2006;79:137–141.

71. Iijima M, Brantley WA, Baba N, et al. Micro-XRD study of beta-titanium wires and infrared soldered joints. Dent Mater 2007;23: 1051–1056.

72. Iijima M, Brantley WA, Yuasa T, Muguruma T, Kawashima I, Mizoguchi I. Joining characteristics of orthodontic wires with laser welding. J Biomed Mater Res B Appl Biomater 2008;84:147–153.

73. Iijima M, Brantley WA, Yuasa T, Kawashima I, Mizoguchi I. Joining characteristics of beta-titanium wires with electrical resistance welding. J Biomed Mater Res B Appl Biomater 2008;85:378–384.

74. Geurtsen W. Biocompatibility of dental casting alloys. Crit Rev Oral Biol Med 2002;13:71–84.

75. Kaneko K, Yokoyama K, Moriyama K, Asaoka K, Sakai J, Nagumo M. Delayed fracture of beta titanium orthodontic wire in fluoride aqueous solutions. Biomaterials 2003;24:2113–2120.

76. Kaneko K, Yokoyama K, Moriyama K, Asaoka K, Sakai J. Degradation in performance of orthodontic wires caused by hydrogen absorption during short-term immersion in 2.0% acidulated phosphate fluoride solution. Angle Orthod 2004;74:487–495.

77. Kwon YH, Seol HJ, Kim HI, Hwang KJ, Lee SG, Kim KH. Effect of acidic fluoride solution on β titanium alloy wire. J Biomed Mater Res B Appl Biomater 2005;73:285–290.

78. Walker MP, Ries D, Kula K, Ellis M, Fricke B. Mechanical properties and surface characterization of beta titanium and stainless steel orthodontic wire following topical fluoride treatment. Angle Orthod 2007;77:342–348.

79. Krishnan V, Krishnan A, Remya R, et al. Development and evaluation of two PVD-coated β-titanium orthodontic archwires for fluoride-induced corrosion protection. Acta Biomater 2011;7:1913–1927.

80. Krishnan V, Ravikumar KK, Sukumaran K, Kumar KJ. In vitro evaluation of physical vapor deposition coated beta titanium orthodontic archwires. Angle Orthod 2012;82:22–29.

81. Kusy RP, Whitley JQ. Effects of sliding velocity on the coefficients of friction in a model orthodontic system. Dent Mater 1989;5:235–240.

82. Kusy RP, Whitley JQ. Effects of surface roughness on the coefficients of friction in model orthodontic systems. J Biomech 1990;23: 913–925.

83. Kusy RP, Tobin EJ, Whitley JQ, Sioshansi P. Frictional coefficients of ion-implanted alumina against ion-implanted beta-titanium in the low load, low velocity, single pass regime. Dent Mater 1992;8:167–172.

84. Jia W, Beatty MW, Reinhardt RA, et al. Nickel release from orthodontic arch wires and cellular immune response to various nickel concentrations. J Biomed Mater Res 1999;48:488–495.

85. Kusy RP, Whitley JQ, de Araújo Gurgel J. Comparisons of surface roughnesses and sliding resistances of 6 titanium-based or TMA-type archwires. Am J Orthod Dentofacial Orthop 2004;126:589–603.

86. 3M Unitek 2010 Product Catalog. Section 7: Archwire Products. http://solutions.3m.com/wps/portal/3M/en_US/orthodontics/Unitek/products/catalog. Accessed 2 March 2012.

87. Ormco Orthodontic Products Catalog. Section 5: Archwires. http://www.ormco.com/ormco/ormcocatalog-7mb.pdf. Accessed 2 March 2012.

88. Dentaurum Wire Manual. http://www.dentaurum.de/files/989-561-20.pdf. Accessed 2 March 2012.

89. Wang Y, Jian F, Lai W, et al. Initial arch wires for alignment of crooked teeth with fixed orthodontic braces. Cochrane Database Syst Rev 2010;4:CD007859.

90. Cobb NW 3rd, Kula KS, Phillips C, Proffit WR. Efficiency of multi-strand steel, superelastic Ni-Ti and ion-implanted Ni-Ti archwires for initial alignment. Clin Orthod Res 1998;1:12–19.

91. Evans TJW, Jones ML, Newcombe RG. Clinical comparison and performance perspective of three aligning arch wires. Am J Orthod Dentofacial Orthop 1998;114:32–39.

92. O'Brien K, Lewis D, Shaw W, Combe E. A clinical trial of aligning archwires. Eur J Orthod 1990;12:380–384.

93. Jones M, Chan C. The pain and discomfort experienced during orthodontic treatment: A randomized controlled clinical trial of two initial aligning arch wires. Am J Orthod Dentofacial Orthop 1992;102:373–381.

94. West AE, Jones ML, Newcombe RG. Multiflex versus superelastic: A randomized clinical trial of the tooth alignment ability of initial arch wires. Am J Orthod Dentofacial Orthop 1995;108:464–471.

95. Fernandes LM, Øgaard B, Skoglund L. Pain and discomfort experienced after placement of a conventional or a superelastic NiTi aligning archwire. A randomized clinical trial. J Orofac Orthop 1998;59:331–339.

96. Pandis N, Polychronopoulou A, Eliades T. Alleviation of mandibular anterior crowding with copper-nickel-titanium vs nickel-titanium wires: A double-blind randomized control trial. Am J Orthod Dentofacial Orthop 2009;136:152.e1–152.e7.

97. Ong E, Ho C, Miles P. Alignment efficiency and discomfort of three orthodontic archwire sequences: A randomized clinical trial. J Orthod 2011;38:32–39.

98. Pandis N, Bourauel CP. Nickel-titanium (NiTi) arch wires: The clinical significance of super elasticity. Semin Orthod 2010;16:249–257.

Peter G. Miles
BDSc, MDS

Daniel J. Rinchuse
DMD, MS, MDS, PhD

5

Class II Malocclusions: Extraction and Nonextraction Treatment

Introduction

We now practice in an evidence-based era, and one of the most highly researched areas of clinical orthodontics is the treatment of Class II malocclusion. An evidence-based clinical practice should integrate scientific or evidence-based orthodontics with patient preferences, clinical or patient circumstances, and clinical experience and judgment.[1,2] The scope of this chapter limits the discussion to human trials and avoids case reports and opinion papers. The best available evidence can then be applied to enhance efficiency in the clinical treatment of Class II malocclusion in orthodontic practice.

Extraction Treatment

The specialty of orthodontics has witnessed the pendulum swing from a nonextraction treatment philosophy initially advocated by Edward Angle to high extraction rates influenced by practitioners such as Charles Tweed and Raymond Begg and back again to nonextraction. Extraction cases now average only about 18% of cases.[3] The purpose of this section is not to define when extraction should or should not be undertaken but to discuss the various options available once that decision has been made after consultation with the patient.

Canine tie-backs

During initial leveling and alignment in extraction cases and some nonextraction cases, the suggestion has been made to use passive canine tie-backs or laceback ligatures from the molars to the canines to support anterior anchor-age by preventing forward tipping of the canines.[4] The evidence regarding lacebacks demonstrates a large interoperator variation in the forces produced, ranging from 0 to 11.1 N (about 1,130 gram-force).[5] The effectiveness of canine lacebacks on preventing an increase in maxillary incisor proclination at the start of treatment was about 0.9 mm, and their effect on mesial molar movement was insignificant.[6] It is up to the clinician to determine if this potential 1-mm effect on overjet is clinically significant for an individual case. The authors also found that if the canine was more distally inclined at the start of treatment, the incisors were more likely to procline, whether canine lacebacks were used or not.[6] In the mandibular arch, it has been demonstrated that the use of laceback ligatures conveys no difference in the anteroposterior or vertical position of the mandibular anterior segment.[7] However, it did create a statistically and clinically significant increase in the loss of posterior anchorage (0.8 mm). The use of tiebacks on a routine basis therefore seems to be deleterious in the mandibular arch and of limited (1-mm) benefit in the maxillary arch.

Canine versus en-masse retraction

In extraction cases, the clinician can choose to either retract the canines prior to retraction of the remaining incisors or retract all the incisors and canines en masse. Some would argue that separate retraction of canines conserves anchorage, while others would suggest that there is no difference in anchorage loss. In a comparison of en-masse retraction and two-step retraction of canines followed by the maxillary incisors in 30 adult women with a Class I malocclusion, approximately 4 mm of the retraction of the maxillary incisal edges resulted in 1 mm of anchorage loss in the maxillary molars in both groups.[8] Although not statistically significant, the average times needed to close

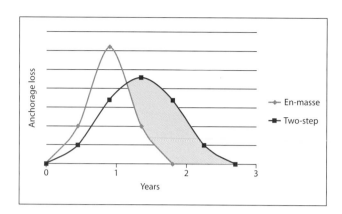

Fig 5-1 Plotting normal curves based on the average and standard deviation data from Heo et al.[8] Note that a sizeable proportion of the two-step cases moved slower than the en-masse cases (shaded area under the pink two-step curve). En-masse space closure saved an average 4.8 months (0.4 years) of treatment time with no noticeable difference in anchorage loss.

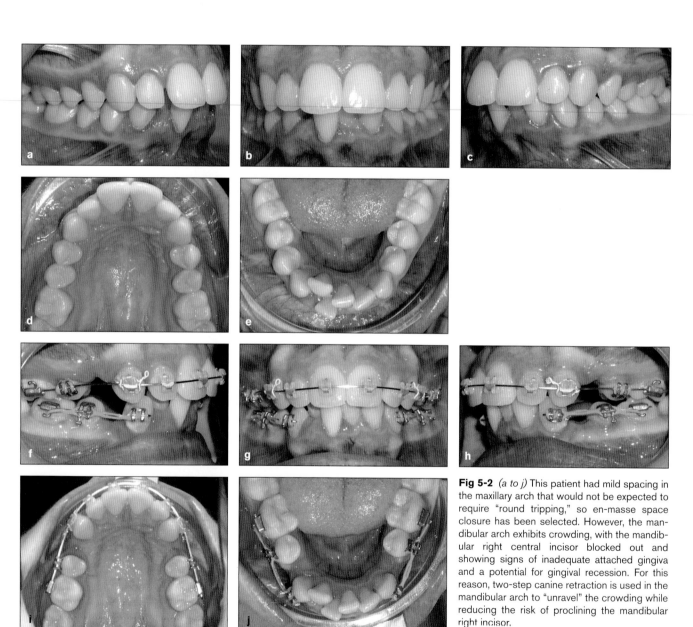

Fig 5-2 *(a to j)* This patient had mild spacing in the maxillary arch that would not be expected to require "round tripping," so en-masse space closure has been selected. However, the mandibular arch exhibits crowding, with the mandibular right central incisor blocked out and showing signs of inadequate attached gingiva and a potential for gingival recession. For this reason, two-step canine retraction is used in the mandibular arch to "unravel" the crowding while reducing the risk of proclining the mandibular right incisor.

Fig 5-3 The width of the bracket determines the size of the moment arm (one-half the bracket width) and the contact angle between the wire and the bracket corner. The wider bracket thereby requires less force to generate the moment necessary to upright the root. (Adapted from Proffit.[13])

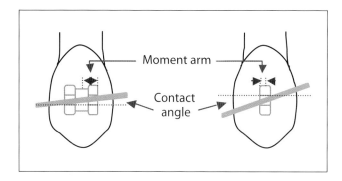

the spaces were 0.9 years (1 standard deviation = 0.6 to 1.3 years) in the en-masse group versus 1.3 years (1 standard deviation = 0.6 to 2.0 years) in the two-step retraction group (Fig 5-1). Two-step retraction demonstrated no benefit in terms of anchorage loss and a tendency to take longer than en-masse retraction. No difference in anchorage loss was also found in a pilot randomized controlled trial (RCT) comparing en-masse retraction with two-step retraction.[9] Therefore, en-masse retraction is the treatment of choice for efficiency. However, there are individual cases in which initial sectional canine retraction or a trapped coil on a continuous archwire is preferred to alleviate anterior crowding (Fig 5-2), such as when not "unraveling" the crowded anterior teeth first would "round trip" them and possibly create periodontal concerns. This treatment philosophy is supported by Burstone,[10] who argued that separating the retraction of canines from that of the incisors makes little sense because all six teeth can be retracted at once with relatively low forces; the only patients for whom separate canine retraction is appropriate, he continued, are those with anterior crowding as a result of arch-length problems. With the trend toward longer treatment times with two-step retraction, there may be an associated risk of greater root resorption. However, in a clinical trial investigating this, no clinically or statistically significant difference could be found.[11]

Some believe that tipping mechanics during canine retraction may be more efficient than bodily retraction. However, a split-mouth study in 14 subjects found that bodily retraction was faster than tipping because of less time spent uprighting the roots, with anchorage loss similar in both groups (17% to 20% or 1.2 to 1.4 mm).[12] The authors also found that the use of a Nance button did not provide absolute anchorage. A previous study had found no difference in the rate of canine retraction but did not measure tipping or time spent uprighting.[13] The split-mouth study also recorded a greater anchorage loss with the tipping mechanics. Another option when retracting canines is to use either a single wing or a twin (also called a *Siamese*) bracket. The advantage of a wider bracket in this situation is that it allows better tip control because it is easier to generate the required moments needed to bring the roots parallel to one another at extraction sites.[14]

When sliding mechanics are used, a wider bracket has a smaller contact angle and requires less force to generate the moment during space closure (Fig 5-3). Conversely, single wing and narrow brackets, including some self-ligating bracket designs, potentially require more force or demonstrate a greater resistance to sliding because of the greater contact angle and smaller moment arm. This is supported by two clinical trials evaluating the rate of maxillary canine retraction and en-masse space closure.[15,16] Both studies found a conventional twin bracket resulted in a slightly faster rate of space closure (1.2 mm/month) compared with the slightly narrower self-ligating brackets (1.1 mm/month and 0.9 mm/month).

Anchorage

As previously described, it appears from the best evidence available that there is no advantage to two-step retraction over en-masse retraction when it comes to anchorage. However, there are other options available for reinforcing anchorage, such as transpalatal arches (TPAs), headgear, and, more recently, temporary skeletal anchorage devices (TSADs) or miniscrews. When examining the effect of the TPA during extraction treatment, Zablocki et al[17] found no significant effect on either the anteroposterior or vertical position of the maxillary first molars. In a study comparing TPAs, headgears, and TSADs, the TSADs and headgears helped to control anchorage during leveling and alignment while the TPA group experienced anchorage loss (mean of 1.0 mm; $P < .001$).[18] However, during the space closure phase, only the TSAD group was stable. Overall, the anchorage loss per incisor retraction was 2% for the TSAD group, 15% for the headgear group, and 54% for the TPA group. A potential confounder in this study was that compliance with headgear wear was not measured, so compliance was assumed when molars remained stable and noncompliance suspected when they were not, representing what would happen clinically. Other authors found a similar 1.2-mm anchorage saving with 1.4 mm greater retraction of the anterior teeth when using skeletal anchorage (miniplates, miniscrews, or microscrews),[19] while others have found palatal implants to be at least as effective as headgear in reinforcing anchorage.[20] When TSADs were compared with anchorage preparation, as in the Tweed-Merrifield technique that involved wearing a high-pull J-hook headgear, there was less anchorage loss in the TSAD group and 1.5 mm greater retraction of the cephalometric landmark A-point.[21] In this study, headgear compliance was rated as excellent by the authors. Therefore, it seems that when maximum anchorage is required, TSADs are the method of choice, with headgear relegated to a moderate anchorage role and reliant upon cooperation. TPAs provide no benefit in terms of anchorage, although they do help maintain transverse width of the attached teeth as well as control molar rotation, which preserves the final interdigitation when maintaining a Class I molar relationship.

When considering the anchorage requirements in the extraction treatment of Class II malocclusions, we have the option of removing either two or four premolars. In a retrospective study examining the occlusion achieved during the treatment of complete Class II malocclusions corrected with two or four premolar extractions, it was demonstrated that the treatment with two premolar extractions achieved a better occlusal success rate than treatment with four premolar extractions.[22] This was attributed to the lower demand on anchorage and compliance in the two premolar extraction group. When feasible, therefore, this treatment option is preferred over the extraction of four premolars. However, when four premolars require removal, then the anchorage demands need to be considered, and if maximum or absolute anchorage is required, miniscrews seem to be the more predictable choice in terms of the occlusal outcome.

Most efficient space closure

For en-masse space closure, the clinician has a number of possible mechanotherapies available, such as closing loops or sliding mechanics with stretched modules, elastic chain, or springs. In a study comparing the intermittent force of closing loops with a continuous force for canine retraction, it was demonstrated that the rate of movement can be up to twice as fast with the continuous force.[23] When lacebacks (which apply an intermittent force) were compared with nickel-titanium (Ni-Ti) springs (considered continuous) for canine retraction, the continuous force from the Ni-Ti springs retracted the teeth about 2.5 times faster.[24] Some of the extra tipping in this study could be attributed to the use of small (0.012- to 0.016-inch) Ni-Ti archwires rather than stiffer, steel archwires used in other studies; therefore, to maintain control during retraction, a stiffer wire is recommended. Similarly, when Ni-Ti springs were compared with intra-arch Class I elastics for canine retraction, the springs achieved twice the rate of movement, which the author attributed to the ability of the springs to maintain a relatively constant force level compared with the elastics and the elimination of the need for

patient cooperation.[25] When discussing a theoretical model of efficiency versus duration of force, Proffit stated, "Theoretically, there is no doubt that light continuous forces produce the most efficient tooth movement."[26]

Another concern with space closure is the risk of orthodontically induced inflammatory root resorption (OIIRR). In a study evaluating OIIRR in patients consecutively assigned to either a continuous arch sliding mechanics group or a sectional closing loop prior to retraction of the remaining anterior teeth, similar levels of OIIRR were found in both groups.[27] The author concluded that variations in the amount of OIIRR may be due to individual variation rather than round tripping. Another study comparing continuous and discontinuous forces on first premolars found that the application of discontinuous forces resulted in less OIIRR than the continuous force.[28] Conversely, another study comparing continuous versus intermittent forces found that the continuous force was more effective for tooth movement, with no difference in the amount or severity of OIIRR.[29] Overall, these results indicate that there appears to be minimal clinical difference in terms of OIIRR between continuous and intermittent forces.

A systematic review of sliding mechanics concluded that Ni-Ti coil springs (Fig 5-4) were faster than active ligatures (a ligature tied to a stretched elastic module), while elastomeric chain produced similar rates of movement to the Ni-Ti springs.[30] In two of the reviewed studies comparing active ligatures with Ni-Ti coil springs in sliding mechanics, the coil springs were found to have a significantly higher and more consistent rate of space closure than the active ligatures.[31,32]

Another split-mouth study compared Ni-Ti springs with elastomeric chain tied from the molar bracket hook to an archwire post distal to the lateral incisor.[33] The patients were seen every 4 to 6 weeks, and the calculated rates of space closure were 0.21 mm/week (0.91 mm/month) for the elastomeric chain versus 0.26 mm/week (1.13 mm/month) for the Ni-Ti spring (not statistically significant). In a randomized clinical trial comparing three methods of space closure (active ligatures, powerchain, and Ni-Ti springs, all tied from the molar hook to a post), Dixon et al[34] found that the active ligatures/stretched module was the least effective method of space closure at 0.35 mm/month. The powerchain closed space at 0.58 mm/month and the Ni-Ti spring at 0.81 mm/month. In this study, the chain and ligatures were replaced at each visit, approximately every 4 to 6 weeks, whereas the Ni-Ti spring was left in place and reactivated to a 9-mm stretch if required.

The difference demonstrated between the Ni-Ti springs and elastomeric chain in these two latter studies was about 0.2 mm/month. As a clinical application, this means that the difference in treatment time between Ni-Ti springs and elastomeric chain would be about 1 to 1.5 months for a 3-mm space; for a larger space such as 6 mm, the time saving becomes 1.4 to 2.9 months, which is more clinically meaningful. Therefore, for small residual spaces, the chain

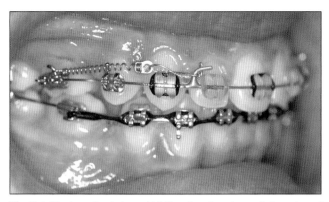

Fig 5-4 Elastomeric chain and Ni-Ti coil springs have similar rates of movement for space closure with sliding mechanics. Chain is less expensive, but coil springs are more likely to remain effective over longer appointment intervals.

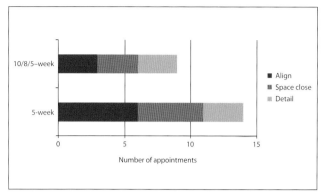

Fig 5-5 In a hypothetical Class II maxillary premolar extraction case treated over a 16-month period, modifying the appointment interval to match the expected biologic response of the patient with the mechanics applied allows the total number of adjustment appointments required to be reduced from 14 to 9. (Reprinted from Miles[35] with permission.)

may be a better option because it is cheaper, but for larger spaces, the Ni-Ti spring is more efficient. The other benefit of the Ni-Ti spring is the ability to choose longer appointment intervals because it can be expected to maintain a relatively constant force compared with an elastomeric chain. As noted above, the chain in the previous studies was replaced at each visit (every 4 to 6 weeks); longer intervals (and therefore fewer appointments) are possible with Ni-Ti springs, which are equally efficient in terms of the rate of space closure because of their constant unloading force.

Appointment efficiency

A hypothetical Class II case involving extractions of maxillary first premolars allows for the clinical application of the information from chapter 4 on alignment and this chapter on space closure. The appointment intervals can be correlated with the properties of the archwires and mechanics being used while the expected physiologic response of the patient's tissues is considered.

If a regular 5-week appointment protocol were to be compared with a 10/8/5–week appointment protocol, the end results would be the same; however, the 10/8/5–week protocol would require fewer appointments[35] (Fig 5-5). For example, if an initial round Ni-Ti or heat-activated (HA) Ni-Ti wire is placed as the first archwire and the appointments are scheduled at regular 5-week intervals, retying would likely be done at 5 weeks. Then perhaps an evaluation for repositioning of brackets and retying would be done at 10 weeks, progressing in another 5 weeks (15 weeks) to the second wire, a rectangular HA Ni-Ti. After an additional 5 weeks (20 weeks), retying would be done again, and then perhaps repositioning of the brackets in another 5 weeks (25 weeks). After a further 5 weeks (30 weeks), the teeth would be ready for the working archwire. On the other hand, if the appointments were scheduled at

10-week intervals during this alignment phase, 10 weeks after initial wire placement the brackets would be repositioned and retied or treatment would progress to the second rectangular HA Ni-Ti wire. After another 10 weeks (20 weeks), any final repositioning would be done and treatment would either progress to the HA Ni-Ti wire or, if this was done at the previous visit, the brackets would be retied; in another 10 weeks, the teeth would be ready for the working archwire. Therefore, the same alignment would be achieved within the same 30 weeks but with fewer appointments.

Then, during the space closure phase in this hypothetical example, a posted wire with sliding mechanics using Ni-Ti springs is chosen to close a residual 5-mm space on each side. Again, with 5-week intervals and the expectation of 1 mm of space closure per month, this closure would take five visits. However, using an 8-week interval (8-week instead of 10-week to monitor space closure and overjet more closely), the same space closure can be achieved within the same 25 weeks but with only three visits. Then would follow the detailing/finishing phase of treatment, where minor adjustments would not be expected to be active over a longer appointment interval, so appointments are scheduled at 5-week intervals to complete treatment. With either the conventional 5-week protocol or the 10/8/5–week protocol, this phase would take three visits. In the end, the 10/8/5–week protocol would accomplish the same result in the same amount of time but with fewer office visits. In Fig 5-5, for example, although both treatment plans took approximately 16 months to complete, the number of appointments required was reduced by five with the 10/8/5–week protocol compared with the 5-week protocol, which is a benefit for both the patient and the orthodontist.

In summary, when spaces are to be closed in premolar extraction cases, en-masse space closure is more efficient than two-step retraction (canines and then incisors). The exception to this is the patient with a significant arch length discrepancy that would require separate canine retraction first. For anchorage, Nance buttons and TPAs offer minimal benefit, and headgear offers moderate anchorage, while miniscrews offer the best option for maximum or absolute anchorage cases. Space closure using sliding mechanics is most efficiently achieved for moderate to large spaces with Ni-Ti coil springs, whereas smaller spaces can be closed with springs or chain. As with initial alignment in the archwire chapter, to improve efficiency during treatment, appointment intervals should be matched with the expected biologic response of the patient. A modified appointment interval, a 10/8/5–week protocol, was suggested for differing stages of treatment to achieve the desired movement while keeping the number of required adjustment visits to a minimum. These intervals, however, can be modified based on the initial alignment and observed rate of movement of the individual during treatment.

Nonextraction Treatment

The literature provides some of the more common factors associated with longer treatment times. Apart from missed appointments and appliance breakages/bond failures, these include the initial alignment, poor cooperation with elastics and hygiene, Class II malocclusion, extractions, and especially delayed extractions (starting nonextraction and changing to extraction during treatment).[36–38] In this section, the current evidence regarding the nonextraction treatment of Class II cases is discussed.

Maxillary incisor proclination, overjet, and initial molar relationship have been suggested as indicators of Class II treatment success.[39,40] In other words, the more severe the molar relationship and overjet, the lower the likelihood of achieving an ideal final molar and incisor relationship with a nonextraction protocol. This explains the finding that full Class II relationships were more predictably corrected with an extraction approach while ½-unit relationships were equally resolved with either an extraction or nonextraction protocol.[41] It also supports the finding that starting nonextraction and then reverting to an extraction approach is a significant factor in extended treatment duration.[38] Therefore, prior to orthodontic treatment, various options and alternative treatments such as orthognathic surgery, camouflage, extractions, and compromises need to be discussed so that patient/parents can make informed decisions/consent, have autonomy, and be made aware of the possibilities of other options becoming available as treatment progresses—ie, a therapeutic diagnosis.

Timing of Class II treatment

The issue of the timing of nonextraction Class II treatment is one of the best-researched areas within orthodontics. The highest level of evidence is considered to be the systematic review,[42] and one source of these is the Cochrane Library

(www.thecochranelibrary.com). Despite the amount of published literature on the treatment of Class II cases, one such Cochrane review concluded that for the treatment of Class II, division 2 cases in children, it is not possible to provide any evidence-based guidance to recommend or discourage any type of orthodontic treatment.[43] However, for division 1 cases with protrusion, the evidence is more lucid. Another Cochrane review concluded that providing early orthodontic treatment for children with prominent maxillary anterior teeth is no more effective than providing one course of orthodontic treatment when the child is in early adolescence.[44] A systematic review of the cephalometric facial soft tissue changes with the activator and bionator appliances in Class II cases concluded that a significant amount of controversy regarding the soft tissue changes exists and that the soft tissue changes that were reported as being statistically significant were of questionable clinical significance.[45] Randomized clinical trials in both the United States and the United Kingdom have found that the benefits of early phase I treatment disappeared when both groups (early treatment and no early treatment) received comprehensive fixed appliance treatment during a second phase of treatment in adolescence.[46,47] This indicates that two-phase treatment started before adolescence in the mixed dentition is no more clinically effective than one-phase treatment started during adolescence in the early permanent dentition. Therefore, for many nonextraction Class II patients, the selection of treatment may well constitute a practice-management rather than a biologic decision.[48]

Early treatment at the age of 9 to 10 years with functional appliances (eg, bionator or twin block) and headgear appears to be inefficient because it produced no reduction in the average time a child was in fixed appliances during a second stage of treatment. Additionally, it did not decrease the proportion of complex treatments involving extractions or orthognathic surgery.[45] Interestingly, the UK study also found that there was no statistically significant difference (8% in the early treatment group versus 14% in the late treatment group) in the incidence of new incisor trauma, with much of the incisor trauma having occurred prior to the commencement of phase I.[47] In the University of North Carolina (UNC) study, on the other hand, there was a statistically significant difference, with new incisor trauma being approximately two times more common in the untreated control group.[49] The Florida RCT comparing early treatment with a bionator versus a headgear or bite plane found no statistically significant difference in the early treatment groups versus the control.[50] However, when phase II treatment was commenced, once again the incidence of maxillary incisor trauma in the control group was about 7% to 8% (or 3 times) higher than the early treatment groups (10.9% versus 3.2% and 2.9%; $P = 0.13$). When broken down by sex, this higher incidence of trauma was observed in the boys but not in the girls. Cross-sectional studies have demonstrated an association between an increased overjet and maxillary incisor trauma.[51] One could then make the argument that orthodontic intervention aimed at reducing trauma should begin very soon after the eruption of the maxillary incisors, although the estimated cost of incisor trauma treatment is small compared with the additional cost of two-phase treatment.[49] In the Florida study, 80% of the trauma was in enamel only and would be considered minor by most. Of the remaining 20%, most patients (19%) had fractures that extended into dentin, and less than 1% (one patient) had a pulpal involvement. Based on the UK and Florida studies and accepting that there is a 7% to 8% elevated risk of incisor trauma with later treatment, the potential additional risk of a fracture involving dentin is 19% of 8%, which is about 1.5%, while the risk of a pulpal involvement is 1% of 8%, or less than 0.1%. The decision to treat early at the age of 9 to 10 years or to wait until early adolescence is affected by an individual family's values and the relative risk they are willing to bear, with some choosing to spend additional time and money for an early phase of treatment. As long as this low risk, increased cost, and time difference is disclosed to the family, they can make an informed choice.

What could be considered a significant benefit from an early phase of treatment is a psychosocial improvement in self-esteem and a reduction in negative social experiences.[52] However, this difference has been shown to be transient and disappeared after the second phase of treatment.[47] Once again, it is up to the individual patient and family to determine if the effect of reducing the overjet would be a significant benefit. For example, if a child is being teased because of protrusive anterior teeth and suffering from low self-esteem, the child and the family may consider an early phase of treatment worthwhile.

Another factor to be considered is the risk of OIIRR. In the UNC study, the percentage of children with more than one incisor with moderate to severe OIIRR (≥ 2 mm) in the two-phase group was 5% in the functional group and 12.5% in the headgear group.[53] In the single-phase treatment group, the incidence was 20.4%. The reduction in overjet during phase II treatment and the duration of fixed appliance treatment were significantly associated with OIIRR. Therefore, this finding may also apply to other nonextraction single-phase approaches to Class II treatment, such as molar distalization.

Some minimal OIIRR is a normal consequence of orthodontic therapy, but in those that do experience moderate to severe OIIRR, does this affect the longevity of the affected teeth? In a long-term evaluation (average of 14.1 years) of longevity of teeth with severe OIIRR (> ⅓ loss of root length), it was found that even the most severely affected teeth were functioning in a reasonable manner many years after orthodontic intervention.[54] This is not surprising because the apical portion of the tooth plays only a minor role in overall periodontal support. It has been reported that 3 mm of apical root loss is equivalent to 1 mm of crestal bone loss.[55] Although resorption stops once the active appliances are removed, the longevity of severely resorbed teeth might be compromised in patients susceptible to marginal periodontal breakdown.[54] Needless to say, the goal in this situation would be to keep OIIRR to a minimum. Patients

at risk of severe OIIRR can be identified according to the amount of resorption during the initial treatment stages.[56] Routine radiographic examinations after about 6 months of treatment and additional examinations after 12 months for those with visible signs of resorption could be a predictable means to identify high-risk patients. A detailed explanation of root resorption can be found in chapter 10.

Another finding in the UNC study was that the functional group experienced more than twice the extraction rate (about 38%) compared with the control (about 18%) and headgear (about 15%) groups.[46] The authors concluded that this was not statistically significant ($P = .02$) because they selected .01 as the cutoff, but many studies would consider a P value of .02 (or $P < .05$) statistically significant, and most clinicians would consider a doubling in the extraction rate as clinically significant. However, when examining a large number of variables, having the lower P value reduces the risk of a type I error, ie, finding a difference by random chance when one does not actually exist. The UK study also found no statistically significant difference, but, conversely, the early treatment groups had fewer extractions (27%) compared with the adolescent (late) treatment group (37%). These results should be valid for other Class II children, as indicated in this study (overjet ≥ 7 mm, normal facial height), but should not be extended to those with combined anteroposterior and vertical problems or to those with skeletal asymmetries.

The timing of functional appliance treatment can be difficult because skeletal and dental development are not synchronized. Chronologic age is also not a reliable indicator of skeletal maturation. Hand-wrist films have been used to attempt to identify the pubertal growth spurt and perhaps the best timing for the functional appliance treatment of Class II malocclusions. However, this involves an additional radiograph and only identifies the peak and end of pubertal growth and is therefore of minimal use to predict the onset of pubertal growth.[57] An alternative cervical vertebral maturation (CVM) method uses the maturational stages of the cervical vertebrae on the lateral cephalogram. These cervical vertebral stages are closely related to mandibular growth changes during puberty.[58] Clinical trials assessing the response of Class II treatment in prepubertal and pubertal subjects assessed by the CVM method suggest a more favorable growth response in the patients treated in the pubertal growth spurt.[59,60] The early treatment (prepubertal) patients were on average about 10 years old, while those in pubertal growth groups were on average 12 to 13 years old. This supports the prospective RCTs discussed earlier, in which the early treatment groups (about 10 years old) demonstrated no long-term advantage over the late treatment groups (about 12 years old).[46,47] Based on the CVM method, the cervical vertebrae stage 3 is closest to the onset of peak statural height.[61] However, the chronologic age closest to this stage varies greatly, from 8½ years to 11 years 5 months in girls and from 10 to 14 years in boys. This large variability makes it more difficult to determine the ideal timing for treatment for an individual, and multiple radiographs may be required to determine this. The

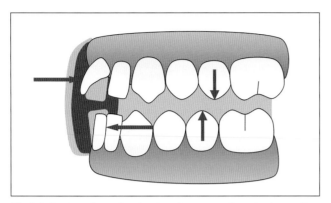

Fig 5-6 Elastomeric myofunctional appliances can tip protrusive maxillary incisors back and retroclined mandibular incisors forward to reduce the overjet while disocclusion of the posterior teeth allows vertical eruption to reduce the overbite.

previous studies comparing prepubertal and pubertal timing of treatment also used a literature control group, which may not be a valid comparison.[59,60] When the Herbst appliance was used at the ideal time, according to the CVM method, a 1.9-mm advancement in pogonion (pogonion to nasion perpendicular) was recorded compared with untreated controls, whereas it has been demonstrated that a 1.3-mm advancement in pogonion (pogonion to occlusal line perpendicular) can still be obtained with the Herbst in nongrowing adult patients.[60,62] Therefore, the timing of treatment seems to have minimal impact (0.6 mm) on the treatment outcome. For a method such as the CVM to be clinically useful, it needs to be reproducible, with the same and different clinicians able to reliably identify each particular stage. When examining this reproducibility, interobserver agreement between 10 orthodontists was found to be below 50%, and intraobserver agreement, where clinicians agreed with their own staging, occurred only 62% of the time.[63] Skeletal age has also been found to be an unreliable predictor of peak mandibular growth.[64] A more recent study evaluating the pattern of mandibular growth and stages of vertebral maturation concluded that the CVM method cannot predict the onset of peak mandibular growth.[65]

In addition to traditional functional appliances such as the bionator, Fränkel, twin block, and headgear, others have recommended the use of "myofunctional" appliances in very young children (ages 5 to 8 years old) to mitigate increased overjet and deep bite. It has been proposed that such very early intervention is more stable because of the early correction of aberrant muscle function. Little data exists, but studies evaluating the use of eruption guidance appliances, such as the Occlus-o-Guide (Ortho-Tain) and the Trainer for Kids (T4K) appliance (Myofunctional Research), have found limited improvement in the overjet and overbite (about 2 mm each), with treatment times of 13 months[66,67] to as long as 3.6 years.[68,69] These changes are not skeletal but dentoalveolar, with retroclination of the maxillary incisors and proclination of the mandibular

incisors to reduce the overjet.[67] The appliances disocclude the posterior teeth, allowing some vertical posterior eruption to reduce the overbite (Fig 5-6). There are substantial limitations to these studies, bringing the results into question, with a strong potential for selection bias because many cases were dropped from the final evaluation. The compliance rate with such appliances also seems poor, with at least 31% not wearing the appliances.[68] As to the claim that these appliances are more stable because of earlier correction, when monitored over 2 years, the overjet relapsed slightly from 2 mm to 1.5 mm, while the overbite correction relapsed from a 1.9-mm improvement to a final 0.5-mm change after 3.6 years of treatment.[69] Interestingly, there was also a transient improvement in crowding of about 2 mm, which relapsed completely over the 2-year observation period.[69] Because of the low quality of evidence and poor compliance rate, even when the appliance is worn properly, the risks, cost, and burden seem to significantly outweigh the small potential benefits, especially when the probability of success with the use of myofunctional appliances appears suspect.

There are also limitations to the conclusions drawn from the RCT studies presented[46,47] in that the authors chose patients with overjets of 7 mm or more and excluded those patients with extreme vertical disproportions. Some would argue that the treatment intervention in these trials had not been individualized for the phenotype of Class II malocclusion for each patient. Based on the results of these studies, those with smaller overjets (< 7 mm) would also not benefit from early intervention of the Class II component of their malocclusion, and, because disproportionally vertical growers were excluded, growth is unlikely to have been significantly different or predictable in subgroups. A case could be made for patients with a reasonable dental alignment that may avoid a second phase of treatment once their overjet and Class II relationship had been corrected. Taking this philosophy one step further, a partial appliances option to improve the dental alignment in conjunction with treatment for Class II correction may avoid a second phase of comprehensive treatment, assuming that the patients achieved a favorable outcome after the functional appliance or first phase of treatment. In the UK trial, almost 15% of the patients receiving an early phase of treatment accepted their occlusion and did not proceed with a second phase of treatment.[47] This percentage would vary with cultural and individual preferences, with some being more or less discerning about what they consider to be an acceptable alignment and occlusion.

The question then looms: Can we predict which cases will avoid a second phase of treatment? Those with mild to moderate crowding (4 to 6 mm) may benefit sufficiently from leeway space preservation and possibly partial maxillary appliances, but the eruption of the remaining permanent teeth into an acceptable alignment is not guaranteed, and an extended retention period is required while they erupt. If the patient then does require a second phase of treatment, the overall cost is now significantly more than if treatment had been done in one phase. It then becomes a personal choice whether to play the odds and wait until all teeth are erupted or consider an early phase, knowing that a second phase may still be required. The patient and the family need to have an informed discussion with the orthodontist about whether early intervention is justified for a child with a Class II, Division 1 malocclusion. It is easy to criticize these trials in retrospect, but proponents of other modalities also need to supply evidence for their claims, and in the absence of new data, these still remain the highest quality of research. The highest level of evidence, the systematic review from the Cochrane library, concluded that "The evidence suggests that providing orthodontic treatment, for children with prominent upper front teeth, in two stages does not have any advantages over providing treatment in one stage, when the children are in early adolescence."[44]

It seems from the above discussion that early intervention should be avoided. However, there are unquestionably patients who would benefit from or elect for an early phase of treatment after being informed of their treatment options. Special circumstances such as psychosocial distress, accident potential, or general convenience to the family can all indicate that an early phase of treatment might be beneficial to the patient[46] (see chapter 2).

Distalization mechanics

An alternative option in two-phase nonextraction treatment of Class II cases is molar distalization appliances, which involve palatal and/or dental anchorage with various forms of intra-arch springs or loops. These often still involve a two-phase approach, with distalization occurring prior to the full fixed phase of treatment. But how effective and efficient are they?

In a review of the effectiveness of maxillary molar distalization appliances, it was concluded that no more than 2 to 2.5 mm of distal maxillary molar movement could be achieved, and the quality of evidence for any method of moving maxillary molars distally was not high.[70] In a follow-up clinical trial of two techniques for molar distalization, only 1.2 to 1.3 mm of molar distalization was achieved.[71] In a randomized clinical trial comparing cervical headgear with Ni-Ti springs anchored against a Nance button for molar distalization, it was found that the springs distalized the molars an average of 3 mm during a period of 5.2 months, while the headgear distalized the molars 1.7 mm ($P < .001$) over 6.4 months ($P < .01$).[72] However, moderate anchorage loss was produced with the Nance/springs, resulting in an increased overjet (0.9 mm), while the headgear reduced the overjet by 0.9 mm. Although 1.3 mm more molar distalization was achieved with the springs, because of the difference in the overjet change, these appliances appear to be equally effective overall. A similar finding was found in a randomized clinical trial comparing the pendulum appliance with a cervical headgear.[73] In this study of 30 patients, the pendulum appliance achieved 4.1 mm of molar distalization, while the headgear achieved only 1.7 mm of molar distalization. However, the pendulum appliance resulted in 15 degrees of distal molar tipping and 1.1 mm of incisor protrusion, while the headgear achieved more bodily movement (1-degree tipping) with 0.6 mm of incisor retraction. The potential additional gain in molar distalization/tipping with the distalization can be lost in the second phase of fixed appliances. This is supported by a retrospective study that compared use of the pendulum appliance followed by fixed appliances with extraction of two maxillary premolars followed by fixed appliances. This study found the average treatment time to be 45.7 months with the pendulum/fixed approach in less severe Class II cases compared with 23.0 months with the extraction/fixed approach in full Class II cases.[74] This also highlights another important issue: All of these distalization studies found molar changes of about 1.5 to 3 mm, which would not allow correction of full Class II molar relationships, so are therefore more applicable to ½-unit cases.

The advantage of headgear and interarch appliances, such as the Forsus Fatigue Resistant Device (FRD) (3M Unitek) and Jasper Jumper (American Orthodontics), is that they can be used simultaneously with fixed appliances, whereas the spring and pendulum appliances are used prior to braces, which increases the overall treatment time associated with two-phase treatment. This ability to use headgear and elastics or spring Class II correctors during fixed appliance treatment rather than using headgear as an early first phase of treatment, as in the UNC trial, potentially makes treatment more efficient, correcting the alignment while simultaneously correcting the overjet/Class II malocclusion (Fig 5-7). Of course, as with any removable appliance, compliance with headgear or elastics can be an issue, with patients overestimating the actual hours of wear and some not wearing the appliances at all. Open and honest communication with the patient as well as an objective measure of progress during treatment, such as the use of appliances incorporating timers or the recording of overjet and maximal protrusion at each appointment to monitor a decrease, allow a more objective assessment of cooperation. Then if there is minimal or no recorded improvement or wear, the treatment approach can be modified to a non–compliance-reliant approach, such as a spring corrector (eg, Forsus FRD or Jasper Jumper). As discussed earlier, the advent of miniscrews/TSADs also allows implant-anchored distalizing appliances and mechanics to be implemented with less risk of anchorage loss.

To achieve the goal of simultaneous overjet correction and alignment, a component approach can be taken to fixed appliances, similar to that which has been described for removable functional appliances.[75] Functional appliances can be broken into some basic components: a bite plane to disocclude the dentition; mandibular repositioning that results in a distal force applied to the maxillary dentition and a mesial force on the mandible and/or the mandibular dentition; additional components such as shields, screens, or screws for expansion; a labial bow to retract the anterior teeth; and the trimming of acrylic to allow selective erup-

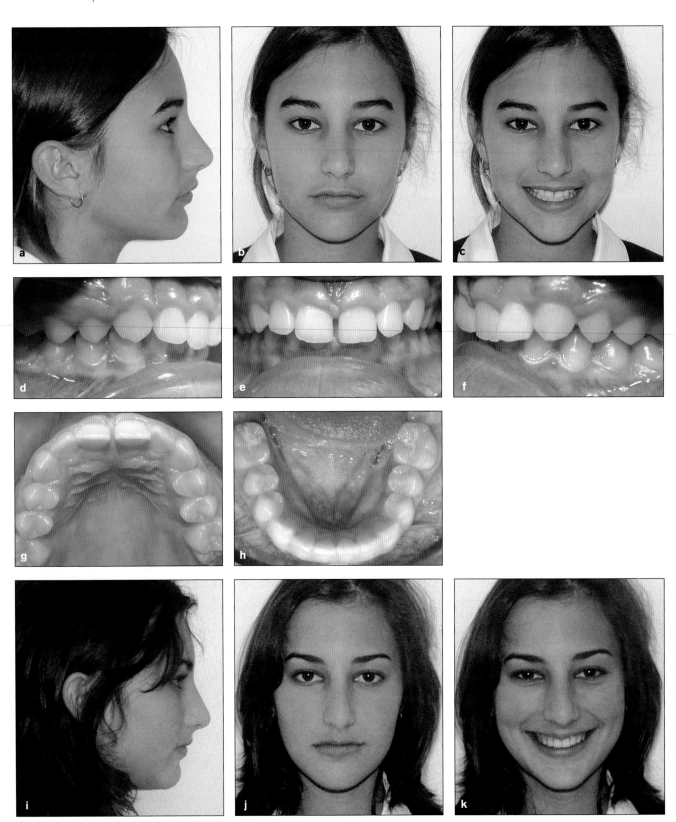

Fig 5-7 This patient had a mildly spaced Class II malocclusion *(a to h)* and was treated with a combination of fixed appliances and a Class II spring corrector (Forsus FRD) over a period of 18.5 months *(i to p)*. Her records 3.5 years later show her occlusion and alignment to have remained stable *(q to x)*.

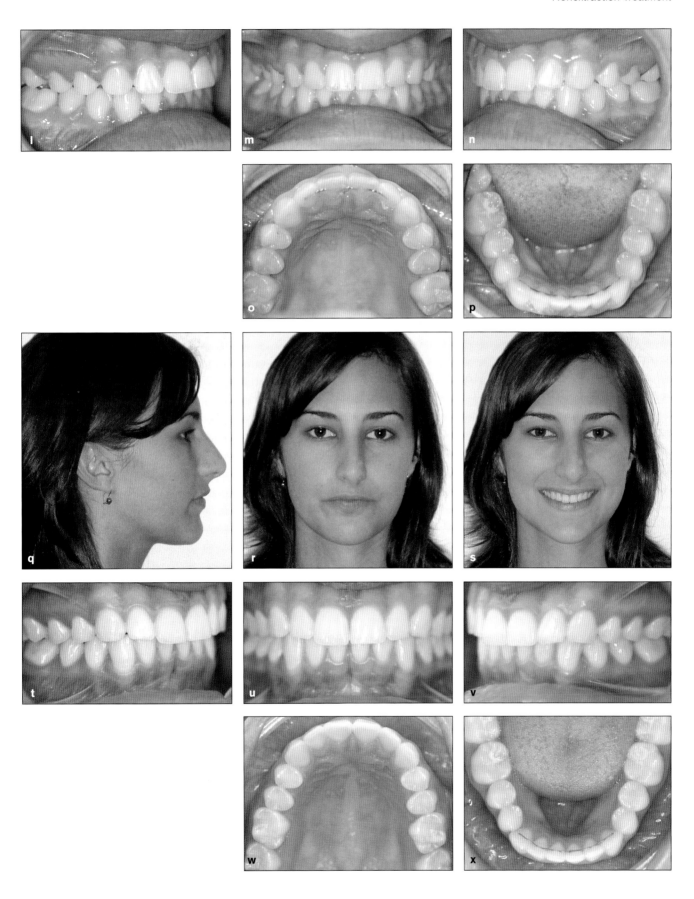

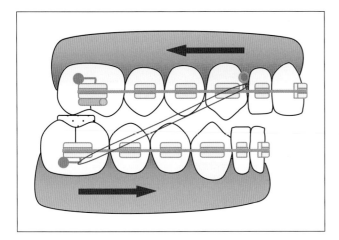

Fig 5-8 Fixed appliances can be designed to apply forces similar to those of functional appliances. A composite bite ramp helps to disocclude the occlusion, as do the bite blocks on functional appliances. Headgear, springs, or, in this example, elastics help to provide a distalizing force to the maxillary dentition and a mesially directed force to the mandibular dentition. Any arch form changes or expansion can be achieved by adjusting or expanding the archwire.

tion. These same components can be mimicked in fixed appliances (Fig 5-8) as follows:

- The dentition can be disoccluded with bite planes or bite wedges on the palatal surface of the maxillary central incisors (when the overjet is smaller and no open bite is present) or on the posterior molars (when the overjet is too large or in open bite cases).
- A distal force can be applied to the maxillary dentition with headgear, elastics, fixed springs, or miniscrew/ TSAD–anchored mechanics.
- A mesial force on the mandibular dentition can similarly be applied with elastics or fixed inter-arch appliances such as springs.
- Any additional adjustments such as retraction of teeth, expansion, or selective eruption can be done with conventional fixed appliances, bracket positioning, and archwire adjustments.

This approach to fixed appliance treatment allows single-phase correction of overjet, molar and canine relation-ships, and alignment, as achieved in previous RCTs in a manner that is potentially shorter and more cost-effective because of the elimination of a first phase of treatment. Some would suggest starting the maxillary arch first in deep bite Class II cases to intrude the maxillary anterior teeth because the use of wedges on anterior teeth results in a backward rotational effect on the mandible. This would be suitable in patients with a high smile line but is less ef-ficient because it delays alignment in the mandibular arch. From an esthetic perspective, in most cases intrusion of the mandibular anterior teeth is preferred to maintain the maxillary dental display during speech and when smiling.

Conclusion

The goal of this chapter was to provide an evidence-based perspective on how to make your orthodontic practice more efficient, but by no means is it intended as a "cook-book" for orthodontic practice. Although there are some specific guidelines, orthodontists must still tailor these guidelines to (1) their particular practices, training, clini-cal experiences, and skills; (2) particular patient situations and circumstances; and (3) patient preferences and auton-omy. With so many books and websites offering advice on, for instance, wire sequencing, this chapter provides a less-biased, evidence-based view. Even though orthodontics has been described as an art and a science, perhaps the art has dwarfed the science. With the overwhelming volume of orthodontic literature published, the busy clinician has little time to read and make sense of the available evidence and then apply it to daily practice. Therefore, this chap-ter offers the clinician a synthesis and application of the best available evidence on specific clinical issues related to Class II malocclusion.

Summary points

- When appropriate for extraction space closure, en-masse retraction is more efficient than two-step retraction.
- When extraction spaces are to be closed, Ni-Ti springs allow a potentially longer appointment interval with possibly slightly more rapid space closure than elastic chain.

- Appointment scheduling efficiency can be improved by basing appointment intervals on the properties of the materials used, the mechanics applied, and the expected biologic response of the patient rather than using a fixed appointment interval approach.
- In the absence of valid reasons for earlier intervention, the nonextraction treatment of Class II malocclusions can be more efficiently treated in one phase in early adolescence.

References

1. Forrest JL, Miller SA. Evidence-Based Decision Making: A Traditional Guide for Dental Professionals. Philadelphia: Lippincott, Williams & Wilkins, 2008.
2. Keim RC. The editor's corner: The power of the pyramid. J Clin Orthod 2007;41:587–588.
3. Keim RC, Gottlieb EL, Nelson AH, Vogels DS 3rd. 2008 JCO study of orthodontic diagnosis and treatment procedures, part 1: Results and trends. J Clin Orthod 2008;42:625–640.
4. McLaughlin R, Bennett JC, Trevisi HJ. Systemized orthodontic treatment mechanics. New York: Mosby, 2005:15,100–101.
5. Khambay BS, McHugh S, Millet DT. Magnitude and reproducibility of forces generated by clinicians during laceback placement. J Orthod 2006;33:270–275.
6. Usmani T, O'Brien KD, Worthington HV, et al. A randomized clinical trial to compare the effectiveness of canine lacebacks with reference to canine tip. J Orthod 2002;29:281–286.
7. Irvine R, Power S, McDonald F. The effectiveness of laceback ligatures: A randomized controlled clinical trial. J Orthod 2004;31:303–311.
8. Heo W, Nahm D, Baek S. A comparison of en-masse retraction and two-step retraction of maxillary anterior teeth in adult class I women: A comparison of anchorage loss. Angle Orthod 2007; 77:973–978.
9. Xu TM, Zhang X, Oh HS, Boyd RL, Korn EL, Baumrind S. Randomized clinical trial comparing control of maxillary anchorage with 2 retraction techniques. Am J Orthod Dentofacial Orthop 2010; 138:544.e1–544.e9.
10. Burstone CJ. The segmented arch approach to space closure. Am J Orthod 1982;82:361–378.
11. Huang Y, Wang X, Zhang J, Liu C. Root shortening in patients treated with two-step and en masse space closure procedures with sliding mechanics. Angle Orthod 2010;80:492–497.
12. Shpack N, Davidovitch M, Sarne O, Panayi N, Vardimon AD. Duration and anchorage management of canine retraction with bodily versus tipping mechanics. Angle Orthod 2008;78:95–100.
13. Lotzof LP, Fine HA, Cisneros GJ. Canine retraction: A comparison of two preadjusted bracket systems. Am J Orthod Dentofacial Orthop 1996;110:191–196.
14. Proffit WR. Mechanical principles in orthodontic force control. In: Proffit WR, Fields HW, Sarver DH (eds). Contemporary Orthodontics. St Louis: Mosby, 2007:376.
15. Burrow SJ. Canine retraction rate with self-ligating brackets vs conventional edgewise brackets. Angle Orthod 2010;80:626–633.
16. Miles PG. Self-ligating vs conventional twin brackets during en-masse space closure with sliding mechanics. Am J Orthod Dentofacial Orthop 2007;132:223–225.
17. Zablocki HL, McNamara JA, Franchi L, Baccetti T. Effect of the transpalatal arch during extraction treatment. Am J Orthod Dentofacial Orthop 2008;133:852–860.
18. Feldmann I, Bondemar L. Anchorage capacity of osseointegrated and conventional anchorage systems: A randomized controlled trial. Am J Orthod Dentofacial Orthop 2008;133:339.e19–339.e28.

19. Yao CJ, Lai EH, Chang JZ, Chen I, Chen Y. Comparison of treatment outcomes between skeletal anchorage and extraoral anchorage in adults with maxillary dentoalveolar protrusion. Am J Orthod Dentofacial Orthop 2008;134:615–624.
20. Sandler J, Benson PE, Doyle P, et al. Palatal implants are a good alternative to headgear: A randomized trial. Am J Orthod Dentofacial Orthop 2008;133:51–57.
21. Park H, Yoon D, Park C, Jeoung S. Treatment effects and anchorage potential of sliding mechanics with titanium screws compared with the Tweed-Merrifield technique. Am J Orthod Dentofacial Orthop 2008;133:593–600.
22. Janson G, Brambilla Ada C, Henriques JF, de Freitas MR, Neves LS. Class II treatment success rate in 2- and 4-premolar extraction protocols. Am J Orthod Dentofacial Orthop 2004;125:472–479.
23. Daskalogiannakis J, McLachlan KR. Canine retraction with rare earth magnets: An investigation into the validity of the constant force hypothesis. Am J Orthod Dentofacial Orthop 1996;109:489–495.
24. Sueri MY, Turk T. Effectiveness of laceback ligatures on maxillary canine retraction. Angle Orthod 2006;76:1010–1014.
25. Sonis AL. Comparison of NiTi coil springs vs. elastics in canine retraction. J Clin Orthod 1994;28:293–295.
26. Proffit WR. The biological basis of orthodontic therapy. In: Proffit WR, Fields HW, Sarver DH (eds). Contemporary Orthodontics. St Louis: Mosby, 2007:341.
27. Alexander SA. Levels of root resorption associated with continuous arch and sectional arch mechanics. Am J Orthod Dentofacial Orthop 1996;110:321–324.
28. Acar A, Canyürek U, Kocaaga M, Erverdi N. Continuous vs. discontinuous force application and root resorption. Angle Orthod 1999; 69:159–163.
29. Owman-Moll P, Kurol J, Lundgren D. Continuous versus interrupted continuous orthodontic force related to early tooth movement and root resorption. Angle Orthod 1995;65:395–400.
30. Barlow M, Kula K. Factors influencing efficiency of sliding mechanics to close extraction space: A systematic review. Orthod Craniofac Res 2008;11:65–73.
31. Samuels RHA, Rudge SJ, Mair LH. A comparison of the rate of space closure using a nickel-titanium spring and an elastic module: A clinical study. Am J Orthod Dentofac Orthop 1993;103:464–467.
32. Samuels RH, Rudge SJ, Mair LH. A clinical study of space closure with nickel-titanium closed coil springs and an elastic module. Am J Orthod Dentofac Orthop 1998;114:73–79.
33. Nightingale C, Jones SP. A clinical investigation of force delivery systems for orthodontic space closure. J Orthod 2003;30:229–236.
34. Dixon V, Read MJ, O'Brien KD, Worthington HV, Mandall NA. A randomized clinical trial to compare three methods of orthodontic space closure. J Orthod 2002;29:31–36.
35. Miles PG. Self-ligation: Evidence versus claims. In: McNamara JA Jr, Hatch N, Kapila SD (eds). Effective and Efficient Orthodontic Tooth Movement, vol 48. Craniofacial Growth Series. Ann Arbor: University of Michigan, 2001;27–43.
36. O'Brien KD, Robbins R, Vig KW, Vig PS, Shnorhokian H, Weyant R. The effectiveness of Class II, Division 1 treatment. Am J Orthod Dentofacial Orthop 1995;107:329–334.
37. Beckwith FR, Ackerman RJ Jr, Cobb CM, Tira DE. An evaluation of factors affecting duration of orthodontic treatment. Am J Orthod Dentofacial Orthop 1999;115:439–447.
38. Skidmore KJ, Brook KJ, Thomson WM, Harding WJ. Factors influencing treatment time in orthodontic patients. Am J Orthod Dentofacial Orthop 2006;129:230–238.
39. Burden DJ, McGuinness N, Stevenson M, McNamara T. Predictors of outcome among patients with Class II Division 1 malocclusion treated with fixed appliances in the permanent dentition. Am J Orthod Dentofacial Orthop 1999;116:452–459.
40. King GJ, McGorray SP, Wheeler TT, Dolce C, Taylor M. Comparison of peer assessment ratings (PAR) from 1-phase and 2-phase treatment protocols for Class II malocclusions. Am J Orthod Dentofacial Orthop 2003;123:489–496.

41. Janson G, Valarelli FP, Cançado RH, de Freitas MC, Pinzan A. Relationship between malocclusion severity and treatment success rate in Class II nonextraction therapy. Am J Orthod Dentofacial Orthop 2009;135:274.e1–274.e8.

42. Ismail A, Bader J. Evidence-based dentistry in clinical practice. J Am Dent Assoc 2004;135:78–83.

43. Millett DT, Cunningham SJ, O'Brien KD, Benson P, Williams A, de Oliveira CM. Orthodontic treatment for deep bite and retroclined upper front teeth in children. Cochrane Database Syst Rev 2006; 4:CD005972.

44. Harrison JE, O'Brien KD, Worthington HV. Orthodontic treatment for prominent upper front teeth in children. Cochrane Database Syst Rev 2007;3:CD003452.

45. Flores-Mir C, Major PW. A systematic review of cephalometric facial soft tissue changes with the Activator and Bionator appliances in Class II division 1 subjects. Eur J Orthod 2006;28:586–593.

46. Tulloch JFC, Proffit WR, Phillips C. Outcomes in a 2-phase randomized clinical trial of early Class II treatment. Am J Orthod Dentofacial Orthop 2004;125:657–667.

47. O'Brien K, Wright J, Conboy F, et al. Early treatment for Class II Division 1 malocclusion with the Twin-block appliance: A multicenter, randomized, controlled trial. Am J Orthod Dentofacial Orthop 2009;135:573–579.

48. Livieratos FA, Johnston LE. A comparison of one-stage and two-stage nonextraction alternatives in matched Class II samples. Am J Orthod Dentofacial Orthop 1995;108:118–131.

49. Koroluk L, Tulloch JF, Phillips C. Incisor trauma and early treatment for Class II Division 1 malocclusion. Am J Orthod Dentofacial Orthop 2003;123:117–126.

50. Chen DR, McGorray SP, Dolce C, Wheeler TT. Effect of early Class II treatment on the incidence of incisor trauma. Am J Orthod Dentofacial Orthop 2011;140:e155–e160.

51. Burden DJ. An investigation of the association between overjet size, lip coverage and traumatic injury to the maxillary incisors. Eur J Orthod 1995;17:513–517.

52. O'Brien K, Wright J, Conboy F, et al. Effectiveness of early orthodontic treatment with the Twin-block appliance: A multicenter, randomized, controlled trial. Part 2: Psychosocial effects. Am J Orthod Dentofacial Orthop 2003;124:488–495.

53. Brin I, Tulloch JF, Koroluk L, Phillips C. External apical root resorption in Class II malocclusion: A retrospective review of 1- versus 2-phase treatment. Am J Orthod Dentofacial Orthop 2003;124:151–156.

54. Remington DN, Joondeph DR, Årtun J, Riedel RA, Chapko MK. Long-term evaluation of root resorption occurring during orthodontic treatment. Am J Orthod Dentofacial Orthop 1989;96:43–46.

55. Kalkwaf KL, Krejci RF, Pao YC. Effect of apical root resorption on periodontal support. J Prosthet Dent 1986;56:317–319.

56. Årtun J, Hullenaar RV, Doppel D, Kuijpers-Jagtman AM. Identification of orthodontic patients at risk of severe apical root resorption. Am J Orthod Dentofacial Orthop 2009;135:448–455.

57. Hägg U, Taranger J. Maturation indicators and the pubertal growth spurt. Am J Orthod 1982;82:299–309.

58. O'Reilly MT, Yanniello GJ. Mandibular growth changes and maturation of cervical vertebrae. Angle Orthod 1988;58:179–184.

59. Baccetti T, Franchi L, Toth LR, McNamara JA Jr. Treatment timing for Twin-block therapy. Am J Orthod Dentofacial Orthop 2000;118:159–170.

60. Baccetti T, Franchi L, Stahl F. Comparison of 2 comprehensive Class II treatment protocols including the bonded Herbst and headgear appliances: A double-blind study of consecutively treated patients at puberty. Am J Orthod Dentofacial Orthop 2009;135:698.e1–698.e10.

61. Franchi L, Baccetti T, McNamara JA Jr. Mandibular growth as related to cervical vertebral maturation and body height. Am J Orthod Dentofacial Orthop 2000;118:335–340.

62. Ruf S, Pancherz H. Orthognathic surgery and dentofacial orthopedics in adult Class II Division 1 treatment: Mandibular sagittal split osteotomy versus Herbst appliance. Am J Orthod Dentofacial Orthop 2004;126:140–152.

63. Gabriel DB, Southard KA, Qian F, Marshall SD, Franciscus RG, Southard TE. Cervical vertebrae maturation method: Poor reproducibility. Am J Orthod Dentofacial Orthop 2009;136:478.e1–478.e7.

64. Hunter WS, Baumrind S, Popovich F, Jorgensen G. Forecasting the timing of peak mandibular growth in males by using skeletal age. Am J Orthod Dentofacial Orthop 2007;131:327–333.

65. Ball G, Woodside D, Tompson B, Hunter WS, Posluns J. Relationship between cervical vertebral maturation and mandibular growth. Am J Orthod Dentofacial Orthop 2011;139:e455–e461.

66. Methenitou S, Shein B, Ramanathan G, Bergersen EO. Prevention of overbite and overjet development in the 3 to 8 year old by controlled nighttime guidance of incisal eruption: A study of 43 individuals. J Pedod 1990;14:219–230.

67. Usumez S, Uysal T, Sari Z, Basciftci FA, Karaman AI, Guray E. The effects of early preorthodontic trainer treatment on Class II, Division 1 Patients. Angle Orthod 2004;74:605–609.

68. Keski-Nisula K, Hernesniemi R, Heiskanen M, Keski-Nisula L, Varrelae J. Orthodontic intervention in the early mixed dentition: A prospective, controlled study on the effects of the eruption guidance appliance. Am J Orthod Dentofacial Orthop 2008;133:254–260.

69. Janson G, Nakamura A, Chiqueto K, Castro R, de Freitas MR, Henriques JF. Treatment stability with the eruption guidance appliance. Am J Orthod Dentofacial Orthop 2007;131:717728.

70. Atherton GJ, Glenny AM, O'Brien K. Development and use of a taxonomy to carry out a systematic review of the literature on methods described to effect distal movement of maxillary molars. J Orthod 2002;29:211–216.

71. Paul LD, O'Brien KD, Mandall NA. Upper removable appliance or Jones Jig for distalizing first molars? A randomized clinical trial. Orthod Craniofac Res 2002;5:238–242.

72. Bondemark L, Karlsson I. Extraoral vs intraoral appliance for distal movement of maxillary first molars: A randomized controlled trial. Angle Orthod 2005;75:699–706.

73. Toy E, Enacar A. The effects of the Pendulum distalising appliance and cervical headgear on the dentofacial structures. Aust Orthod J 2011;27:10–16.

74. Pinzan-Vercelino CR, Janson G, Pinzan A, de Almeida RR, de Freitas MR, de Freitas KM. Comparative efficiency of Class II malocclusion treatment with the Pendulum appliance or two maxillary premolar extractions and edgewire appliances. Eur J Orthod 2009;31:333–340.

75. Vig PS, Vig KW. Hybrid appliances: A component approach to dentofacial orthopedics. Am J Orthod Dentofacial Orthop 1986;90:273–285.

Peter Ngan
DMD

Timothy Tremont
DMD, MS

CHAPTER

6 | Treatment of Class III Malocclusions

Per accepted orthodontic protocol, objectives for the treatment of Class III malocclusions include maintaining or improving a patient's facial esthetics, smile esthetics, function, and periodontal health, as well as a stable outcome. Recognition of the extent to which a condition is dentally and/or skeletally based is fundamental to the process. Clear comprehension of this aids in consideration of optimal or compromise treatment goals for the individual patient—and whether these goals are attainable and defendable. Because treatment objectives are rhetorically generalized, the specificity of treatment goals must clarify the course of action.

In this chapter, the authors propose the use of Andrews's Six Elements of Orofacial Harmony as a diagnostic tool to discern the underlying dental and skeletal components of a Class III malocclusion and as a basis for establishing optimal or compromise treatment goals. Treatment plans that target teeth and jaws in either optimal or compromise positions can be quantified using the referents and landmarks unique to the Six Elements. Effective clinical strategies can then be devised to attain these goals. It is beyond the scope of this chapter to provide a comprehensive presentation of the Six Elements. Interested readers are advised to seek a thorough study of the Six Elements through the cited references[1–10] and through courses sponsored by the Andrews Foundation (www.andrewsfoundation.org).

Children with Class III malocclusions can often benefit from early orthodontic or orthopedic treatment. Anterior crossbites can be dental or skeletal in nature. Whether these problems should be addressed in the mixed or permanent dentition depends on the nature of the problem.

Class III malocclusions with a dental origin in the permanent dentition can often be resolved in an optimal or compromise manner through successful orthodontic tooth movement.

A nongrowing patient presenting with a mild to moderate anteroposterior skeletal disharmony may be a candidate for a compromise treatment through orthodontic tooth movement alone. This may involve either an extraction or nonextraction approach. There is evidence supporting the limits of compromise orthodontic treatment for Class III patients.[11,12]

Often a Class III malocclusion exceeds the limits of a compromise approach, and a surgical correction of the underlying skeletal disharmony can be provided. It is essential to decompensate the teeth to permit optimal repositioning of the jaws. Orthognathic surgery may address the maxilla, mandible, or both, depending on the skeletal etiology of the malocclusion.

Differential Diagnosis of Class III Malocclusions

Fundamental to a differential diagnosis is clarity regarding the etiology of the malocclusion, whether it is disharmony in tooth position, jaw position, or both. The Six Elements philosophy[13] defines many unique landmarks (points or lines that can be used to measure the quality of the position of teeth and jaws) and referents (points or lines representing anatomy, the positions of which are measured relative to landmarks). Using these landmarks and referents, the Elements define optimal positions for the teeth and jaws. Comparing the position of the patient's teeth and jaws to the optimal allows for recognition of the dental and/or skeletal nature of the problem.

According to Andrews and Andrews,[13] use of the Six Elements philosophy will suggest a treatment plan not based

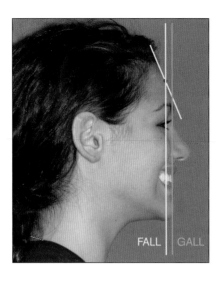

Fig 6-1 The maxilla is Element II when the maxillary incisor is in an optimal position within the jaw and falls on the GALL line. For every degree of forehead inclination greater than 7, the GALL is 0.6 mm more anterior than the FALL but not exceeding glabella. The FALL is a frontal plane of the head passing through the FFA point of the forehead. The GALL indicates the optimal anteroposterior position of the maxillary incisors and jaw. The FALL and GALL are coincident when the forehead inclination is 7 degrees or less.

on norms but one customized to each individual's face. It is proposed that the Elements are universal, meaning that they work equally well for all patients regardless of race, age, or sex. For the purpose of addressing the specific topic of this chapter, the discussion of the Six Elements is limited to Element II.

Element II: Anteroposterior jaw positions

An optimal anteroposterior position of the maxilla is recognized when the maxillary incisor is at an optimal inclination and centered over basal bone and the crown's FA point is on the Goal Anterior Limit Line (GALL). The referent for the maxilla is the optimal incisor FA point, and the landmark is the GALL. In turn, an optimal anteroposterior position of the mandible is recognized when the mandibular incisors are at an optimal inclination and centered over basal bone and the mandibular incisors couple in an ideal overjet with the maxillary incisors[1-3,13] (Fig 6-1). Andrews and Andrews[13] found that in individuals with facial harmony there is a correlation between the prominence and inclination of the forehead and the anteroposterior position of the teeth and jaws; the more inclined and/or prominent the forehead, the more anterior an optimal maxilla. Foreheads are classified as round, straight, or angular, with the FA point of the forehead (FFA) as the midpoint. In essence, anteroposterior treatment goals are based on incisor/jaw position viewed in a smiling profile.

Dental etiology

Figure 6-2 illustrates three types of dental malocclusions in which the maxillary and mandibular jaws are in optimal anteroposterior Element II position. However, the occlusion is Class III because of anteroposterior disharmony of tooth position within the jaws. Treatment strategies would

be designed to move teeth to attain either an optimal or compromise occlusion. Note that a green outline indicates optimal tooth position within a jaw, a red outline indicates excessively positive incisor inclination or mesial version of the dentition within a jaw, and a black outline indicates excessively negative incisor inclination or distal version of the dentition within a jaw.

Skeletal etiology

Figure 6-3 illustrates four types of anteroposterior skeletal disharmony of the maxilla and/or mandible resulting in Class III malocclusions. By measuring from the optimal maxillary incisor to the GALL and from the optimal mandibular incisor to the optimal maxillary incisor, the anteroposterior position of the jaws can be determined.

Thus, a Class III malocclusion can have both dental and skeletal etiologic components judged by using referents and landmarks identified for optimal tooth position and jaw position. In a study of Class III skeletal and dental relationships in adolescents, maxillary retrusion was found in 25% of the sample, mandibular protrusion in 19% of the sample, and a combination of maxillary retrusion and mandibular protrusion in 22% of the sample.[14] While 60% of the children had the maxilla and the mandible positioned within normal range, only 14% of the adults did. The authors surmised that with continued growth, the mandible outgrew the maxilla or that the proportion of individuals exhibiting mandibular protrusion increased from childhood to adulthood. It is therefore important to note that Class III malocclusion does not indicate some typical facial skeletal pattern. Rather, it can result from several aberrations in the craniofacial complex, including longer posterior cranial bases, larger mandibular plane angles, larger gonial angles, longer mandibular bodies, maxillary incisor protrusion, and mandibular incisor retrusion.

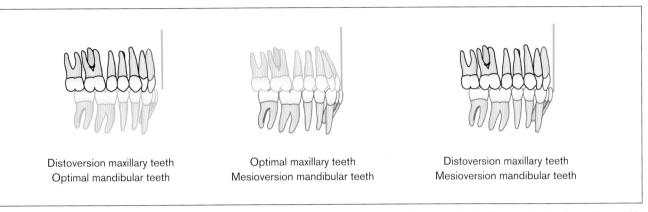

Distoversion maxillary teeth
Optimal mandibular teeth

Optimal maxillary teeth
Mesioversion mandibular teeth

Distoversion maxillary teeth
Mesioversion mandibular teeth

Fig 6-2 Optimal skeletal relationships with Class III occlusions from various dental etiologies. *Green outlines* indicate optimal tooth positions within a jaw, *red outlines* indicate excessively positive incisor inclination or mesioversion of the dentition within a jaw, and *black outlines* indicate excessively negative incisor inclination or distoversion of the dentition within a jaw.

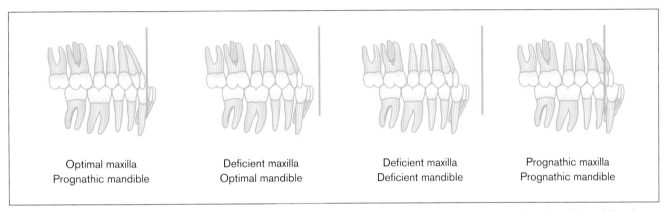

Optimal maxilla
Prognathic mandible

Deficient maxilla
Optimal mandible

Deficient maxilla
Deficient mandible

Prognathic maxilla
Prognathic mandible

Fig 6-3 Identical Class III occlusions reflecting various underlying skeletal dysplasias. *Green outlines* indicate optimal tooth positions within a jaw.

Treatment plans can be devised to attain optimal goals for the teeth and jaws using Six Elements referents and landmarks. At times, treatment plans that are more attainable, defendable, and acceptable to the patient can set compromise goals for the teeth and jaws.

Pseudo skeletal Class III malocclusions

Patients with pseudo skeletal Class III malocclusions[15] may only appear facially to have a prognathic mandible because of an anterior shift of the mandible. With the condyles seated, the incisors meet in an end-to-end relationship, and upon closure to maximal intercuspation the mandible shifts forward into an anterior crossbite. Properly defined, a *pseudo skeletal Class III malocclusion* does not have a skeletal etiology but is the result of disharmony in tooth position. This condition may be related to lack of vertical occlusal support from the posterior teeth caused by carious primary molars. It can also be related to palatal eruption of the maxillary incisors or palatal tipping of the maxillary incisors because of arch perimeter collapse, as in

the case of small lateral incisors or impacted or congenitally absent maxillary anterior teeth.

Lateral cephalometric radiographs should be taken in centric relation. Rotation of the traced mandible until the posterior teeth touch will permit accurate interpretation of the anteroposterior jaw positions. Patients with pseudo skeletal Class III malocclusions usually have harmonious facial profiles in centric relation.

Kwong and Lin[16] conducted a cephalometric study comparing the characteristics of patients with Class I, pseudo skeletal Class III, and true skeletal Class III malocclusions. Although their use of the term *pseudo* is not descriptively correct, most of the cephalometric measurements from the study suggested that pseudo skeletal Class III malocclusions are an intermediate form between Class I and skeletal Class III malocclusions. The only exception was the gonial angle, which was generally more obtuse in the skeletal Class III sample. Measurement of the gonial angles in the pseudo skeletal Class III sample was found to be rather similar to the Class I sample, making this measurement a feature in the differential diagnosis between pseudo skeletal and skeletal Class III malocclusions.

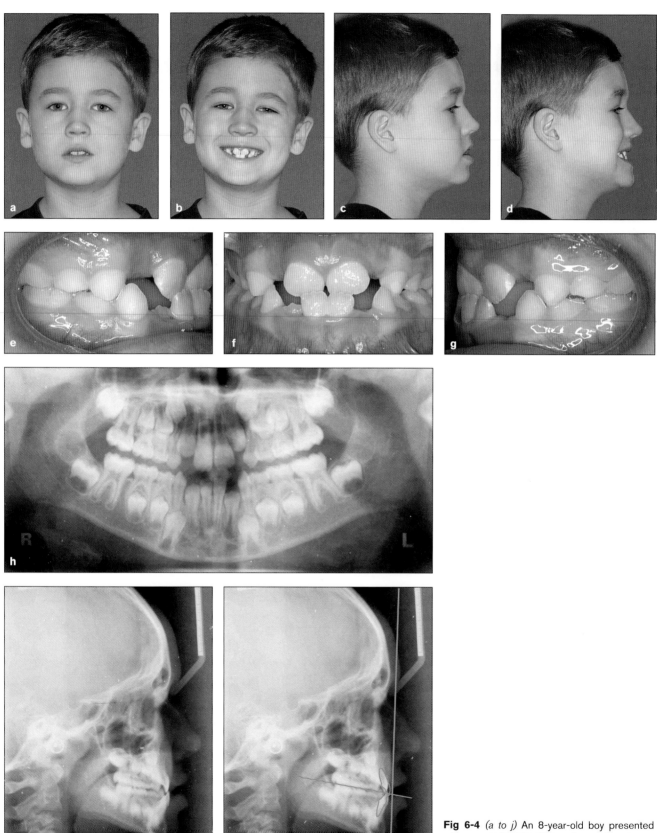

Fig 6-4 *(a to j)* An 8-year-old boy presented with an anterior crossbite and a maxillary transverse deficiency. *Green outlines* indicate optimal tooth positions within the jaws.

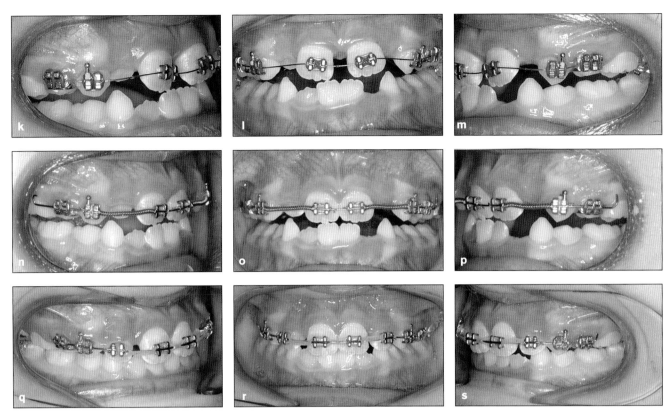

Fig 6-4 *(cont) (k to s)* Treatment with a Hyrax expander and fixed appliances.

Early Orthodontic Treatment

Indications

Objectives of early Class III treatment may include *(1)* preventing progressive hard or soft tissue damage, such as enamel abrasion and bony or gingival dehiscence; *(2)* improving skeletal discrepancies and possibly avoiding orthognathic surgery; *(3)* improving occlusal function; *(4)* developing arch length; and *(5)* improving dental and facial esthetics.[17] Common conditions warranting early treatment are anterior or posterior crossbites with or without functional shifts and blocked-out maxillary lateral incisors. Favorable factors for successful early treatment include mild to moderate skeletal disharmony, no familial mandibular prognathism, a convergent facial type, symmetric condylar growth, and expected good cooperation. Patients and parents should be informed that unpredictable dysplastic skeletal growth in the future may necessitate orthognathic surgery despite early intervention.

Borrie and Bearn[18] published a systematic review of 45 articles to identify the appropriate method for anterior crossbite correction. The authors found low-level evidence, and no statistical methods were employed for the analysis. They stated that higher-level studies are necessary before definitive conclusions can be made.

Maxillary expansion and partial fixed appliances

Figure 6-4 shows a patient who presented with an anterior crossbite and a maxillary transverse deficiency. Associated with the transverse discrepancy is inadequate arch length for the unerupted maxillary lateral incisors. This particular patient had a near optimal anteroposterior positioning of the maxilla and mandible, as indicated by the relationship of the optimal incisors to the GALL (Fig 6-4j). The panoramic radiograph (Fig 6-4h) showed that the lateral incisors were ready to erupt but were blocked out of the arch. The primary first molars had minimal root resorption and, along with the permanent first molars, provided good anchor units for rapid maxillary expansion (RME).

A Hyrax expander was inserted, and brackets were bonded to the central incisors and primary canines (maxillary premolar brackets were used on the primary canines) (Figs 6-4k to 6-4m). Skeletal expansion was accomplished with two turns per day for 10 days. The expander was tied off, and a 0.012-inch nickel-titanium (Ni-Ti) wire was inserted from the right primary first molar through the right canine, central incisors, left canine, and left primary first molar. Six weeks later, a 0.018-inch Ni-Ti wire was inserted, and a Ni-Ti open coil was compressed between the incisors and the primary canines (Figs 6-4n to 6-4p). The archwire was cinched distal to the primary first molar brackets to direct

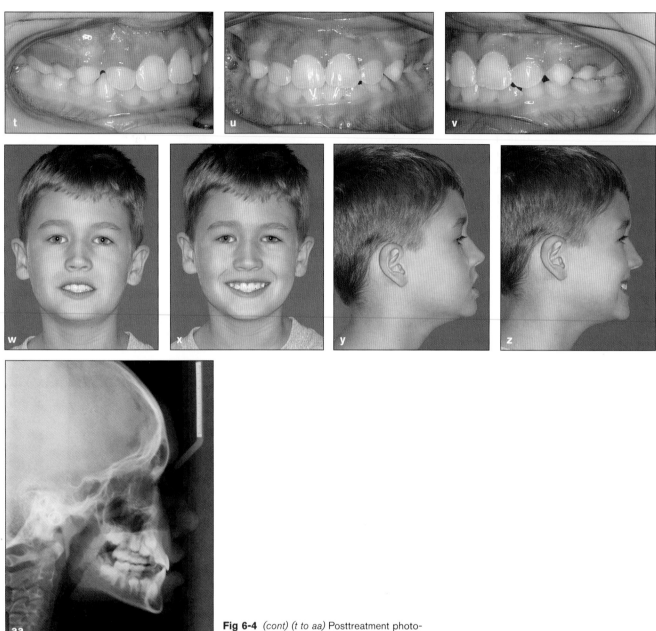

Fig 6-4 *(cont)* *(t to aa)* Posttreatment photographs and lateral cephalometric radiograph.

the incisors mesially, taking advantage of the central diastema to gain arch length for the unerupted lateral incisors. Once the central incisors were closed, the coil spring was increased on a new 0.018 Ni-Ti wire. Because the new archwire was not cinched at the primary first molar brackets, the coil springs proclined the central incisors out of the crossbite. Space was maintained until the lateral incisors erupted. The lateral incisors were then bracketed, and following successive 0.012 Ni-Ti, 0.018 Ni-Ti, and 0.018 stainless steel (SS) archwires, chain elastic was used to consolidate the four incisors (Figs 6-4q to 6-4s). Figures 6-4t to 6-4aa show the posttreatment results after correction of the anterior crossbite and alignment of the maxillary inci-

sors. No retention was used, and the patient was placed on recall to monitor his future dentofacial development.

Protraction face mask therapy

Protraction face mask therapy has been used in the treatment of Class III patients with maxillary deficiency in both the sagittal and vertical dimensions. In 1944, Oppenheim[19] argued that one could not control the growth or anterior displacement of the mandible and suggested moving the maxilla forward in an attempt to counterbalance mandibular protrusion. In 1960, Delaire and others[20] revived the interest in using a face mask for maxillary protraction. Petit[21] modified the Delaire face mask concept by increasing the amount of force generated by the appliance, thus decreasing the overall treatment time. In 1987, McNamara[22] introduced the use of a bonded expansion appliance with acrylic occlusal coverage as anchorage for maxillary protraction. Turley[23] suggested that expansion of the maxilla prior to protraction can help in "disarticulating" the maxilla and thus facilitate the forward movement of the maxilla. However, two studies found no difference in the forward movement of the maxilla with or without the use of an expansion appliance.[24,25] To date, short-term results show promising skeletal, dental, and profile improvements with treatment. The long-term benefits of early face mask treatment need further substantiation from prospective clinical trials.

Treatment effects

Meta-analysis has shown that the treatment effects of protraction face mask therapy are a combination of skeletal and dental changes of the maxilla and mandible.[26] The maxilla moves downward and forward, with a slight upward movement in the anterior and downward movement in the posterior palatal plane as the result of the protraction force; at the same time, posterior teeth extrude somewhat. As a consequence, downward and backward rotation of the mandible improves the maxillomandibular skeletal relationship in the sagittal dimension but results in an increase in lower anterior facial height. This rotation is a major contributing factor in establishing an anterior overjet improvement. A force exerted by the chin cup has been speculated to help in redirecting the mandibular downward and backward growth. Maxillary incisor labial inclination increased, although mandibular incisor inclination decreased. It is postulated that maxillary incisor proclination is a result of mesial dental movement, and mandibular incisor uprighting occurs as the result of pressure by the chin cup and soft tissue.

Expansion versus no expansion

In the mixed dentition, a banded or bonded expansion appliance can be fabricated as anchorage for maxillary protraction. Patients with an increased lower face height may benefit from using a bonded expansion appliance, which provides a temporary bite plane effect. Additionally, a bonded maxillary appliance can be used in patients with a deep overbite and overclosure of the mandible to facilitate the "jumping" of the anterior crossbite.[27] The expansion appliance can be activated once or twice daily (0.25 or 0.5 mm per turn) by the patient or parent for 7 to 10 days. In patients with a more constricted maxilla, activation of the appliance is carried out for 2 weeks or more.

Several facial sutures play an important role in the development of the nasomaxillary complex, including the frontomaxillary, nasomaxillary, zygomaticotemporal, zygomaticomaxillary, pterygopalatine, intermaxillary, ethmo-

maxillary, and the lacrimomaxillary sutures.[15] Animal studies have shown that the maxillary complex can be displaced anteriorly with significant changes in the facial sutures.[28] Maxillary protraction, however, does not always result in forward movement of the maxilla. With the same line of force, different midfacial bones were displaced in different directions depending on the moments of force generated at the sutures. The center of resistance of the maxilla was found to be located at the distal contacts of the maxillary first molars, one-half the distance from the functional occlusal plane to the inferior border of the orbit.[29] Protraction of the maxilla below the center of resistance produces counterclockwise rotation of the maxilla, which may not be favorable for patients with open bite tendency.[30] The face mask has an adjustable anterior wire that can accommodate a downward and forward pull on the maxilla with elastics. To minimize the tipping of the palatal plane, the protraction elastics are attached near the maxillary canines with a downward and forward pull of 30 degrees from the occlusal plane. Maxillary protraction usually requires 300 to 600 g of force per side, depending on the age of the patient. Patients are instructed to wear the appliance for 12 hours per day.

Sutural expansion and/or protraction induces new bone growth by mechanically stretching the sutures. The craniofacial sutures are osteogenic tissues between opposing membranous bones. Experimental separation of craniofacial sutures in animals, with traction forces, resembles the sutural activity noted during normal growth, though more marked.[31–33] The response to mechanical traction includes a widening of the sutures, changes in the orientation of fiber bundles, an increase in the number of osteoblasts, and deposition of osteoid on both sutural bone surfaces.[34] Clinically, it has been shown that maxillary expansion can disarticulate the maxilla to allow a more favorable forward movement of the maxilla.[33–35] A well-disarticulated maxilla seems to be critical when using tooth-borne devices for orthopedic effects. A protocol of repetitive weekly alternate RME and constriction of the maxilla to disarticulate the maxilla without overexpanding has been proposed.[34] Usually, it requires 7 to 9 weeks to loosen the maxilla. An average of 5.8 mm of forward movement of the maxilla at A-point was noted when using this method. This protocol was used to protract cleft lip and cleft palate patients with maxillary deficiency during early adolescence.[36] The sutures were loosened by alternating weekly expansion with constriction for 8 weeks, a face mask was used at night to pull the maxilla forward, and Class III elastics were used during daytime to hold the result of the protraction.

Figure 6-5 shows a 7-year-old girl who presented with the chief concern that her "bite was not right." Clinically, she presented with an obtuse nasolabial angle, a deficient maxilla, and a relatively normal mandible, as evidenced by the optimally positioned incisors relative to the GALL. Intraorally, she had an anterior crossbite and crowding in the maxillary arch. The maxillary left and right permanent canines were blocked out because of crowding. The maxillary incisors were proclined, and the mandibular incisors

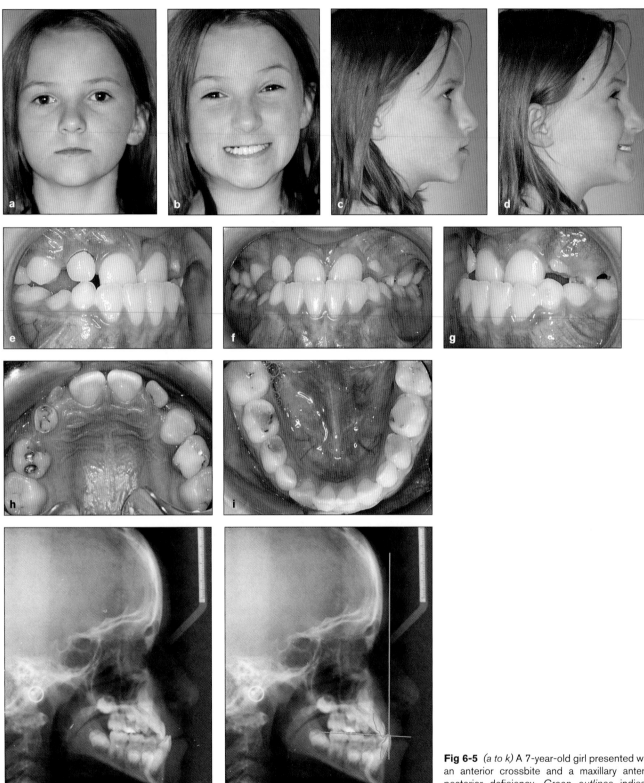

Fig 6-5 *(a to k)* A 7-year-old girl presented with an anterior crossbite and a maxillary antero-posterior deficiency. *Green outlines* indicate optimal tooth positions within the jaws.

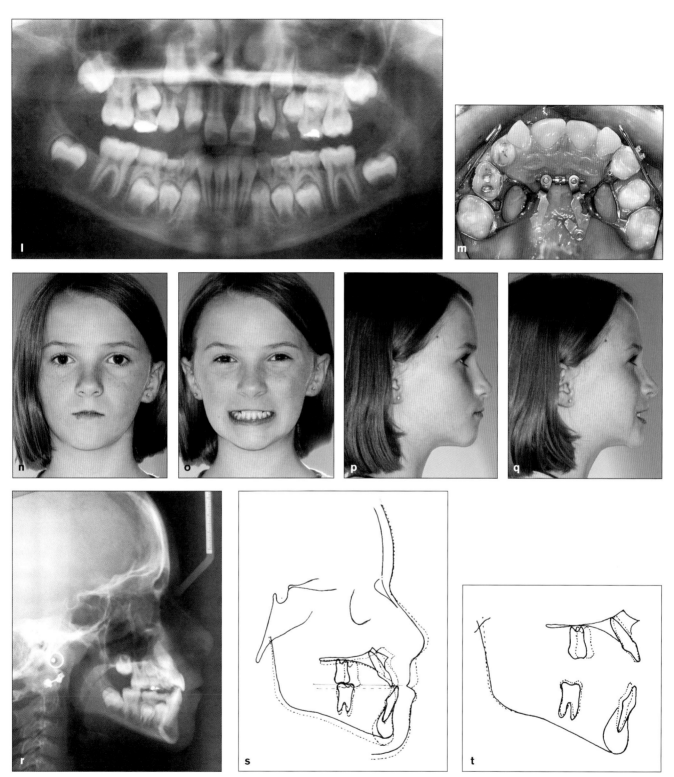

Fig 6-5 *(cont)* *(l)* Pretreatment panoramic radiograph. *(m)* Treatment with a double hinge expander, face mask at night, and Class III elastics during the daytime. *(n to q)* Posttreatment photographs. *(r to t)* Posttreatment lateral cephalometric radiograph and superimpositions to show skeletal and dental changes after treatment.

were retroclined, compensating for the skeletal malocclusion. There was no family history of mandibular prognathism.

Two treatment options were proposed. The first option was an early phase of orthopedic treatment to induce harmonious skeletal growth and improve facial esthetics followed by phase II treatment to correct the remaining crowding, overjet, and overbite problems. This option would preferably eliminate the necessity for orthognathic surgery. The patient would be followed to determine the stability of treatment. The second option was to wait until all growth was completed and determine whether the malocclusion could be camouflaged by orthodontic treatment or a combination of surgical and orthodontic treatment. The patient and family agreed to the first option of treatment.

A Hyrax rapid palatal expansion appliance was constructed by using bands on the posterior teeth (Fig 6-5m). Bands were fitted on the maxillary primary second molars and on the maxillary permanent first molars. The bands were soldered to heavy wires (0.045-inch), which were connected to a jackscrew that centered along the midline of the maxillary palate. Bilaterally, a 0.045-inch wire was soldered to the buccal aspects of the molar bands and extended anteriorly to the canine area. This buccal wire had a curve at the canine area so that elastics could be used to connect the appliance to a protraction face mask. The sutures that connect the maxilla to the surrounding bones were loosened via rapid expansion and contraction on an alternating weekly basis for 7 weeks.[34] The maxilla was expanded or contracted 1 mm per day (two turns in the morning and two turns in the evening). The amount of expansion was checked after the first, second, and fifth week. The mobility of the maxilla was checked before proceeding to maxillary protraction. The maxilla was clinically examined for mobility by holding the patient's head with one hand and rocking the anterior segment of the maxilla up and down with the other hand. The Petit protraction face mask (Ormco) is a one-piece construction with adjustable forehead padding, an adjustable chin cup, and an adjustable anterior bar. The adjustable components of the protraction face mask and appropriate positioning of the anterior bar (to which elastics were attached to both right and left sides) allowed for proper positioning of the chin cup for comfort upon both opening and closing of the mandible. To avoid an opening of the bite as the maxilla was protracted, the elastics were attached near the maxillary canines with a downward and forward pull of 30 degrees to the occlusal plane. A Correx Gauge (Haag-Streit) was used to measure the elastic force to ensure that approximately 450 g of force was generated on each side. A ³/₈-inch, 14-oz elastic can usually provide 12 oz or 400 g of

force from the maxillary canine area to the face mask. The patients was instructed to wear the protraction face mask for 10 to 12 hours at night.

On the mandibular arch, bands were fitted on the mandibular first molars, and brackets were placed on the mandibular four incisors. A 0.019 × 0.025–inch posted archwire with a stop-loop in front of the mandibular first molar was placed so that the patient could wear Class III elastics during the day for 8 hours. Figures 6-5n to 6-5q shows the correction of the anterior crossbite after 4 months of maxillary protraction with the face mask at night and Class III elastics during the daytime. Superimposition of the pre- and posttreatment lateral cephalometric radiographs (Fig 6-5s) shows a 4.5-mm forward movement of the A-point. The patient was placed on retention with a Fränkel III regulator for 1 year.

Treatment timing for maxillary protraction

A question of clinical importance in maxillary protraction is when to start face mask treatment. The main objective of early face mask treatment is to enhance forward displacement of the maxilla by sutural growth. Histologic studies have shown that the midpalatal suture is broad and smooth during the "infantile" stage (8 to 10 years of age), and the suture becomes more squamous and overlapping in the "juvenile" stage (10 to 13 years).[37] Biologically, the circummaxillary sutures are smooth and broad before age 8 years and become more heavily interdigitated around puberty. These findings related to observations in clinical studies that have shown that maxillary protraction was effective in the primary, mixed, as well as early permanent dentitions. Several studies suggested that a greater degree of anterior maxillary displacement can be found when treatment is initiated in the primary or early mixed dentition.[38,39] The optimal time to intervene in a Class III malocclusion is at the time of the initial eruption of the maxillary incisors. A positive overjet and overbite at the end of face mask treatment appears to maintain the anterior occlusion.

An additional question worth addressing is whether the results of early protraction treatment can be sustained when subsequent mandibular growth occurs during puberty. In a prospective clinical trial, protraction face mask treatment starting in the mixed dentition was found to be stable 2 years after the removal of the appliances.[30] This probably resulted from the overcorrection and the use of a functional appliance as a retainer for 1 year. When these patients were followed for another 2 years, 15 of the 20 patients maintained a positive overjet.[30] In patients that relapsed back to a reverse overjet, the mandible outgrew the maxilla in the horizontal direction. When these patients were followed for another 4 years (8 years after treatment, until about 17.5 years of age), 14 out of 20 patients (67%) maintained a positive overjet.[40] For the patients that relapsed back into a reverse overjet, the mandible outgrew the maxilla by four times compared with two times in the stable group. These results suggest that in a randomized clinical trial in which patients are followed until after completion of pubertal growth, two out of three patients (or 67%) will have a favorable outcome. About one-third of the patients might be candidates for orthognathic surgery later in life because of an unfavorable growth pattern. A study in which patients were treated with protraction face mask therapy either in the early mixed dentition or in the late mixed and permanent dentitions and followed up after a second phase of fixed appliance therapy demonstrated ongoing improvements in the former group but not in the latter group at the end of phase II treatment.[41] Specifically, a 1.8-mm additional forward movement of the maxilla was noted in the early treatment group compared with the controls. In the late mixed dentition group, no significant difference in forward movement of the maxilla was found after puberty compared with the controls.

Utility of maxillary protraction therapy

Clinically, anterior crossbite can be corrected with 3 to 4 months of maxillary expansion and protraction therapy, depending on the severity of the malocclusion. Improvement in overbite and molar relationships can be expected with an additional 4 to 6 months of treatment. In a prospective clinical trial, overjet correction was found to be the result of forward maxillary movement (31%), backward movement of the mandible (21%), labial movement of the maxillary incisors (28%), and lingual movement of the mandibular incisors (20%).[27] Overcorrection of the overjet and molar relationships was highly recommended to anticipate unfavorable mandibular growth. Overbite was improved by eruption of the posterior teeth. The total facial height was increased by inferior movement of the maxilla and downward and backward rotation of the mandible. According to several clinical studies, the mean forward movement of the maxilla with 6 to 8 months of maxillary protraction is about 1 to 3 mm.[22–25,27] A meta-analysis on the effectiveness of protraction face mask treatment found that the average change in Wits appraisal was 4 to 6 mm, and the average horizontal A-point movement was 1 to 3 mm.[25] The average forward movement of the A-point with 8 to 12 months of maxillary protraction was 2 to 4 mm. The increase in the ANB angle ranged from 0.9 to 4.4 degrees, with a mean value of 2.8 degrees. This is well over the expected growth changes for 1 year, but variability exists among individual subjects.

Mandall et al[39] reported on a 15-month, multicenter, randomized controlled trial investigating the effectiveness of early Class III protraction face mask treatment in children under 10 years of age. The authors concluded that this therapy was skeletally and dentally effective in the short-term and does not result in temporomandibular joint dysfunction. Seventy percent of patients had successful treatment, defined as achieving a positive overjet. However, early treatment does not seem to confer a clinically significant psychosocial benefit.

Chin cup therapy

Skeletal Class III malocclusion with a relatively normal maxilla and a moderately protrusive mandible can be treated with the use of a chin cup. This treatment modality is popular among Asian populations because of its favorable effects on the sagittal and vertical dimensions. The objective of early treatment with the use of a chin cup is to provide growth inhibition or redirection and posterior positioning of the mandible.

The orthopedic effects of a chin cup on the mandible include *(1)* redirection of mandibular growth vertically, *(2)* backward repositioning (rotation) of the mandible, and *(3)* remodeling of the mandible with closure of the gonial angle. To date, there is no agreement in the literature as to whether chin cup therapy can inhibit the growth of the mandible.[42–44] However, chin cup therapy has been shown to produce a change in the mandible associated with a downward and backward rotation and a decrease in the angle of the mandible.[43–45] In addition, there is less incremental increase in mandibular length together with posterior movement of B-point and pogonion.

Protrusive mandibles can usually be recognized in the primary dentition despite the fact that the mandible appears retrognathic in the early years for most children. Evidence exists that treatment to reduce mandibular protrusion is more successful when it is started in the primary or early mixed dentition.[43–45] The treatment time varies from 1 year to as long as 4 years, depending on the severity of the skeletal malocclusion. However, the stability of chin cup treatment remains unclear. Several studies reported a tendency to return to the original growth pattern after the chin cup was discontinued.[46–48] Patients who started treatment at an earlier age had a catch-up mandibular displacement in a forward and downward direction before growth was completed. In a study by Deguchi and Kitsugi,[49] several patients complained of temporary soreness of the temporomandibular joint after chin cup therapy.

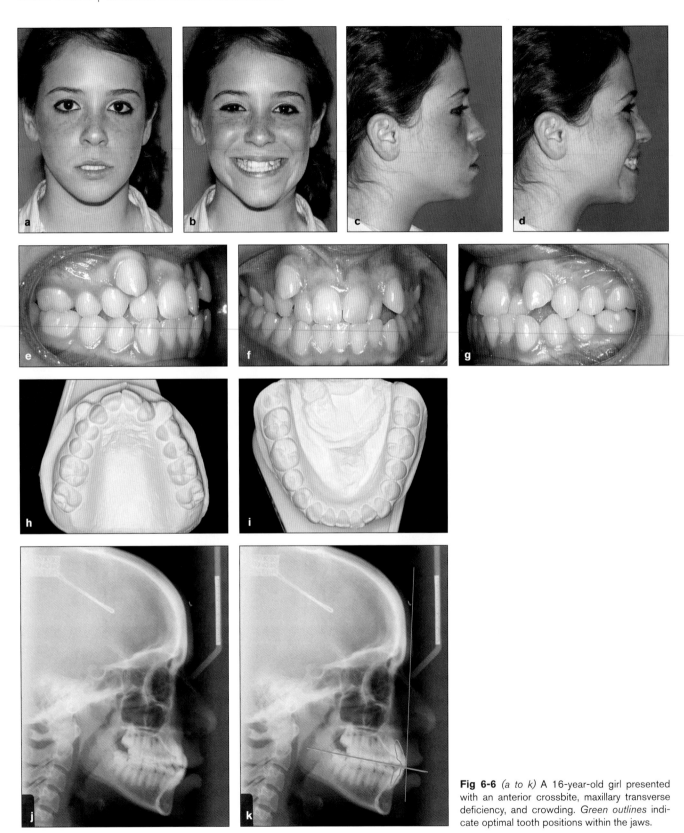

Fig 6-6 *(a to k)* A 16-year-old girl presented with an anterior crossbite, maxillary transverse deficiency, and crowding. *Green outlines* indicate optimal tooth positions within the jaws.

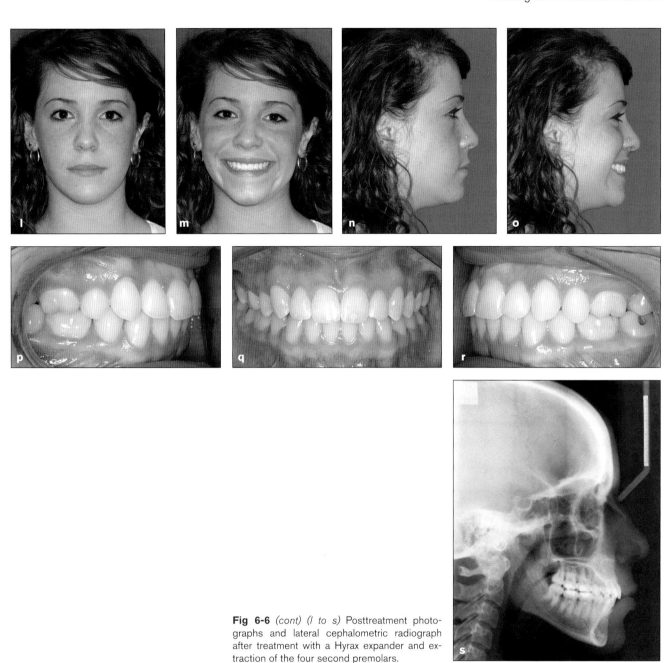

Fig 6-6 *(cont) (l to s)* Posttreatment photographs and lateral cephalometric radiograph after treatment with a Hyrax expander and extraction of the four second premolars.

Nonsurgical Orthodontic Treatment

Extraction – optimal

The patient in Fig 6-6 presented with an anterior crossbite, maxillary transverse deficiency, and crowding. Hypothetical optimal maxillary and mandibular incisors were coupled, and the maxillary incisor fell on the GALL (Fig 6-6k). Diagnostically, the patient did not have an underlying anteroposterior skeletal dysplasia but indeed had an optimal anteroposterior jaw relationship. A treatment plan involving RME and four second premolar extractions was concluded from quantifying the targeted optimal tooth positions. A posttreatment lateral cephalometric radiograph and photographs showed that a Key I occlusion was successfully attained, with the patient demonstrating a harmonious profile.

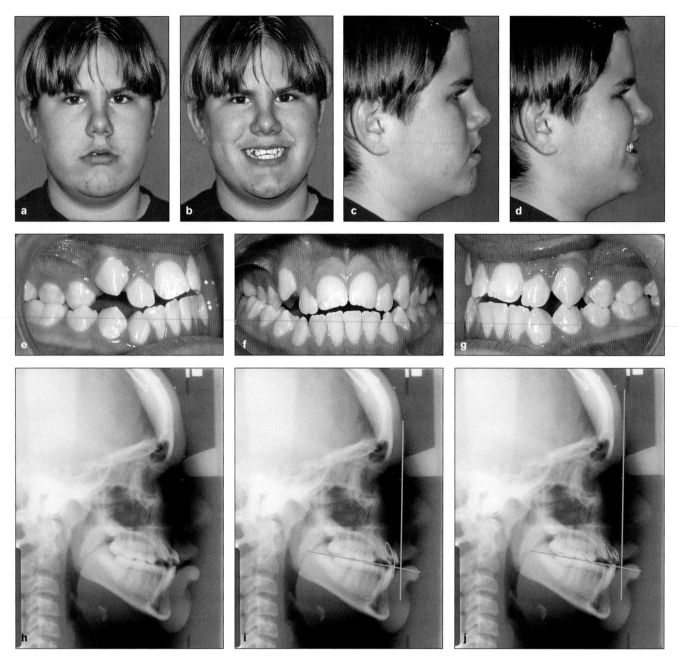

Fig 6-7 *(a to j)* A 14-year-old boy presented with a Class III malocclusion, crowding, and open bite tendency. *Green outlines* indicate optimal tooth positions within the jaws, and *red outline* indicates proclined tooth position.

Extraction – compromise

The patient in Fig 6-7 presented with a Class III molar relationship, open bite, mandibular crowding, and posterior crossbite. Optimal maxillary and mandibular incisors indicated an anteroposterior discrepancy between the maxilla and mandible. Relating the optimal maxillary incisors to the GALL showed that both jaws were anteroposteriorly deficient, with the maxilla more deficient than the mandible (Fig 6-7i). If the optimal position of the teeth were quantified, the optimal treatment plan would involve RME and four first premolar extractions. Additionally, both the

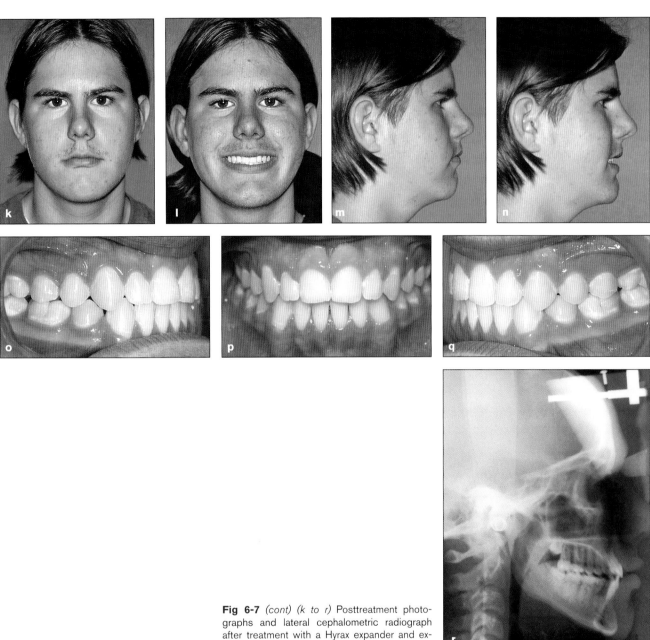

Fig 6-7 *(cont) (k to r)* Posttreatment photographs and lateral cephalometric radiograph after treatment with a Hyrax expander and extraction of the mandibular first premolars.

maxilla and the mandible would be advanced surgically. A defendable compromise treatment was accepted by the patient/parents involving RME, extraction of the mandibular first premolars, and maintenance of the maxillary incisor proclination. Posttreatment records demonstrate that the compromise treatment goals were successfully attained. The canines were finished in Key I occlusion, with the molars in a Class III relationship. The occlusion was gnathologically functional. Relative to the GALL, the patient showed a moderate jaw deficiency.

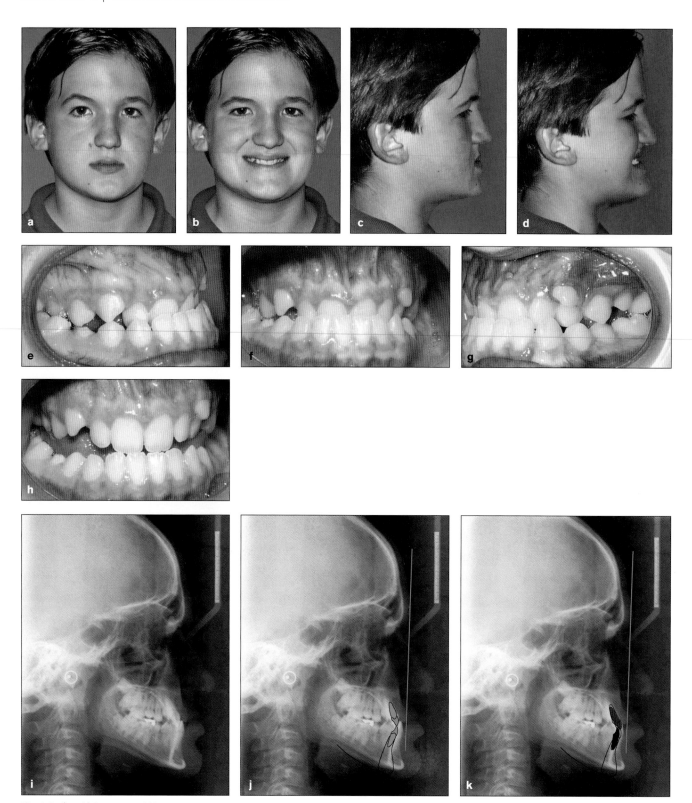

Fig 6-8 *(a to k)* A 12-year-old boy presented with anterior and posterior crossbites together with a maxillary anteroposterior deficiency and mandibular prognathism. *Green teeth* indicate optimal tooth positions within the jaws, *red tooth* indicates proclined tooth position, and *black tooth* indicates retroclined tooth position.

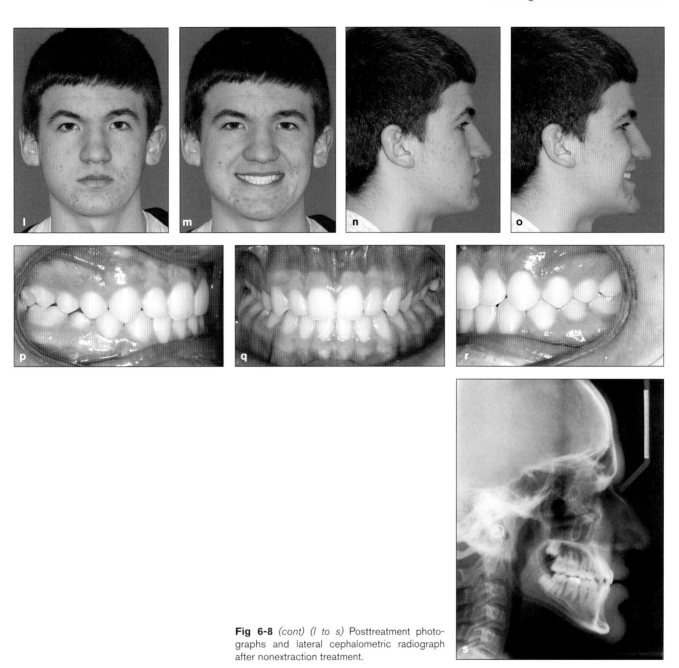

Fig 6-8 *(cont) (l to s)* Posttreatment photographs and lateral cephalometric radiograph after nonextraction treatment.

Nonextraction – compromise

The patient in Fig 6-8 presented with an anterior and posterior crossbite. Facially he demonstrated a maxillary anteroposterior deficiency, mandibular prognathism, excessive pogonion prominence, and an overclosed vertical dimension. With the condyles seated, the occlusion was edge-to-edge with the facial height improved. Analysis of optimal incisors and the GALL indicated a maxillary skeletal deficiency (Fig 6-8j). A compromise treatment was devised to slightly procline the maxillary incisors, upright the mandibular incisors, and erupt the posterior teeth (Fig 6-8k). Future disharmony in facial growth would necessitate orthognathic surgery. Posttreatment records indicate a successful com-

promise outcome. The occlusion was nearly optimal, and the face displayed a deficient maxilla and prognathic mandible, particularly in the smiling profile view.

The patient in Fig 6-9 presented with a Class III molar relationship, crowding in both arches, open bite, and posterior crossbite. Facially she appeared to have a maxillary and mandibular deficiency. Cephalometric analysis of optimal incisors and the GALL indicated that both jaws were deficient, with the maxilla more deficient than the mandible (Fig 6-9k). A compromise nonextraction treatment involved RME and interarch elastics to distalize the mandibular teeth and slightly procline the maxillary teeth (Fig 6-9l). Posttreatment records demonstrate that the compromise goals were successfully attained.

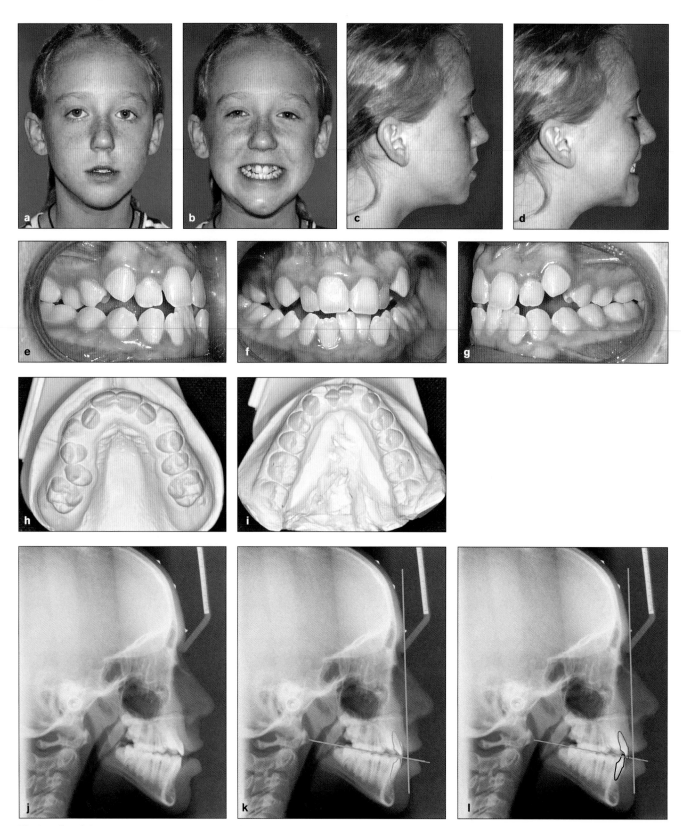

Fig 6-9 *(a to l)* A 13-year-old girl presented with a Class III malocclusion, maxillary transverse deficiency, and crowding of both arches. *Green outlines* indicate optimal tooth positions within the jaws, *red outline* indicates proclined tooth position, and *black outline* indicates retroclined tooth position.

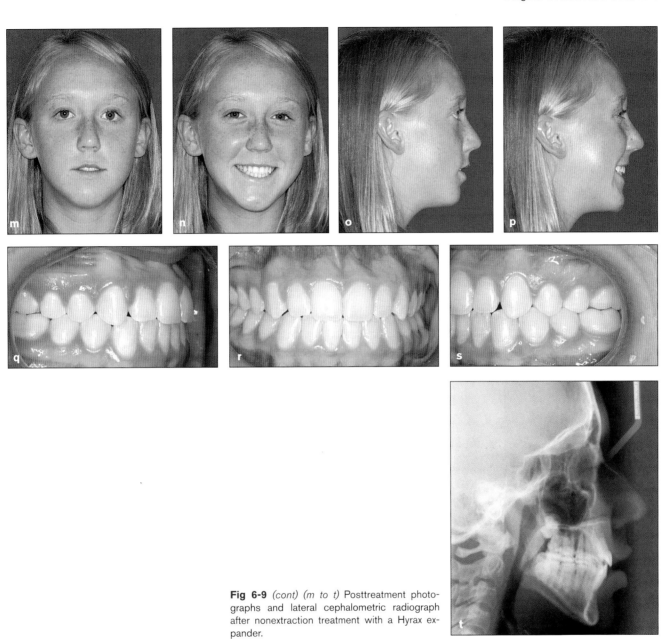

Fig 6-9 *(cont) (m to t)* Posttreatment photographs and lateral cephalometric radiograph after nonextraction treatment with a Hyrax expander.

Surgical Orthodontic Treatment

Planning teeth and jaws in three dimensions

A chapter pertaining to Class III problems is self-limiting because malocclusions, particularly those with underlying skeletal dysplasias, may encompass dental and/or skeletal discrepancies in the vertical and transverse dimensions as well as the anteroposterior dimension. With use of the Six Elements approach to diagnosis and treatment planning, all parameters can be addressed in a precise and comprehensive manner. Similar to quantifying the tooth position goals, the planned position of the jaws can be quantified for either optimal or compromise goals. Treated to optimal tooth and jaw positions, a patient's profile will be harmoni-

ous in both repose and during smiling. Compromise treatment plans should be defendable in regards to facial and smile esthetics, function, periodontal health, and stability.

Presurgical orthodontics

The dentition and jaws should be viewed as parts of the face, just like the eyes, nose, and lips. A useful concept is to think of optimizing the parts. Treatment plans should decompensate the position of the teeth within their respective jaws. Surgically repositioning the jaws to optimal positions will result in facial harmony. Often decompensation involves proclination of mandibular incisors, transverse expansion of the maxilla, or retraction of maxillary incisors. The referents and landmarks provided by the Six Elements are reliable guides for setting treatment goals.

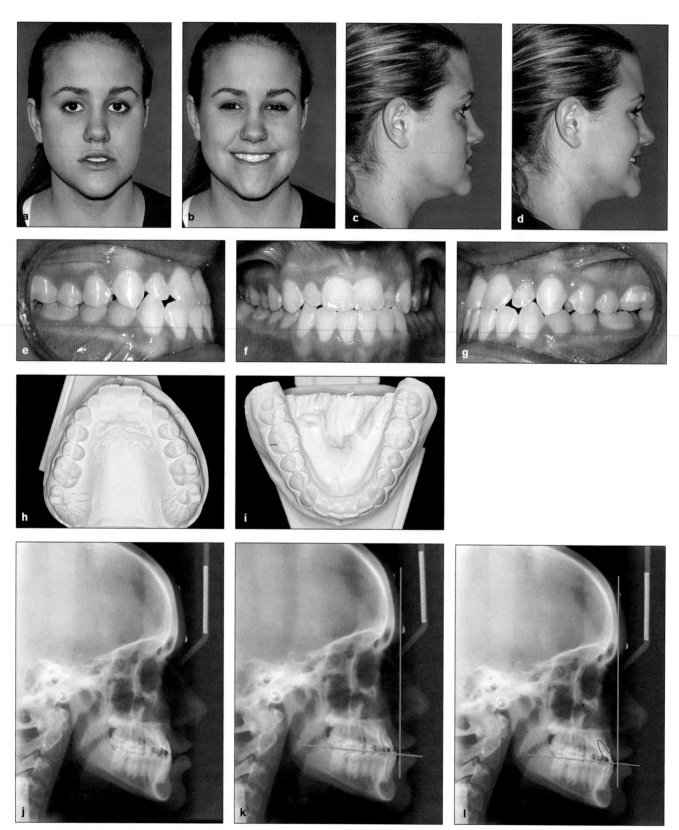

Fig 6-10 *(a to l)* A 16-year-old girl presented with a Class III malocclusion and a severe anteroposterior deficiency of the maxilla. *Green outlines* indicate optimal tooth positions within the jaws, and *red outline* indicates proclined tooth position.

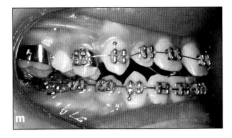
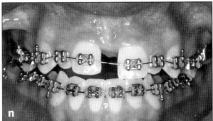
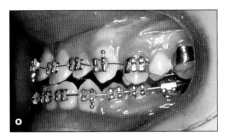

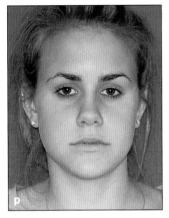
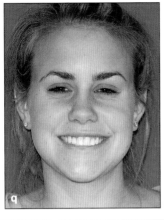
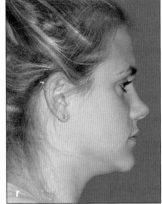
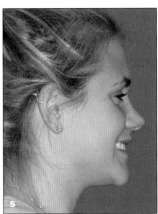

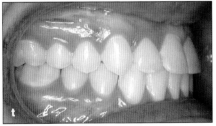
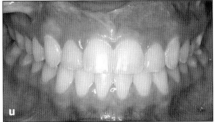
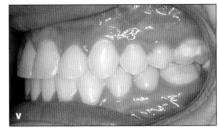

Maxillary surgery

The patient in Fig 6-10 presented with a Class III dental relationship with a posterior crossbite, edge-to-edge incisors, negatively inclined mandibular incisors, and positively inclined maxillary incisors. The maxillary lateral incisors were small, creating a tooth size discrepancy. Presurgical orthodontics included RME and a nonextraction approach. The increased maxillary arch length allowed for some palatal uprighting of the maxillary incisors. Optimal uprighting of the incisors would have required premolar extractions. Space was created for enlarging the lateral incisors. Cephalometrically it was determined that surgical advancement of the maxilla to couple with the mandibular teeth would place the maxillary incisors on the GALL (Figs 6-10k and 6-10l). Diagnostically this confirmed an anteroposterior skeletal dysplasia caused by a maxillary deficiency alone. Posttreatment records document that the treatment goals were successfully attained. Both repose and smiling profiles were harmonious, and the occlusion was gnathologically functional.

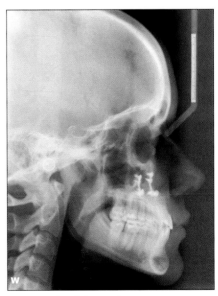

Fig 6-10 *(cont) (m to w)* Treatment and posttreatment photographs and lateral cephalometric radiograph after treatment with a Hyrax maxillary expander and maxillary surgical advancement.

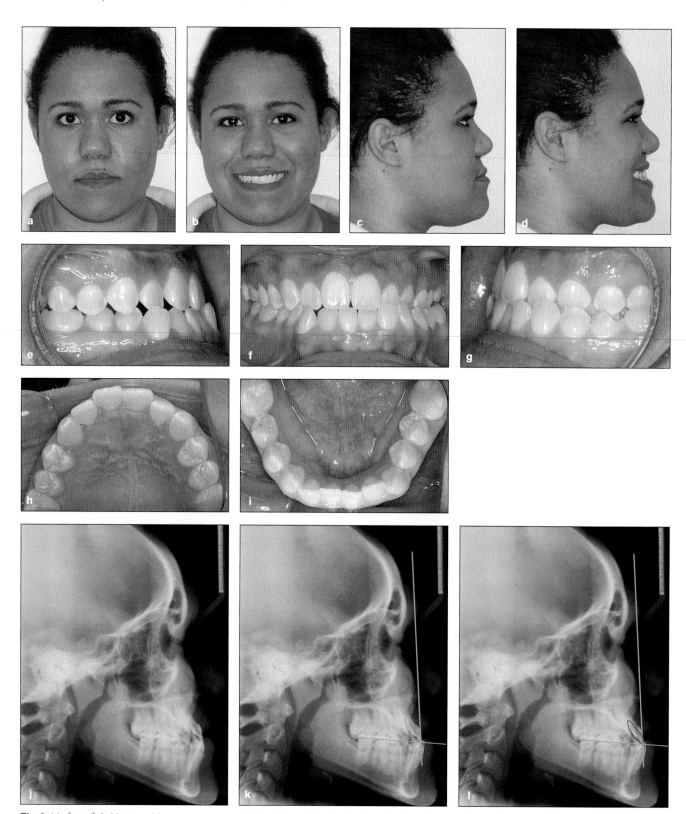

Fig 6-11 *(a to l)* A 20-year-old woman presented with a Class III malocclusion, anterior and posterior crossbites, maxillary deficiency, and severe mandibular prognathism. *Green outlines* indicate optimal tooth positions within the jaws, and *red outline* indicates proclined tooth position.

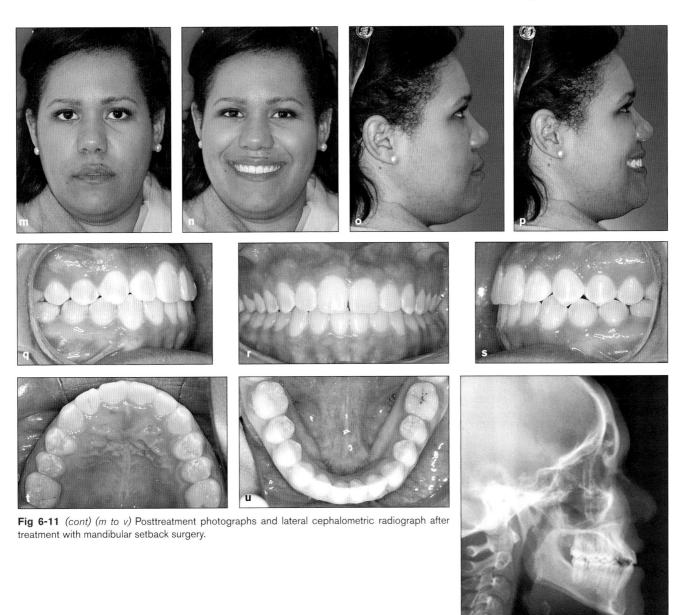

Fig 6-11 *(cont) (m to v)* Posttreatment photographs and lateral cephalometric radiograph after treatment with mandibular setback surgery.

Mandibular surgery

Figure 6-11 shows a 20-year-old woman with anterior and posterior crossbites. The maxilla was deficient and the mandible prognathic, as evidenced by the optimal incisors relative to the GALL. The maxillary incisors were proclined, and the mandibular incisors were retroclined.

There was no family history of mandibular prognathism. A compromise treatment plan consisted of maintaining the inclination of the maxillary incisors and proclining the mandibular incisors to an optimal inclination followed by a mandibular setback surgery. The profile was improved together with a correction of the anterior and posterior crossbites.

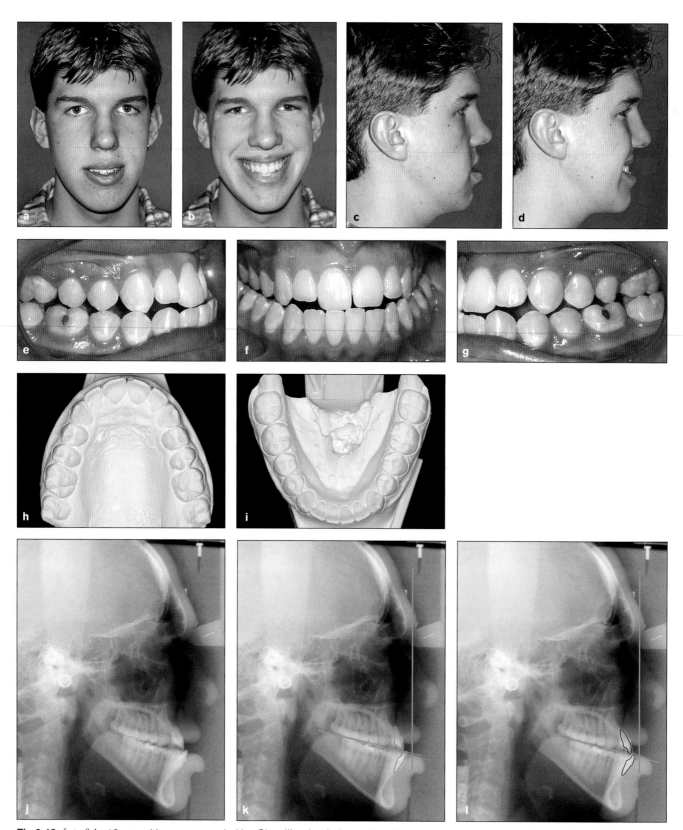

Fig 6-12 *(a to l)* An 18-year-old man presented with a Class III malocclusion and maxillary transverse discrepancies. *Green outlines* indicate optimal tooth positions within the jaws, and *red outlines* indicate proclined tooth positions.

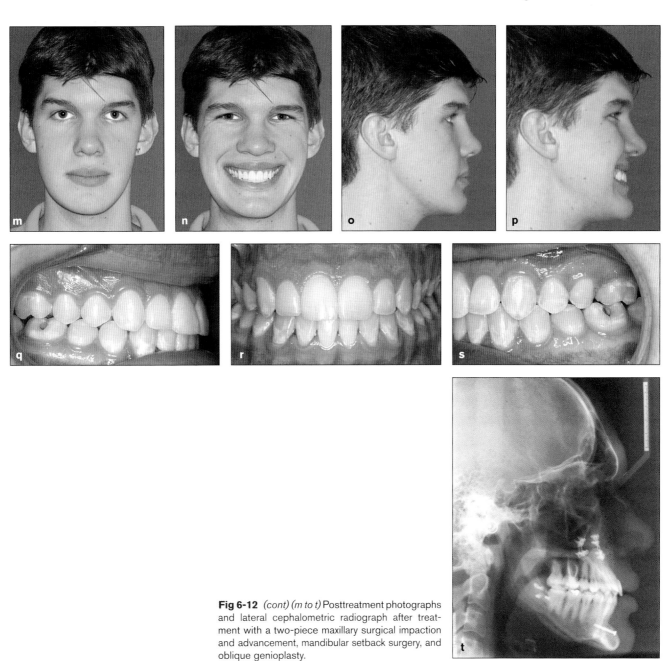

Fig 6-12 *(cont) (m to t)* Posttreatment photographs and lateral cephalometric radiograph after treatment with a two-piece maxillary surgical impaction and advancement, mandibular setback surgery, and oblique genioplasty.

Maxillary and mandibular surgery

The patient in Fig 6-12 demonstrates a Class III dental relationship with anterior and posterior crossbites, open bite, and no crowding. With the maxillary and mandibular incisors placed in optimal positions, the maxilla appears deficient and the mandible prognathic relative to the GALL (Fig 6-12k). A maxillary impaction would result in anterior rotation of the mandible, further accentuating the prognathism. Four premolar extractions would be necessary to reposition the incisors into optimal positions. A defendable nonextraction compromise treatment was planned (Fig 6-12l). Surgically the maxilla was impacted vertically and advanced. A two-piece Le Fort I osteotomy was used to correct the transverse discrepancy. The mandible was set back, and a genioplasty was performed to improve the chin prominence. Posttreatment records demonstrate that the compromise goals were attained. The patient demonstrated dentofacial harmony and a gnathologic occlusion.

Summary Points

- Objectives for the treatment of Class III malocclusions include improving or maintaining a patient's facial esthetics, smile esthetics, function, and periodontal health, as well as a stable outcome.
- Treatment objectives are rhetorically generalized; it is the specificity of treatment goals that clarifies the course of action.
- The Six Elements of Orofacial Harmony can be used as an effective diagnostic tool to discern the underlying dental and/or skeletal components of a Class III maloccclusion.
- Treatment plans can target and quantify teeth and jaws in either optimal or compromise positions using referents and landmarks unique to the Six Elements. Effective clinical mechanics or strategies can be devised to attain these goals.
- Patients with pseudo skeletal Class III malocclusions may only appear facially to have a prognathic mandible because of an anterior shift of the mandible. Properly defined, a *pseudo skeletal Class III malocclusion* does not have a skeletal etiology but is rather the result of disharmony in tooth position.
- Common conditions warranting early treatment are anterior or posterior crossbites with or without functional shifts and blocked-out maxillary lateral incisors.
- Protraction face mask therapy can be used in the treatment of Class III malocclusions with maxillary deficiencies in both the sagittal and vertical dimensions. The optimal time to address a Class III malocclusion is at the time of the initial eruption of the maxillary incisors. Long-term benefits of early face mask treatment need further substantiation from prospective clinical trials.
- To date, there is no agreement in the literature as to whether chin cup therapy can inhibit the growth of the mandible. The stability of chin cup treatment remains unclear. Several studies reported a tendency to return to the original growth pattern after the chin cup was discontinued.
- Depending on the treatment goal specified after accurate diagnostic analysis of the dental and/or skeletal components, Class III malocclusions may be effectively treated with appropriate early phase or adolescent/adult phase treatment using orthopedic, extraction, nonextraction, surgical, and nonsurgical approaches.
- Presurgical orthodontics should decompensate the position of teeth within their respective jaws. Surgical repositioning of the jaws to the optimal location will result in facial harmony.

References

1. Andrews WA. AP relationship of the maxillary central incisors to the forehead in adult white females. Angle Orthod 2008;78:662–669.
2. Schlosser JB, Preston CB, Lampasso J. The effects of computer-aided anteroposterior maxillary incisor movement on ratings of facial attractiveness. Am J Orthod Dentofac Orthop 2005;127:17–24.
3. Cao L, Zhang K, Bai D, Tian Y, Guo Y. Effect of maxillary incisor labiolingual inclination and anteroposterior position on smiling profile esthetics. Angle Orthod 2011;81:121–129.
4. Triviño T, Siqueira DF, Andrews WA. Evaluation of the distances between the mandibular teeth and the alveolar process in Brazilians with normal occlusion. Am J Orthod Dentofacial Orthop 2010;137:308.e1–308.e4.
5. Ronay V, Miner RM, Will LA, Arai K. Mandibular arch form: The relationship between dental and basal anatomy. Am J Orthod Dentofacial Orthop 2008;134:430–438.
6. Gupta D, Miner RM, Arai K, Will L. Comparison of the mandibular dental and basal arch forms in adults and children with Class I and Class II malocclusions. Am J Orthod Dentofacial Orthop 2010;138:10.e1–10.e8.
7. Ball RL, Miner RM, Will L, Arai K. Comparison of dental and apical base arch forms in Class II division 1 and Class I malocclusions. Am J Orthod Dentofacial Orthop 2010;138:41–50.
8. Andrews LF. The Six Keys to Normal (Optimal) Occlusion. Am J Orthod 1972;62:296–309.
9. Andrews LF. Straight-Wire: The Concept and Appliance. San Diego: L.A. Wells, 1989.
10. Weaver K, Tremont T, Ngan P, et al. Changes in dental and basal archforms with preformed and customized archwires during orthodontic treatment. Orthodontic Waves 2012;71:45–50.
11. Burns NR, Musich DR, Martin CA, Razmus T, Gunel E, Ngan P. Class III camouflage treatment: What are the limits? Am J Orthod Dentofacial Orthop 2010;137:9.e1–9.e13.
12. Sugawara J, Mitani H. Facial growth of skeletal Class III malocclusion and the effects, limitation and long-term dentofacial adaptations to chincap therapy. Semin Orthod 1997;3:244–254.
13. Andrews LF, Andrews WA. The Six Elements of Orofacial Harmony. Andrews J 2000;1:13–22.
14. Guyer EC, Ellis E, McNamara JA, RG, Behrents RG. Components of Class III malocclusion in juveniles and adolescents. Angle Orthod 1986;56:7–30.
15. Ngan P. Treatment of Class III malocclusion in the primary and mixed dentitions. In: Bishara S (ed). Textbook of Orthodontics. Philadelphia: WB Saunders, 2001:378–414.
16. Kwong WL, Lin JJ. Comparison between pseudo and true Class III malocclusion by Veterans' General Hospital cephalometric analysis. Clin Dent 1987;7:69–78.
17. Joondeph DR. Early orthodontic treatment. Am J Orthod 1993;104:199–200.
18. Borrie F, Bearn D. Early correction of anterior crossbites: A systematic review. J Orthod 2011;38:175–184.
19. Oppenheim A. A possibility for physiologic orthodontic movement. Am J Orthod Oral Surg 1944;30:277–328,345–368.
20. Delaire VJ, Verdon P, Floor J. Ziele und ergebnisse extraoraler Zuge in postero-anteriorer Richtung in anwendung einer orthopadischen Maske bei der Behandlung von Fallen der Klasse III. Fortschr Kiefer Orthop 1976;37:246–262.

21. Petit H. Adaptations following accelerated facial mask therapy in clinical alteration of the growing face. In: McNamara JA Jr, Ribbens KA, Howe RP (eds). Clinical Alteration of the Growing Face, monograph 14, Craniofacial Growth Series. Ann Arbor, MI: University of Michigan, 1983.

22. McNamara JA Jr. An orthopedic approach to the treatment of Class III malocclusion in growing children. J Clin Orthod 1987;21:598–608.

23. Turley P. Orthopedic correction of Class III malocclusion with palatal expansion and custom protraction headgear. J Clin Orthod 1988;22:314–325.

24. Turley PK, Vaughn GA, Mason B, Moon HB. The effects of maxillary protraction therapy with or without rapid palatal expansion: A prospective, randomized clinical trial. Am J Orthod Dentofac Orthop 2005;128:299–309.

25. Tontop T, Keykubat A, Yuksel S. Facemask therapy with and without expansion. Am J Orthod Dentofac Orthop 2007;132:467–474.

26. Kim JH, Viana MA, Graber TM, Omerza FF, Begole EA. The effectiveness of protraction facemask therapy: A meta-analysis. Am J Orthod Dentofac Orthop 1999;115:675–685.

27. Ngan P, Cheung E, Wei, SH. Comparison of protraction facemask response using banded and bonded expansion appliances as anchorage. Semin Orthod 2007;13:175–182.

28. Kambara T. Dentofacial changes produced by extraoral forward force in Macaca irus. Am J Orthod 1977;71:249–277.

29. Braun S. Extraoral appliances: A twenty-first century update. Am J Orthod Dentofacial Orthop 2004;125:624–629.

30. Ngan PW, Hägg U, Yiu C, Wei SH. Treatment response and long-term dentofacial adaptations to maxillary expansion and protraction. Semin Orthod 1997;4:255–264.

31. Droshl H. The effect of heavy orthopedic forces on the sutures of the facial bones. Angle Orthod 1975;45:26–33.

32. Engström C, Thilander B. Premature facial synostosis: The influence of biomechanical factors in normal and hypocalcemic young rats. Eur J Orthod 1985;781:35–47.

33. Linge L. Tissue reactions incident to widening of facial sutures. An experimental study in the Macaca mulatta. Trans Eur Orthod Soc 1972;48:487–497.

34. Liou EJ. Effective maxillary orthopedic protraction for growing Class III patients: A clinical application simulates distraction osteogenesis. Prog Orthod 2005;6:36–48.

35. Do-Delatore T, Ngan P, Martin CA, Razmus T, Gunel E. Effect of alternate maxillary expansion and contraction on protraction of the maxilla: A pilot study. Hong Kong Dent J 2009;6:72–82.

36. Yen SL. Protocols for late maxillary protraction in cleft lip and palate patients at Children's Hospital, Los Angeles. Semin Orthod 2011;17:138–148.

37. Melsen B, Melsen F. The postnatal development of the palatomaxillary region studied on human autopsy material. Am J Orthod 1982;82:329–342.

38. Franchi L, Baccetti T, McNamara JA. Postpubertal assessment of treatment timing of maxillary expansion and protraction therapy followed by fixed appliances. Am J Orthod Dentofacial Orthop 2004;126:555–568.

39. Mandall N, Dibiase A, Littlewood S, et al. Is early Class III protraction facemask treatment effective? A multicentre, randomized, controlled trial: 15 month follow-up. J Orthod 2010;37:149–161.

40. Hägg U, Tse A, Bendeus M, Rabie AB. Long-term follow-up of early treatment with reverse headgear. Eur J Orthod 2003;25:95–102.

41. Westwood PV, McNamera JA, Baccetti T, Franchi L, Sanver DM. Long-term effects of Class III treatment with rapid maxillary expansion and facemask therapy followed by fixed appliances. Am J Orthod Dentofac Orthop 2003;123:306–320.

42. Sakamoto T, Iwase I, Uka A, Nakamura S. A roentgenocephalometric study of skeletal changes during and after chin cup treatment. Am J Orthod 1984;85:341–350.

43. Wendell PD, Nanda R, Sakamoto T, Nakamura S. The effects of chin cup therapy on the mandible: A longitudinal study. Am J Orthod 1985;87:265–274.

44. Mitani H, Fukazawa H. Effects of chincap force on the timing and amount of mandibular growth associated with anterior reverse occlusion (Class III malocclusion) during puberty. Am J Orthod Dentofac Orthop 1986;9:454–463.

45. Graber LW. Chin cup therapy for mandibular prognathism. Am J Orthod 1977;72:23–41.

46. Ritucci R, Nanda R. The effect of chin cup therapy on the growth and development of the cranial base and midface. Am J Orthod Dentofac Orthop 1984;85:341–350.

47. Uner O, Yuksel S, Ucuncu N. Long-term evaluation after chin cup treatment. Eur J Orthod 1995;17:135-141.

48. Sugawara J, Asano T, Endo N, Mitani H. Long-term effects of chincap therapy on skeletal profile in mandibular prognathism. Am J Orthod Dentofacial Orthop 1990;98:127–133.

49. Deguchi T, Kitsugi A. Stability of changes associated with chin cup treatment. Angle Orthod 1996;66:139–146.

Peter G. Miles
BDSc, MDS

CHAPTER

7 | Subdivisions: Treatment of Dental Midline Asymmetries

Introduction

In this section the diagnosis and correction of dental asymmetries is examined. Discrepancies in the spatial position of the line of the occlusion can occur in three planes: anteroposterior, transverse, and vertical. These have been described in aeronautical terms as *pitch*, *roll*, and *yaw*, respectively.[1] From the perspective of asymmetries, roll would result in an occlusal plane cant, while yaw would skew the midline to one side. In the past, a significant cant could require surgical correction, but the boundary between dental and skeletal correction may have shifted with the advent of miniscrews, or temporary skeletal anchorage devices (TSADs). However, the extent of this is as yet unknown because only lower levels of evidence (case reports) exist for their use in these circumstances. The focus of this chapter is dental yaw deviations, or midline discrepancies. Skeletal asymmetries requiring surgical or TSAD correction are not discussed in this chapter, but if such a case of skeletal asymmetry was being treated via camouflage instead of surgery, then the principles discussed in this chapter would apply.

Asymmetries and midline discrepancies are obviously important to orthodontists; the Peer Assessment Rating (PAR) Index, used to assess treatment outcome, gives the midline a weighting of 3.5, which is only outweighed by the overjet at 4.[2] In fact, if the PAR Index is broken down into the components of severity weighting and difficulty weighting, the midline is perceived as the most difficult to correct, along with the overjet. Many patients will accept a slight midline discrepancy, while others will be extremely discerning (Fig 7-1).

A recent systematic review of smile attractiveness concluded that a limit of 2.2 mm of midline deviation is considered acceptable.[3] One study in that review concluded that 1-mm midline shifts were perceived only by orthodontists, whereas prosthodontists did not perceive a difference until the shift was 3 mm, and laypersons did not notice midline shifts up to 4 mm.[4] Another study found that an orthodontist's threshold for noticing a midline deviation could be as high as 4 mm, while both laypersons and general dentists still did not perceive 4-mm midline deviations.[5] However, when the dental angulation discrepancy was superimposed on top of the midline deviation, the orthodontist's threshold for noticing the midline was 2 mm. Kokich[6] has suggested that if the line that forms the contact between the two central incisors is perpendicular to the incisal plane and parallel to the long axis of the individual's face, then the midline discrepancy seems to be camouflaged. Another study concluded that orthodontic treatment objectives should include correction of the dental midline to within 2 mm of the facial midline where possible.[7] However, in that study a 1-mm facial to dental midline discrepancy was still perceived by 19% of laypersons. The facial to dental midline could become more important to patients during treatment because they may become more discerning when it comes to their own midline, especially as their treatment approaches completion. Therefore, the ideal goal is to have the maxillary dental midline coincident with the facial midline or as close as possible.

When the midline is being corrected, a cant or skew of the arch could result, or the anterior teeth may tilt. So how far can the midline tilt before it is considered unacceptable? Orthodontists are generally more discerning

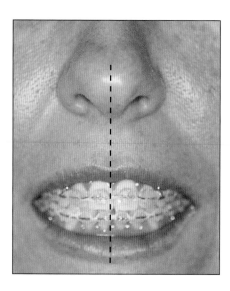

Fig 7-1 Although the dental midlines are coincident in this patient, she was concerned by the 1-mm discrepancy between the dental and facial midlines.

than laypersons, with roughly 70% of orthodontists and 40% of laypersons finding a 10-degree tilt unacceptable.[8] However, even at a 5-degree midline angulation, 10% of laypersons considered this unacceptable compared to no angulation. Therefore, the ideal goal in treatment is to have no tilt or, if a compromise must be accepted, a tilt less than ten degrees. Although this is the goal, patients should be aware that this cannot always be achieved and that a compromise such as a mild midline deviation may need to be accepted to avoid excessive tilting or canting.

Class II Subdivisions

What does it mean when a case is described as a Class II subdivision left? Does the left refer to the Class II side or the Class I side? This may seem obvious, but when a survey was done of orthodontic departments in the United States, only 65% of orthodontic educators agreed on the meaning of *subdivision*, with the subdivision referring to the Class II side.[9] In fact, 12% were unsure or did not teach it one way or the other. For clarity, in this chapter the subdivision always refers to the Class II side for Class II subdivisions and the Class III side for Class III subdivisions.

There are many approaches and appliances to correct dental asymmetries, including differing extraction patterns, elastics, asymmetric distalization, and interarch ap-

pliances, and the choice is governed by the diagnosis as well as the experience the clinician has with each. Diagnosis of a dental asymmetry is best made from looking at the patient or images of the patient and not solely at the patient's study casts. For example, the casts may demonstrate a Class II subdivision malocclusion, and it may seem tempting to extract a single maxillary premolar. However, it has been demonstrated that Class II subdivision dentoalveolar asymmetry is primarily related to the distal positioning of the mandibular first molar on the Class II side and seldom to the more mesial positioning of the maxillary molar.[10–12] More recently, a cone beam computed tomography (CBCT) study found that about 60% of Class II subdivision asymmetries were in the mandibular arch because of a 2-mm mandibular retrusion on the Class II side.[13] For this reason, a single maxillary extraction or an asymmetric maxillary molar distalization is less likely to be suitable for many dental asymmetry cases. When evaluating 44 Class II subdivisions cases, Janson et al[14] described two basic types. A Type 1 Class II subdivision malocclusion demonstrates coincidence of the maxillary dental midline with the facial midline and deviation of the mandibular midline. A Type 2 Class II subdivision malocclusion has the opposite characteristics, demonstrating coincidence of the mandibular dental midline with the facial midline and deviation of the maxillary midline. Of the sample of 44 cases, 61.36% had Type 1, 18.18% had Type 2, and 20.45% had characteristics of both types of Class II subdivision maloc-

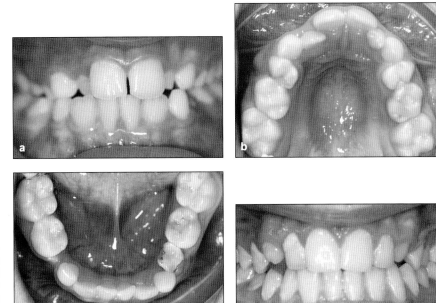

Fig 7-2 *(a to d)* Utility arches, or 2 × 4 appliances, were placed in this patient to regain space where the mandibular right primary first premolar had been lost early while also correcting the anterior crossbite, resulting in an improved midline and simpler final phase of treatment.

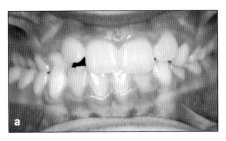
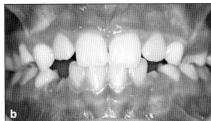

Fig 7-3 *(a)* Before treatment, this patient had a 5-mm slide shift to the right upon closing of the mandible. *(b)* After expansion therapy, the slide shift has resolved, and the dental midlines are coincident.

clusion. Therefore, based on this diagnosis, about 60% of Class II subdivision cases should have asymmetric extractions and/or mechanics directed at the mandibular arch.

Nanda et al[15] have argued that to reduce the risk of potential side effects, a midline discrepancy should be corrected as early as possible. This allows the remainder of treatment to be completed symmetrically, thereby reducing unilateral vertical forces, skewing of the dental arches, and asymmetric anchorage loss.

Early intervention

Some asymmetries may develop because of the early loss of teeth, and this could simply involve space maintenance therapy to regain space (Fig 7-2) or symmetry followed by space maintenance. Another possible cause is a single- or multiple-tooth crossbite, which results in a slide shift upon occluding. Treatment entails correction of the crossbite (Fig 7-3) to remove the occlusal interference that causes the slide shift upon closure.

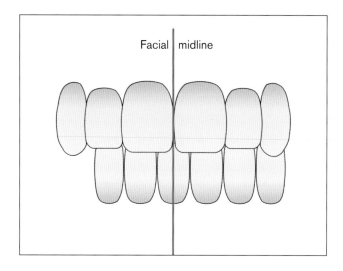

Fig 7-4 Type 1 Class II subdivision where the maxillary dental midline is coincident with the facial midline and the discrepancy arises in the mandibular arch.

Facial | midline

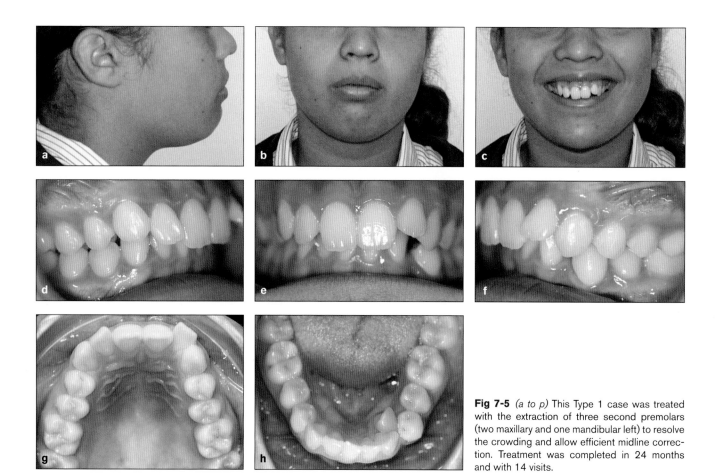

Fig 7-5 *(a to p)* This Type 1 case was treated with the extraction of three second premolars (two maxillary and one mandibular left) to resolve the crowding and allow efficient midline correction. Treatment was completed in 24 months and with 14 visits.

Type 1 Class II subdivision treatment

As stated previously, in the Type 1 Class II subdivision case, the asymmetry is primarily derived in the mandibular arch (Fig 7-4). Any treatment in these Type 1 cases should therefore be aimed at the mandibular arch. This also maintains symmetry in the maxillary arch, where it is most visible to the patient.

For cases with moderate to severe crowding, incisor protrusion, and/or the absence of a passive lip seal, an extraction approach is ideal (Fig 7-5). But should three or four premolars be extracted? To answer this question, Janson and colleagues[16] retrospectively evaluated 51 patients with Class II subdivision malocclusions. Twenty-eight of the patients had four symmetric premolars removed, while the remaining 23 patients had three premolars removed, two in the maxillary arch and one in the mandibular arch on the Class I side. The results showed no real difference for most of the variables assessed. However, the three premolar extraction group had a greater improvement of the initial interdental midline deviation.

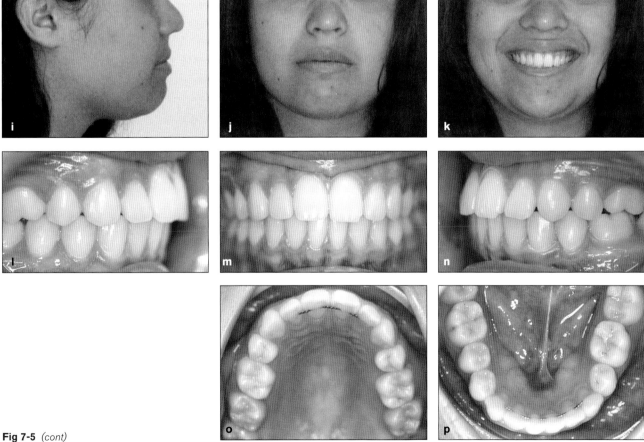

Fig 7-5 *(cont)*

For patients with less crowding and flatter lip profiles, a nonextraction approach is more likely to be considered. Asymmetric Class II or Class III elastics or heavy anterior diagonal elastics supported by Class II elastics can be used. However, these may tilt the maxillary teeth or cant the occlusal plane, and their success relies heavily on patient cooperation. As a general rule of thumb, the author uses elastics in nonextraction cases up to a $^1/_3$ molar Class II subdivision case if it appears that compliance will be good. In Class II subdivisions greater than $^1/_3$, the author places a spring Class II corrector on the asymmetric side once alignment is complete and only uses light elastics to maintain the correction during detailing.

For patients using elastics, the author measures the overjet and maximum protrusion at each visit, and if there is no improvement within 3 months, the elastics are abandoned for a spring corrector. This overcomes the compliance issue with elastics. The use of a spring or elastics treats both arches as though they were a combination rather than a pure Type 1 case, but it also entails less risk of skewing the maxillary arch or tilting the midline compared with extraction of one maxillary premolar. For example, the patient in Fig 7-6 presented with a Class II malocclusion on the right side with a posterior crossbite and a Class I occlusion on the left side. Full fixed appliances were placed, and crossbite elastics were used on the right side. After 6 months of leveling and aligning, a spring Class II corrector was placed on the right side. The mandibular wire was cinched back to prevent incisor flaring, and the maxillary arch was tied with chain elastic to prevent spaces from opening. Within 4 months, the molar relationship was corrected and the spring removed. Light Class II elastics were placed on the right side to maintain the correction during final detailing, and the brackets were removed after a total of 14 months of treatment (Figs 7-6f to 7-6j).

These nonextraction Type 1 cases have been treated in both arches in the past, but with the advent of miniscrews, appropriate cases could possibly be treated by protraction of the mandibular arch on the Class II side.

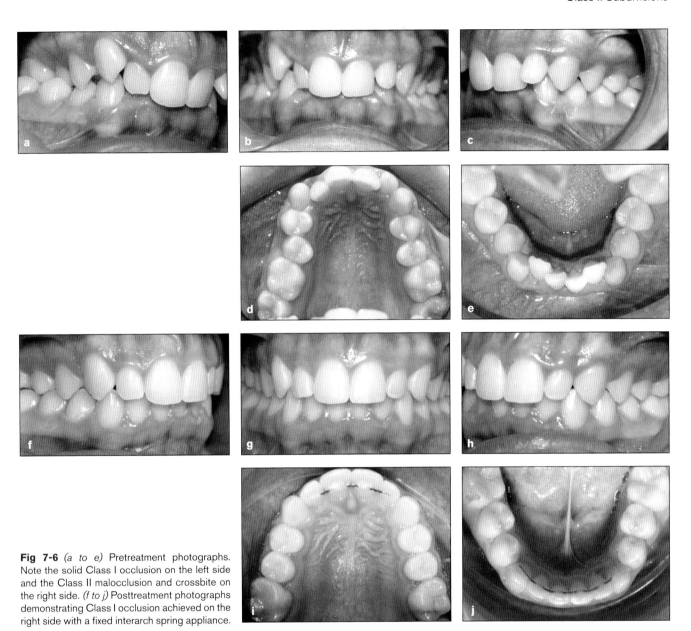

Fig 7-6 *(a to e)* Pretreatment photographs. Note the solid Class I occlusion on the left side and the Class II malocclusion and crossbite on the right side. *(f to j)* Posttreatment photographs demonstrating Class I occlusion achieved on the right side with a fixed interarch spring appliance.

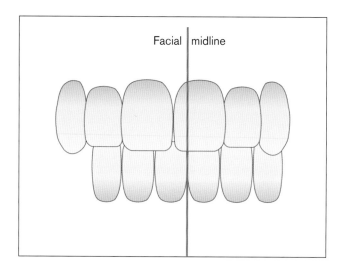

Fig 7-7 Type 2 Class II subdivision where the mandibular dental midline is coincident with the facial midline and the discrepancy arises in the maxillary arch.

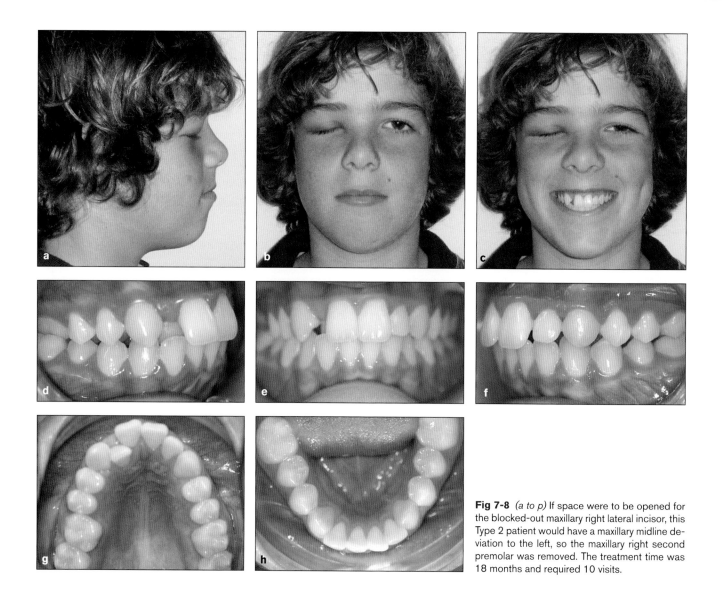

Fig 7-8 *(a to p)* If space were to be opened for the blocked-out maxillary right lateral incisor, this Type 2 patient would have a maxillary midline deviation to the left, so the maxillary right second premolar was removed. The treatment time was 18 months and required 10 visits.

Type 2 Class II subdivision treatment

Type 2 Class II subdivision cases are in the minority (about 20%) and present with the maxillary dental midline off and the mandibular dental midline coincident (Fig 7-7). If extraction is indicated in these cases, then one maxillary premolar may be removed (Fig 7-8). However, care must be taken to avoid tilting the teeth, skewing the arch, or overcorrecting the midline of the highly visible maxillary anterior dentition. The maxillary midline needs to be obviously deviated to one side or else both arches may be treated as a combination case. The amount of crowding and midline discrepancy also influence the decision to extract a first or second premolar.

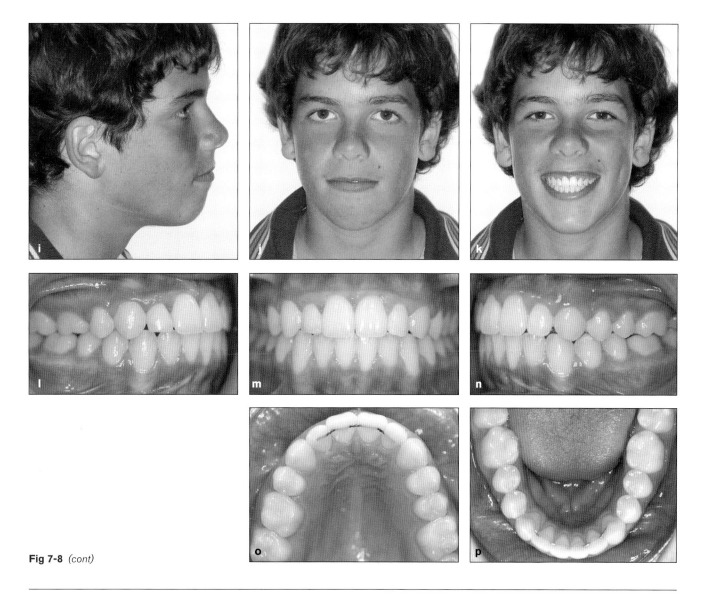

Fig 7-8 *(cont)*

Combination Class II subdivision treatment

The remaining 20% of cases show traits of both Type 1 and Type 2 Class II subdivision malocclusion, with some discrepancy present in both arches. The goal is therefore to aim correction at both arches, so interarch mechanics such as elastics or a spring Class II corrector seem most appropriate (Fig 7-9).

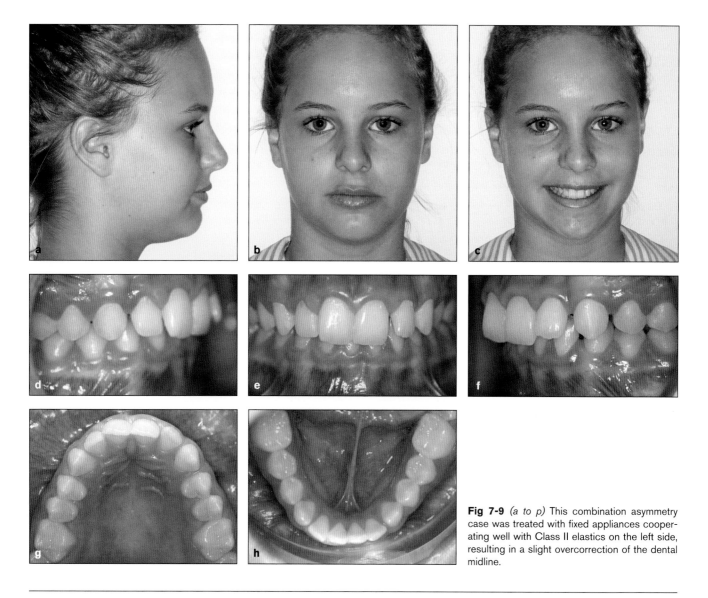

Fig 7-9 *(a to p)* This combination asymmetry case was treated with fixed appliances cooperating well with Class II elastics on the left side, resulting in a slight overcorrection of the dental midline.

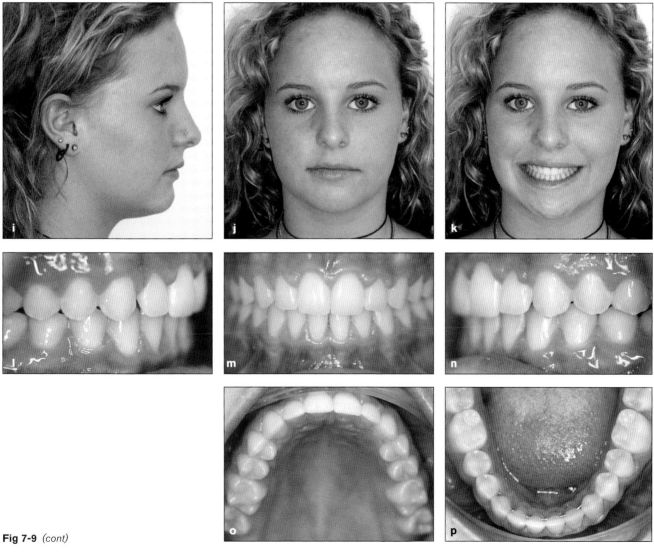

Fig 7-9 *(cont)*

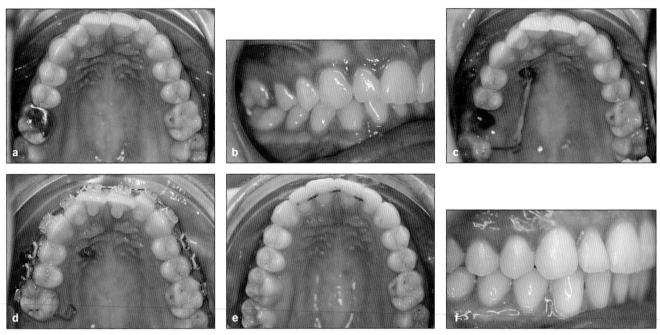

Fig 7-10 *(a to d)* The maxillary right first molar required extraction, so miniscrew anchorage was used to protract the second molar into its place. This was done prior to placement of full fixed appliances to reduce the overall time in full braces. *(e and f)* The second molar has taken the place of the maxillary right first molar, and the third molar erupted and aligned to replace the second molar.

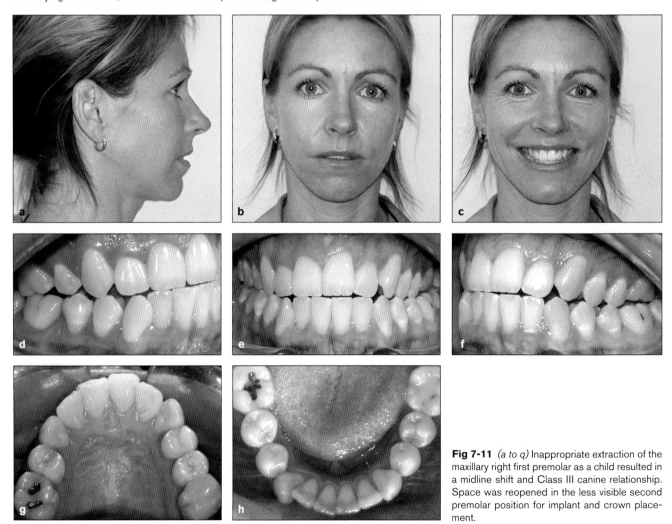

Fig 7-11 *(a to q)* Inappropriate extraction of the maxillary right first premolar as a child resulted in a midline shift and Class III canine relationship. Space was reopened in the less visible second premolar position for implant and crown placement.

Other Asymmetries

Asymmetries can also be created by the inappropriate extraction of teeth in crowded dentitions, by congenitally absent teeth or impacted teeth, or by the loss of teeth. For example, the patient in Fig 7-10 had an internally resorbing maxillary right first molar that required extraction. Because she had only minor crowding in a Class I occlusion, a nonextraction approach was preferred. After consultation with the family, miniscrews were placed to protract the second molar into the first molar space. After 6 months and six visits, the extraction space was closed with no movement of the anterior teeth (Figs 7-10c and 7-10d). Full

braces were then placed to commence aligning the remaining teeth and permit root uprighting on the second molar. Use of the miniscrew maintained the canine relationship, thereby preventing an asymmetry from developing in this case.

Inappropriate removal of a tooth can result in an asymmetry that was not originally present. The patient in Fig 7-11 had a blocked-out maxillary right premolar removed as a child, which resulted in a reasonable alignment but also created a Class III subdivision malocclusion with the maxillary midline skewed to the right side. In this case, treatment would involve either extraction of three other teeth to match or the reopening of the space for prosthetic replacement, which was the option chosen by the patient.

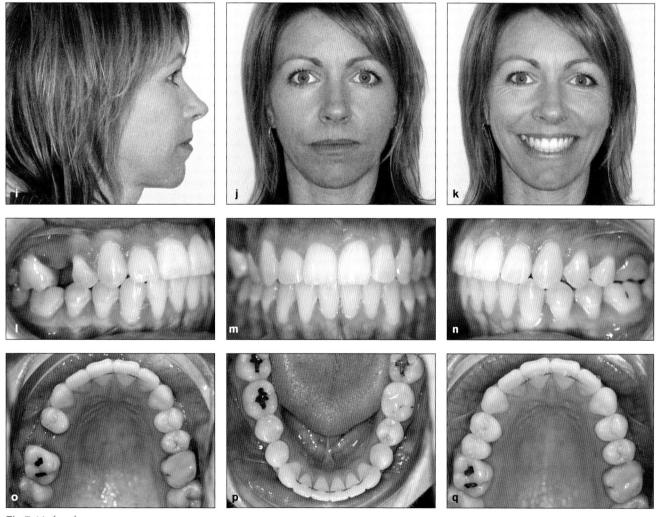

Fig 7-11 (cont)

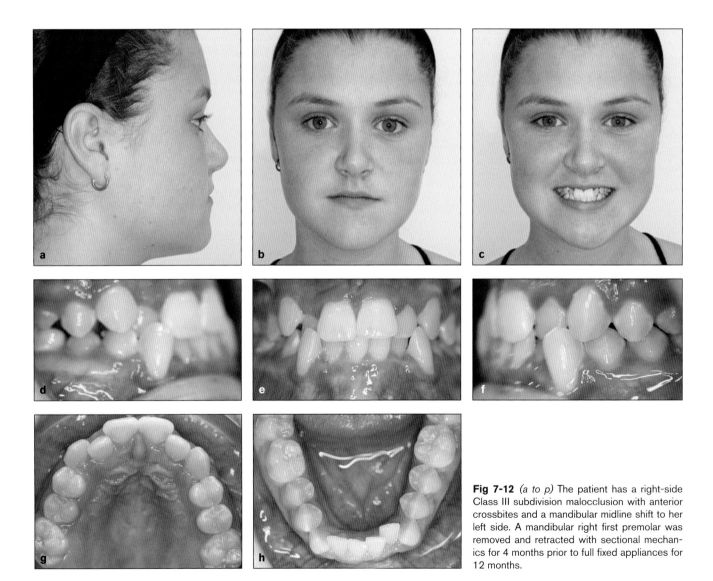

Fig 7-12 *(a to p)* The patient has a right-side Class III subdivision malocclusion with anterior crossbites and a mandibular midline shift to her left side. A mandibular right first premolar was removed and retracted with sectional mechanics for 4 months prior to full fixed appliances for 12 months.

Class III subdivisions

Although studies similar to those for Class II subdivisions have not been conducted in dental Class III subdivision cases, Janson[17] has suggested that an analogous rationale in diagnosis and treatment planning can be applied in these patients. For example, for a patient with crowding and a deviated maxillary midline, extraction of two mandibular premolars and only one maxillary premolar on the Class II side is indicated. However, if only the mandibular midline is deviated, only one mandibular premolar on the Class III side would need to be extracted.[18] This approach is exemplified in Fig 7-12, in which the mandibular first premolar has been removed on the Class III side to allow the canine

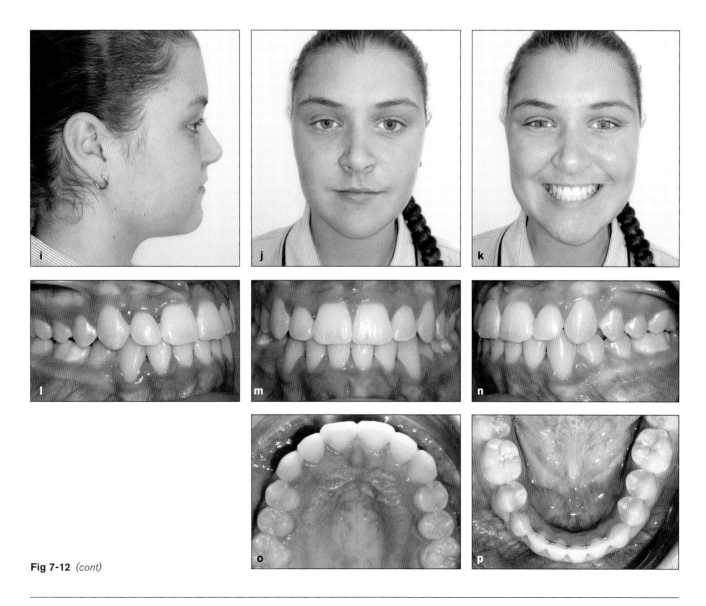

Fig 7-12 (cont)

to be retracted into a Class I relationship. The extraction of only one mandibular tooth instead of two allows for better control over the mandibular midline and reduces the need for asymmetric elastics, which could potentially skew or tilt the more visible maxillary arch. Another option that could be considered in Class III subdivision cases is the extraction of a mandibular incisor (Fig 7-13). When indicated, this can achieve an esthetic and functional result with potentially less dependence on elastic wear.

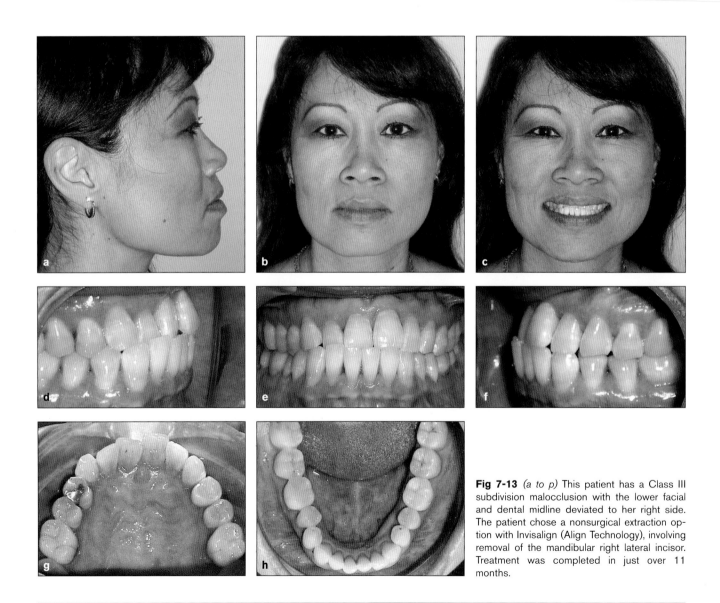

Fig 7-13 *(a to p)* This patient has a Class III subdivision malocclusion with the lower facial and dental midline deviated to her right side. The patient chose a nonsurgical extraction option with Invisalign (Align Technology), involving removal of the mandibular right lateral incisor. Treatment was completed in just over 11 months.

Summary Points

- In Type 1 Class II subdivision malocclusion, the maxillary midline is coincident with the facial midline, and the mandibular arch is skewed (about 60% of cases).
- In Type 2 Class II subdivision malocclusion, the mandibular midline is coincident with the facial midline, and the maxillary arch is skewed (about 20% of cases).
- The remaining 20% of Class II subdivision cases are a combination of Types 1 and 2.

- Functional shifts should be corrected early, if possible. The asymmetry should be corrected early so the remainder of treatment is as symmetric as possible to minimize side effects.
- If the maxillary arch is symmetric, it should be kept symmetric.
- If a compromise is necessary, it should be made where it is least visible (in the mandibular arch).
- Any side effects of asymmetric treatment should be discussed with the patient because these may cause concern. A treatment plan should be formulated that addresses the patient's values while minimizing potential risks.

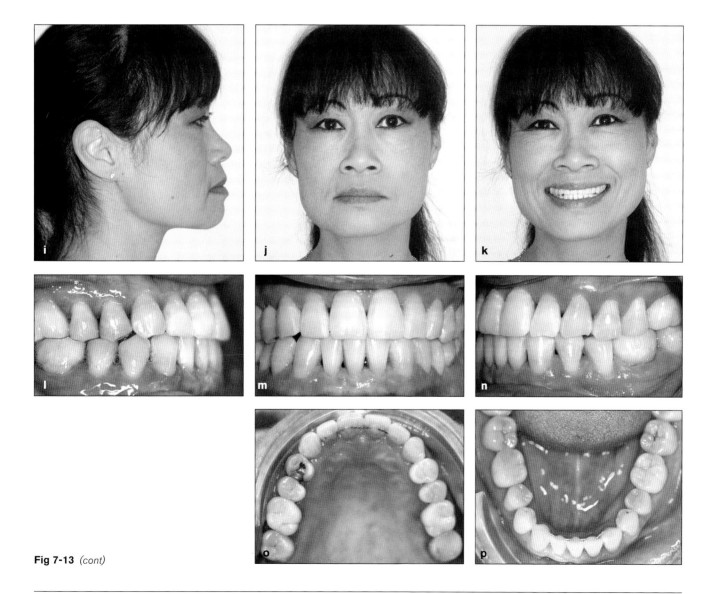

Fig 7-13 (cont)

References

1. Ackerman JL, Proffit WR, Sarver DM, Ackerman MB, Kean MR. Pitch, roll, and yaw: Describing the spatial orientation of dentofacial traits. Am J Orthod Dentofacial Orthop 2007;131:305–310.
2. DeGuzman L, Bahiraei D, Vig KW, Vig PS, Weyant RJ, O'Brien K. The validation of the Peer Assessment Rating index for malocclusion severity and treatment difficulty. Am J Orthod Dentofacial Orthop 1995;107:172–176.
3. Janson G, Branco NC, Fernandes TM, Sathler R, Garib D, Lauris JR. Influence of orthodontic treatment, midline position, buccal corridor and smile arc on smile attractiveness. Angle Orthod 2011;81:153–161.
4. Pinho S, Ciriaco C, Faber J, Lenza MA. Impact of dental asymmetries on the perception of smile esthetics. Am J Orthod Dentofacial Orthop 2007;132:748–753.
5. Kokich V, Kiyak A, Shapiro PA. Comparing the perception of dentists and lay people to altered dental esthetics. J Esthet Dent 1999;11:311–324.
6. Kokich V. Anterior dental esthetics: An orthodontic perspective. III. Mediolateral relationships. J Esthet Dent 1993;5:200–207.
7. Johnston CD, Burden DJ, Stevenson MR. The influence of dental to facial midline discrepancies on dental attractiveness ratings. Eur J Orthod 1999;21:517–522.
8. Thomas JL, Hayes C, Zawaideh S. The effect of axial midline angulation on dental esthetics. Angle Orthod 2003;73:359–364.
9. Siegel MA. A matter of Class: Interpreting subdivision in a malocclusion. Am J Orthod Dentofacial Orthop 2002;122:582–586.
10. Janson GR, Metaxas A, Woodside DG, de Freitas MR, Pinzan AP. Three-dimensional evaluation of skeletal and dental asymmetries in Class II subdivision malocclusions. Am J Orthod Dentofacial Orthop 2001;119:406–418.
11. Alavi DG, BeGole EA, Schneider BJ. Facial and dental arch asymmetries in Class II subdivision malocclusion. Am J Orthod Dentofacial Orthop 1988;93:38–46.
12. Rose JM, Sadowsky C, BeGole EA, Moles R. Mandibular skeletal and dental asymmetry in Class II subdivision malocclusions. Am J Orthod Dentofacial Orthop 1994;105:489–495.
13. Sanders DA, Rigali PH, Neace WP, Uribe F, Nanda R. Skeletal and dental asymmetries in Class II subdivision malocclusions using cone-beam computed tomography. Am J Orthod Dentofacial Orthop 2010;138:542.e1–542.e20.
14. Janson G, de Lima KJ, Woodside DG, Metaxas A, de Freitas MR, Henriques JF. Class II subdivision malocclusion types and evaluation of their asymmetries. Am J Orthod Dentofacial Orthop 2007;131:57–66.
15. Nanda R, Kuhlberg A, Uribe F. Biomechanics basis of extraction space closure. In: Nanda R (ed). Biomechanics and Esthetic Strategies in Clinical Orthodontics. St Louis: Saunders, 2005;199.
16. Janson G, Dainesi EA, Henriques JF, de Freitas MR, de Lima KJ. Class II subdivision treatment success rate with symmetric and asymmetric extraction protocols. Am J Orthod Dentofacial Orthop 2003;124:257–264.
17. Janson G, De Souza JE, Barros SEC, Andrade P Jr, Nakamura AY. Orthodontic treatment alternative to a Class III subdivision malocclusion. J Appl Oral Sci 2009;17:354–363.
18. Janson G, Woodside DG, Metaxas A, Henriques JF, de Freitas MR. Orthodontic treatment of subdivision cases. World J Orthod 2003;4:36–46.

James Noble
BSc, DDS, MSc, FRCD(C)

8 | Evidence-Based Use of Orthodontic TSADs

Introduction

The struggle to control anchorage can be one of the most challenging factors for an orthodontist during the course of treatment. Orthodontists employ numerous techniques to control the unwanted movement of teeth, including the use of Nance appliances, headgear, and maxillomandibular elastics and the splinting of teeth and even pretipping of teeth in the opposite direction, to name just a few. *Absolute anchorage*, or no movement from the reactive forces of teeth, is often required for an orthodontist to improve the clinical outcome and optimize the efficiency and effectiveness of treatment mechanics. Traditionally, absolute anchorage was obtained from an ankylosed tooth or dental implant, which pits the reactive forces against bone. Temporary skeletal anchorage devices (TSADs), or orthodontic miniscrews, have become a simple-to-use, cost-effective, predictable, and successful clinical tool in the orthodontist's armamentarium. TSADs can be used as a vehicle to obtain absolute anchorage without the need for patient compliance and with minimal associated patient morbidity.[1–3] TSADs are particularly indicated when conventional methods of anchorage are very difficult to achieve.[4] Their success rates vary between 80% and 85%; although these rates may be lower than those of dental implants, their advantage lies in their easy removal and reinsertion should they fail.

History

The first published report of screws fixed to bone for absolute anchorage for use in orthodontics was an animal study published in 1945 that used small Vitallium (Dentsply) screws in the ascending ramus of six dogs to retract canines.[5] In 1969, Linkow[6] published a report of an attempt to move teeth against an endosseous blade implant. In 1983, Creekmore and Eklund[7] used a Vitallium bone screw inserted into the anterior nasal spine to treat a patient with a deep overbite.

The concept of miniscrew implants was not immediately embraced by the specialty of orthodontics, and there was a gap in published studies until the late 1990s. During this time, published articles on absolute anchorage focused on the use of onplants,[8,9] palatal implants,[10–13] dental implants,[14–18] and ankylosed teeth.[19] Although other types of implants are effective in obtaining anchorage and have high success rates,[20] they result in osseointegration, are larger in width and length, are more time-consuming and involved, and have more expensive insertion and removal protocols with increased associated patient morbidity. Though numerous case reports describe various osteosynthetic plates used for orthodontic anchorage, similar disadvantages exist.[21–24] For these reasons, the orthodontic community favors orthodontic miniscrews for skeletal anchorage because these devices involve a simpler placement and removal protocol that can easily be performed in the setting of an orthodontic office. Further, TSADs do not fully osseointegrate, have minimal morbidity, and are more cost-effective for the patient.

Only recently have TSADs been popularized for use in orthodontics. Kanomi[1] first described a TSAD specifically designed for orthodontic use in 1997. In 1998, there were articles describing a TSAD with a bracketlike head[2] and zygomatic ligatures used for orthodontic anchorage.[25] In 1999, there was an article published in the *American Journal of Orthodontics* on closure of an anterior open bite using TSADs.[26] Numerous case reports followed.[27–30] In 2005, there was a full issue of the journal *Seminars in Orthodontics* dedicated to the topic of TSADs. From this point forward, there was a dramatic increase in the number of studies, peer-reviewed articles, case reports, and attention at meetings devoted to TSADs.

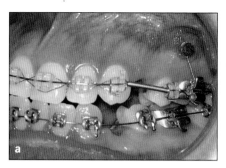 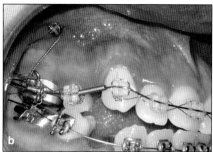

Fig 8-1 TSADs placed by orthodontic (a) and periodontal (b) residents. The orthodontic resident understood the biomechanics required, and the TSAD was placed closer to the center of resistance of the anterior tooth segment that is to be retracted. The periodontal resident was not expected to have an understanding of tooth movement, and the location of TSAD placement is not ideal.

Nomenclature

Terms used to describe a screw placed in bone to be used as anchorage in orthodontic biomechanics include *mini-screw*, *microscrew*, *mini-implant*, *microimplant*, *pin-plant*, *ortho-implant*, and *temporary anchorage device (TAD)*. A meeting among a panel of orthodontists at the 2004 American Association of Orthodontists meeting suggested that the terms *micro* and *screw* be avoided because the former implies a metric measurement of 10^{-6} or something that must be viewed with the aid of a microscope, and the latter can have a negative connotation associated with it.[31] The orthodontic literature has adopted both the terms *orthodontic miniscrew* and *TAD*. In 2005, a *TAD* was defined in the orthodontic literature as a "device that is temporarily fixed to bone for the purpose of enhancing orthodontic anchorage either by supporting the teeth of the reactive unit or by obviating the need for the reactive unit altogether, and which is subsequently removed after use."[32] The term *TAD*, however, is a misnomer in the context of absolute anchorage because other appliances such as headgear and mandibular lingual holding arches can also be a classified as TADs. The term *temporary skeletal anchorage device* (TSAD) is preferred.[33] Ironically, this abbreviation is also pronounced "tad," with the s remaining silent.

Who Places TSADs?

TSADs can be placed by the orthodontist, the general dentist, or other dental specialists such as the oral and maxillofacial surgeon or periodontist. The advantage of having an orthodontist place a TSAD is that it can save the patient from having additional appointments and consultations and thereby increased cost. The orthodontist also understands the ideal location and angulation of placement for optimal biomechanics. Figure 8-1 demonstrates two TSADs placed on the right and left buccal alveolus of a patient to be used for maximum posterior anchorage during the lev-

eling and aligning phase of orthodontic treatment and then for retraction of the anterior segment of teeth during the space closure phase of orthodontic treatment. These TSADs were placed by graduate students at the University of Manitoba, which has graduate programs in orthodontics and periodontics, with both clinics located side by side. The periodontal resident first placed the TSAD on the patient's right side, and then the orthodontic resident placed the TSAD on the patient's left side. The TSAD placed by the periodontal resident was located well above the center of resistance of the anterior segment. This was done despite written and verbal communication from the orthodontic resident to place the TSAD at the mucogingival junction. In a patient with an anterior open bite tendency, proclined and protruded incisors, and a low smile line, a force directed above the center of resistance of the anterior teeth would result in a worsening of the anterior open bite by further proclining and protruding the incisors and also a worsening of the smile line. The orthodontic resident had knowledge of the biomechanics involved in treatment and understood the importance of placing the TSAD in a location closer to the center of resistance of the anterior teeth. The orthodontic resident also understood that a more ideal location in the buccal alveolus is at the mucogingival junction. The orthodontic resident was therefore the most ideal clinician to place the TSADs in this patient.

Orthodontists still may shy away from TSAD placement because they may not be accustomed to performing a surgical procedure and using topical and local anesthetics. They also may not have the necessary instrumentation, equipment, and sterilization and disposal systems available for the procedure. For this reason, surgical stents have been suggested as a means for orthodontists to communicate their desired location for TSAD placement with their surgical colleagues performing the procedure.[34]

A survey of orthodontic residents in the United States published in 2009 found that 92.03% of residents plan to use TSADs and 72.26% plan to place them themselves when in private practice.[35] This suggests that TSADs are being taught in the graduate clinics of orthodontic programs in the United States. Orthodontic residents understand the benefits of placing TSADs, and this may be the future trend in treatment. They are not far displaced from dental school and may be more comfortable with surgical procedures and the use of anesthetics.

In 2008, Buschang[36] published results of a survey of members of the American Association of Orthodontists, which found that 43% of orthodontists place TSADs themselves. A 2010 survey of 47 orthodontists from five US states who graduated from 28 different orthodontic programs found that 91% of respondents used TSADs, and 42% placed them themselves. Surprisingly, a total of 57% of these orthodontists had been in private practice for more than 10 years, suggesting that an extended length of time out of residency or general dentistry practice does not necessarily preclude an orthodontist from placing a TSAD. When those who did not place TSADs were asked why they did not, the reasons included the need to give local anesthetic (58%), longer chair time (25%), a need to manage acute pain (20%), and lack of training (20%).[37]

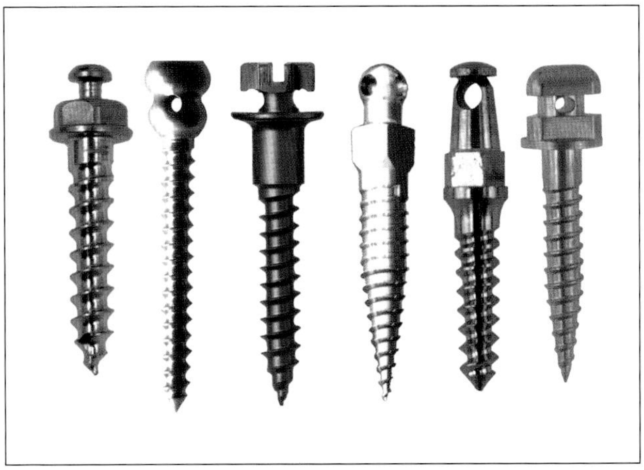

Fig 8-2 Six different commercially available TSADs with different head, thread, and length designs.

Types of TSADs and Design

There are over 40 manufacturers producing over 700 TSADs, with 1 to 154 different screw designs available per system (Fig 8-2). With so many systems and designs available, each with its own nuances and manufacturer claims, the decision to purchase a practical TSAD system can be complicated and confusing to a clinician, similar to making the decision to purchase a particular bracket. Switching systems can be costly and potentially increase office inventory, so the initial decision in purchasing a TSAD system is an important one.

TSADs are mostly made from osteosynthesis technology; they are made with Type IV or Type V titanium and must be biocompatible with human tissue. They are made with a smooth, machine-polished surface to prevent osseointegration and bone ingrowth and to allow for simple removal once they have served their purpose.

Commercially available TSADs vary in their length, diameter, thread depth, thread design, pitch, taper, flute, head design, self-drilling or -tapping characteristics, and material. The diameter usually ranges from 1.0 to 2.3 mm. The length of a TSAD refers to the length of the threaded body, not the entire TSAD. TSADs are typically available in lengths of 6, 8, 10, and 12 mm but can have a range from 4 to 21 mm.[38–41] The length of the neck is typically 1 to 3 mm. Implants smaller than 1.3 mm should be avoided because they are at greater risk of fracture, particularly in the thick cortical bone of the mandible.[42,43] The appropriate TSAD length is determined by the quality of bone, angulation of insertion, transmucosal thickness, and adjacent anatomical structures. Different TSAD lengths are used in different areas of the jaw. A minimum length of 5 to 6 mm is recommended,[44] and longer lengths are recommended where the bone quality is poor. There are no reported studies specifically assessing length and diameter of TSADs with primary stability; however, it makes sense that a lon-

ger length would have more threads in bone and therefore greater primary stability. The body of a TSAD is made available in straight and tapered designs. There are no reported studies comparing stability and fracture rates with straight or tapered TSADs; however, the risk of fracture of the tip is likely greater with tapered TSADs. A small fracture may merely require follow-up to assess for infection to avoid an invasive surgical procedure for removal.

The tip of a TSAD differs depending on whether it is self-drilling or self-tapping. Self-drilling TSADs have a tip that is sharp, with a tapered apex or a notch at the tip to allow it to self-drill through cortical bone. Self-tapping TSADs can have a tip that is thread-forming or thread-cutting. The thread-forming design compresses the bone around the thread as the TSAD moves into bone, and the thread-cutting design has either a notch at the tip parallel to the long axis or a sharpened thread that actually cuts threads into the bone as the TSAD is placed.

The head design usually comes as a button/sphere with an eyelet to accommodate a steel tie or the head of a coil spring or in the shape of a bracket to accommodate an orthodontic archwire; however, a plethora of different head designs are available from different manufacturers.

The design of the length of TSADs is based on principles from the prosthodontic and oral surgery literature. Threads are incorporated to improve initial stability, increase the surface area, and distribute stress more favorably.[45] There are no reported studies in the literature assessing whether a specific type of thread design influences primary stability. Thread design would likely be more of a factor on primary stability in poorer quality bone. The threads result in the TSAD having an outer and inner diameter; the outer diameter is the maximum diameter of the TSAD, and the inner diameter is the outer diameter minus the length of the threads. The threads can be designed in a symmetric or asymmetric pattern. A symmetric thread design is V-

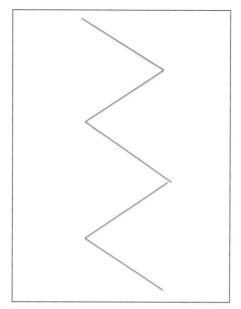

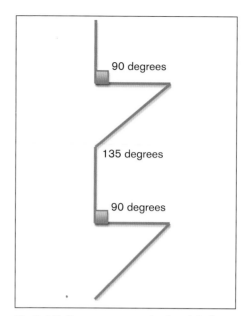

Fig 8-3 V-shaped symmetric thread design.

Fig 8-4 Buttress, or asymmetric, thread design.

shaped, with leading and trailing angles that are congruent (Fig 8-3). An asymmetric, or buttress, thread design is one with a leading angle located toward the tip of the TSAD that is at 45 degrees to the long axis of the shaft and a trailing angle located toward the head of the TSAD that is at 90 degrees to the long axis of the shaft (Fig 8-4).

The *pitch* of the TSAD is the distance between threads, which is typically 0.75 to 1.25 mm. When the threads are spaced far apart, the TSAD has a high pitch; conversely, when the threads are spaced close together, the TSAD has a low pitch. Decreasing the pitch of the TSAD results in an increase in primary stability but may increase torque and stress on the bone. Decreasing the pitch also results in the need for more turning during placement and a slower speed of advancement. Brinley et al[46] compared placement torque and pullout strength of TSADs with a pitch of 0.75, 1.0, and 1.25 mm in both synthetic and cadaver bone models.[46] They found that placement torque of TSADs with a 0.75-mm pitch was higher than that of TSADs with 1.0- and 1.25-mm pitches, but this was only in the synthetic bone model, and the differences were not statistically significant. They also demonstrated that pullout strength significantly increases as pitch decreases from 1.0 to 0.75 mm. There was no difference in pullout strength with a pitch of 1.0 versus 1.25 mm, again only in the synthetic bone model. The results of this study suggest a recommendation of a pitch of 1.0 mm.

Flutes are recessed areas in the cross-sectional area that carry bone chips away from the cutting edge as the screw rotates. The greater depth of the flute can provide more mechanical interlock between the TSAD and bone to assist in primary stability. As flute depth increases, however, there is increased torque and stress on the bone because of an increase in the pressure needed to insert the TSAD as a result of more resistance upon insertion.[47] There is also increased damage to the bone, more bone chips, and the potential for more bony microfractures. The depth of the flute is also a significant factor in the amount of bone chips that are carried away and the mechanical retention obtained. There are no reported studies that quantify the flute of the TSAD with stability. In a cadaver model, Brinley et al[46] demonstrated that pullout strength and placement torque were greater in TSADs that were fluted versus those that were not. The authors suggest that this could have been a result of accumulated bone chips providing greater friction and resistance to insertion.

Pre-drilled versus self-drilling TSADs

Pre-drilled TSADs require that a pilot hole be drilled before placement, whereas self-drilling TSADs can be placed directly without a pilot hole. Pre-drilled TSADs are manufactured with a blunt end, whereas self-drilling TSADs have a sharp end to allow for an initial puncture into cortical bone. There are no reported studies demonstrating differences in success rates between pre-drilled and self-drilling TSADs. A clinical study by Suzuki and Suzuki[48] assessed the torque values of pre-drilled versus self-drilled TSADs using a torquing wrench and found increased maximum insertion torque with self-drilling TSADs.[48] However, this study did not assess the torque and stress applied by the pilot hole and found similar success rates between pre-drilled and self-drilling TSADs.

There are several advantages to using self-drilling TSADs. Because they do not require a pilot hole, the surgical insertion protocol is simpler and takes less time. This also results in less overall stress and heat on the bone, which may increase stability and success and decrease the number of complications resulting from the TSAD.[49]

Site Selection

Soft tissue

When possible, TSADs should be placed in attached keratinized gingiva instead of loose alveolar mucosa. This decreases the risk of tissue overgrowth and inflammation and provides more support and patient comfort.[50]

Hard tissue

The thickness of cortical bone should be adequate to ensure primary stability. The palate is the most suitable site because of its thick and dense cortical bone, the minimal anatomical structures present (apart from the greater palatine nerves, arteries, and veins), and ease of placement.[11,50–52] The disadvantage of TSAD placement in the palate is the potential thickness of the keratinized gingiva in the posterior areas. A tissue punch prior to placement may therefore be required. There is also a need for more profound topical and local anesthesia because of the tightness of the soft tissue.

Gracco et al[52] used digital volumetric tomographs from 162 patients for a quantitative cone beam computed tomography (CBCT) evaluation of palatal bone thickness for TSAD placement. They found that the anterior region is the thickest part of the palate but that the thickness of the cortical bone in the posterior palate is also suitable for primary stability. TSADs placed in the anterior palate should be a short length (no more than 6 mm) to prevent perforation into the nasal cavity, and a thicker and denser bone in this area permits smaller TSADs to be successful.[11,51] The midpalatal suture itself is not a good location for TSAD placement because of the possibility that it is incompletely calcified and the risk of insertion into connective tissue, which would reduce primary stability.[52]

To increase both primary stability and the chances of success, bicortical anchorage should be obtained if possible.[41] Bicortical anchorage is commonly obtained in the buccal alveolus. To obtain bicortical anchorage, the buccolingual width of the alveolus is measured, and a TSAD with a thread length equivalent to or slightly shorter than this measurement is chosen. The TSAD is then inserted toward the buccal while the lingual is palpated. Once the tip of the screw is palpated on the lingual soft tissue, it has perforated the lingual cortical bone, and bicortical anchorage has been obtained. Insertion should be stopped at this point, and the clinician should turn the driver slightly counterclockwise to back the TSAD away from the soft tissue to prevent the risk of inflammation and patient discomfort from contact between the TSAD and the tongue.

There should be sufficient interradicular distance assessed clinically and with radiographs to avoid root damage. Preorthodontic TSAD preparation may be necessary to separate roots. The TSAD should avoid important anatomical landmarks such as the inferior nerve, artery, and vein; the lingual nerve; the long buccal nerve; the greater palatine nerve, artery, and vein; the mental foramen; the maxillary sinus; and the nasal sinus. Failure has been shown to be greater with proximity of a TSAD to a root.[53]

Sites for placement in the maxilla include the nasal spine, the palate, the alveolar process, the infrazygomatic crest, and the tuberosity. Sites in the mandible include the alveolar process, the retromolar pad, and the symphysis. The optimal sites for TSAD insertion based on quality of bone and interradicular space include:

- The maxillary buccal alveolus:
  - Place the TSAD interdentally between the roots of the maxillary second premolar and first molar.[54]
  - Alternatively, place the TSAD interdentally between the roots of the first and second molars.
  - If between the central incisors or between the lateral incisor and the canine, place the TSAD 8 mm from the cementoenamel junction (CEJ) or in attached gingiva; if between the canine and the first premolar, place the TSAD 6 mm from the CEJ or in attached gingiva; if between the first and second premolars, place the TSAD 4 mm from the CEJ or in attached gingiva; if between the second premolar and the first molar, place the TSAD 4 mm from the CEJ or in attached gingiva.[55]
  - Ensure that there is more than 1.5 mm of space between the TSAD and each root when feasible.
- The infrazygomatic crest:
  - The quality of bone is excellent, but loose alveolar gingiva is present.
  - Be careful with the proximity of the soft tissue of the inner cheek, particularly in patients with tight musculature.
  - It is preferable for TSADs to be used here for indirect anchorage.
- The palate:
  - The bone is excellent throughout.
  - Avoid the greater palatine nerve, artery, and vein.
  - In the anterior palate, use TSADs no longer than 6 mm to avoid perforation into the nasal sinus.
  - Avoid placement directly into the midpalatal suture, which can be calcified. Consider tissue punch in the posterior palate, where tissue is not as taut.
  - Use both topical and local anesthesia.
- Various sites in the mandible:
  - If between the first and second premolars or between the second premolar and the first molar, place the TSAD 4 mm from the CEJ or in attached gingiva.[55]
  - Ensure that there is 1.5 mm of space between the TSAD and each root.

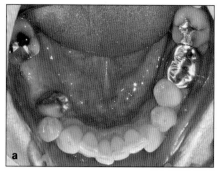
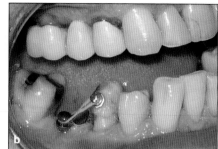
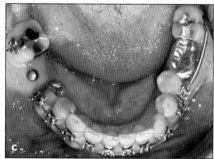
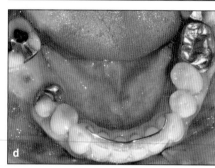

Fig 8-5 *(a)* Patient with a missing mandibular right first molar and a mandibular right second premolar in buccal crossbite. *(b)* Prior to full fixed orthodontic treatment, a TSAD is placed in the extraction site. Direct anchorage is achieved with force from the TSAD to the orthodontic attachment on the mandibular right second premolar. The patient was asked to wear a maxillary Essix retainer full-time with relief at the tooth opposing the mandibular right second premolar to allow for cross occlusion. *(c)* Once the buccal crossbite has been corrected, the mandibular arch is bonded, and a continuous archwire is placed. The TSAD is not removed in case it is required for future mechanics. *(d)* Day of debonding and TSAD removal. Immediately following debonding, the patient saw a general dentist for preparation of a three-unit fixed partial denture.

The maxillary tuberosity has poorer bone and therefore is not an optimal site for placement. The retromolar pad in the mandible has good bone, but access for placement is difficult because of interference of surrounding anatomy and the fact that the TSAD will always be placed on an angle. There is also risk for insertion into the lingual nerve.

Types of Anchorage

Direct anchorage

Direct anchorage is when a TSAD is used directly to move a tooth. In this type of anchorage, it is important to consider the three-dimensional location of the TSAD in relation to the center of resistance of the tooth or teeth to be moved. An example of a case that utilized direct anchorage is demonstrated in Fig 8-5 (see also Fig 8-8).

Indirect anchorage

Indirect anchorage occurs when a tooth or a group of teeth are connected to a TSAD that acts as a periodontal-skeletal anchorage unit, allowing for another tooth or group of teeth to be moved against this stabilized unit. The movement of the stabilized unit is negligible, and it allows for absolute anchorage of the tooth or unit of teeth against the reactive forces of other teeth being moved. Examples of cases utilizing indirect anchorage are demonstrated in Figs 8-6 to 8-8.

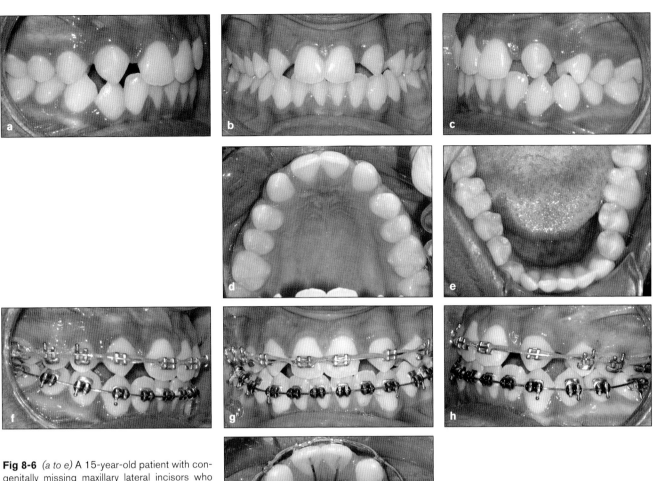

Fig 8-6 *(a to e)* A 15-year-old patient with congenitally missing maxillary lateral incisors who refused the option for dental implants as a replacement. *(f to i)* Indirect anchorage. Two 6-mm TSADs were placed in the anterior palate and bonded together with composite resin. They were also bonded to the palatal of the maxillary central incisors with 19 × 25–inch stainless steel wires to prevent retroclination of the maxillary central incisors as the maxillary space is consolidated to allow for the canines to substitute as lateral incisors.

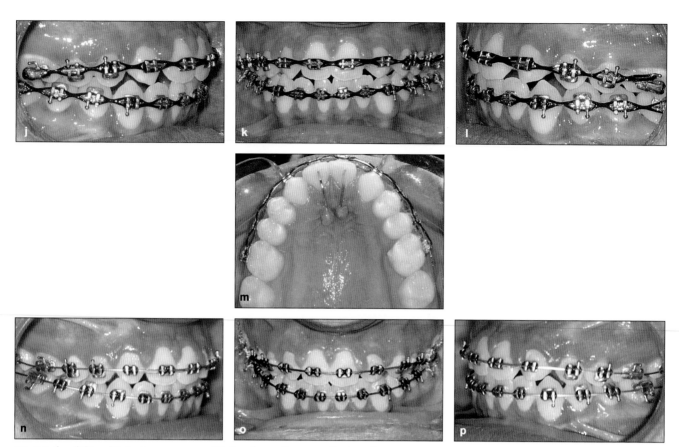

Fig 8-6 *(cont)* *(j to m)* Following space consolidation, the maxillary central incisors have not changed position, and the patient is still in positive overjet. *(n to p)* Final finishing.

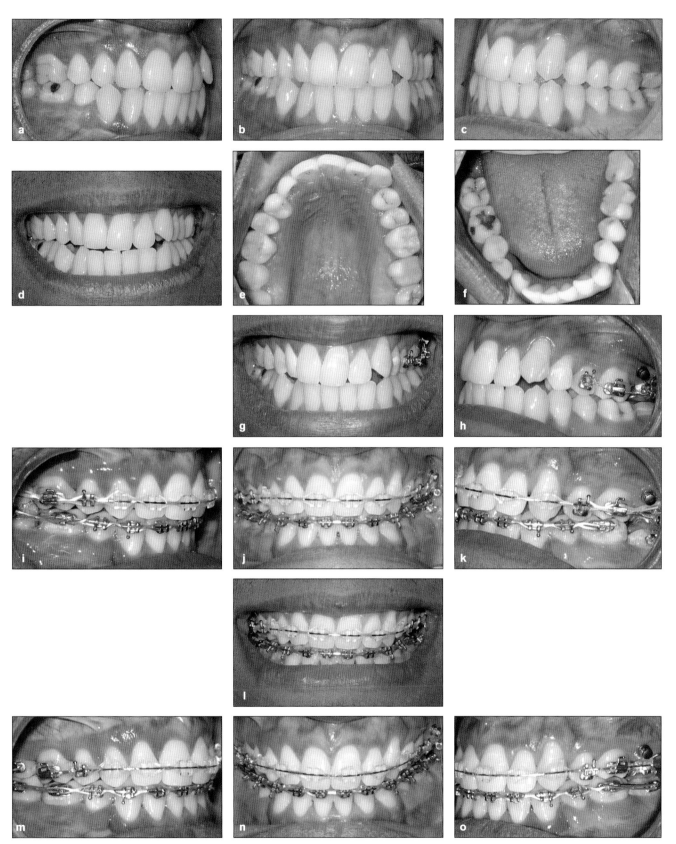

Fig 8-7 *(a to f)* A 22-year-old patient with a chief concern of a midline discrepancy because of a horizontal and palatally impacted maxillary right canine that is treatment planned for extraction. *(g and h)* A TSAD is placed in the maxillary left quadrant and tied to the maxillary left posterior teeth prior to extraction of maxillary right canine, maxillary left first premolar, and mandibular first premolars. The purpose of the TSAD is to provide maximum anchorage to prevent mesial drift of the maxillary left posterior segment, an example of indirect anchorage. *(i to l)* The TSAD is anchoring the maxillary left posterior segment to maximize midline correction during space closure. *(m to o)* Final finishing.

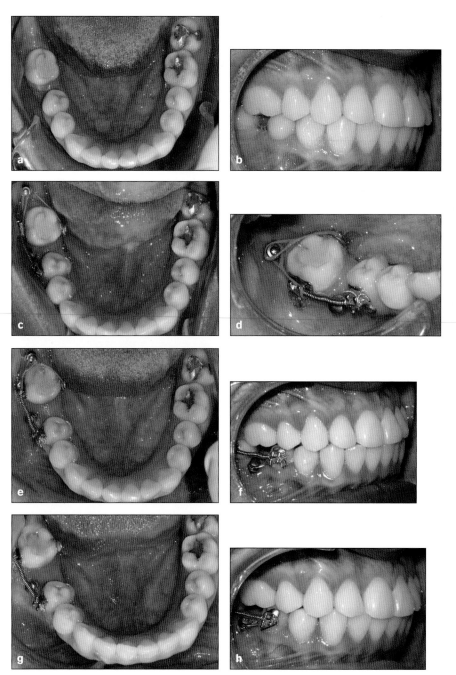

Fig 8-8 *(a and b)* A 32-year-old woman who presented with a mutilated Class I dental malocclusion, missing mandibular right first molar (extracted when she was a teenager) with mesial drift and tipping of the mandibular right second premolar into the space, mild mandibular arch crowding, an overjet of 1 mm, an overbite of 5%, and a mandibular midline discrepancy of 2 mm to the right of the facial midline. The space between the mandibular right second premolar and second molar was 3 mm. *(c and d)* Orthodontic attachments were bonded on these teeth, and a lingual button was bonded on the second molar. Two 8-mm-long TSADs were placed, one in the retromolar pad for distalization (direct anchorage) and one in the area of the missing first molar, which was attached to the bracket on the second molar to prevent its anterior movement (indirect anchorage). A lingual wire was also bonded to the second premolar and second molar to supplement the anchorage. Distalization was achieved with an elastic chain tied from the TSAD in the retromolar pad as well as with an open coil between the orthodontic attachments on the second premolar and second molar. *(e and f)* Clinical photographs 2.5 months after initial bonding showing 2.5 mm of space gained from distalization. The occlusion has not been compromised. *(g and h)* Clinical photographs 4.5 months after initial bonding. The TSAD in the retromolar pad has been removed to prevent contact with the tooth, and 7 mm of space is present between the second premolar and second molar.

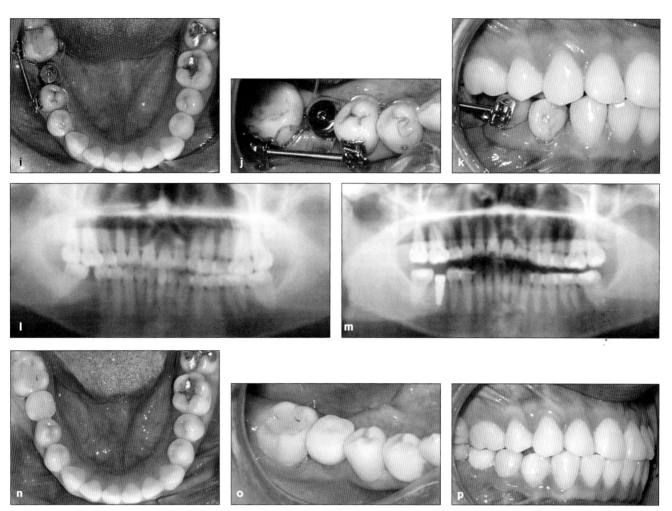

Fig 8-8 *(cont) (i to k)* Day of implant surgery, 7.5 months after initial bonding. The oral surgeon removed the TSAD that was in the area of the missing tooth and placed the dental implant. *(l and m)* Panoramic radiographs before bonding *(l)* and on the day the implant was placed *(m)*. *(n to p)* Day of final crown insertion, 12 months after initial bonding. (Reprinted from Noble and Cassolato[56] with permission.)

TSAD Failure

There are three published systematic reviews that assess the failure rates of TSADs. A systematic review by Reynders et al[57] quantified success and complications with the use of TSADs and factors attributed to success. Another systematic review by Crismani et al[38] also assessed success rates and their relationship to TSAD design, surgery, and loading.[38] A systematic review by Schätzle et al[39] reviewed the literature on the survival rates of palatal implants, onplants, miniplates, and TSADs. There are numerous published clinical trials that assess the success of TSAD placement.[43,58–78] Most of these studies demonstrated a success rate greater than 80%, with a range of 0% to 100%. In the 14 published trials included in the systematic review by Crismani et al,[38] the mean success rate was 83.8% ± 7.4%. However, these studies are inconsistent in their definition of *success* and *failure*, and some studies failed to define them at all. Further, comparisons are difficult between these studies because of different assessment of timing of failure, differences in study methodology and design, uncontrolled variables, and removal and replacement of TSADs in the same patient, which could have introduced underreporting. If a TSAD is loose, and/or if inflammation is present, but it is still being used for its desired purposes, it should not be considered a failure, though some studies reported these as failure. Rather, *failure* should be defined as a TSAD that must be removed prior to fulfillment of its purpose of providing anchorage.

In Crismani's systematic review,[38] the mean success rates were 87.9% ± 7.6% for the maxilla and 80.4% ± 8.5% for the mandible. In three studies that were assessed in this systematic review, the differences between the maxilla and the mandible were significant ($P < .05$), with greater success in the maxilla. The sex of the patient was not found to be correlated to success.[57] There is also a suggestion that TSADs placed in the left side may have higher success rates; however, this may be a function of increased mastication and improved bone density on the left side as well as improved oral hygiene on this side in right-handed patients.[38] Chen et al[44] demonstrated significantly greater success (90% versus 70%) when using 8-mm instead of 6-mm TSADs[47]; other studies have also suggested this trend, though without significance.[63,64,66] Some studies suggest lower success rates in patients with higher mandibular plane angles as a result of reduced cortical bone,[43,59] while other studies found no difference.[60]

Surgery-related factors determining TSAD success include the experience of the surgeon, use of a pre-drilled versus self-drilling technique, angle of insertion, surgical technique, sterilization protocol and techniques, the pressure and torque applied with insertion, and the attainment of monocortical versus bicortical anchorage. It has also been suggested that if the moment of the applied force is generated in the direction to unscrew the TSAD, it could loosen.[2]

Patient-related factors that determine success include age, the quality of the cortical bone present, whether the TSAD is placed in keratinized or nonkeratinized tissue, patient oral hygiene, the force of mastication, and root proximity. TSADs are believed to have a decreased success rate in younger patients because of less dense bone. In these patients, it is suggested to wait 2 weeks before loading the TSAD.

TSAD factors that may influence success include diameter, screw length, and thread design.[67–69] Miyawaki et al[43] concluded that TSADs with a diameter of 1 mm had a significantly reduced success rate compared with those with diameters of 1.5 to 2.3 mm and therefore should be avoided. In his systematic review, Schätzle et al[39] reported that TSADs with a diameter of 2 mm or more showed a significantly (1.8-fold) lower risk (95% confidence interval) of failing compared with TSADs with a diameter of 1.2 mm or less.

In a study assessing the success of midpalatal TSADs for anchorage, Kim et al[40] found that the only clinical variable that showed a significant difference in success rate was the splinting of two TSADs. They believe this is because of the applied force being distributed over more area. These authors found that inflammation surrounding a TSAD did not improve with improved patient oral hygiene. They concluded that inflammation or swelling around a TSAD is likely the result of the TSAD being loose and that inflammation itself does not contribute to TSAD failure. Others, however, believe that soft tissue inflammation contributes to TSAD failure and have shown that TSADs placed in nonkeratinized gingiva are more likely to fail.[61,62,70]

The ability to obtain bicortical anchorage, or positioning the TSAD on both the buccal and lingual alveolar plates, is suggested to increase success because of the stress being distributed over better quality bone, increased resistance, and increased mechanical resistance and primary stability.[41]

Immediate loading

Because TSAD stability is based on *primary stability*, or the interlocking of the threads of the TSAD into bone, immediate loading following placement is possible. A finite element analysis suggested that immediate loading should be limited to 0.5N (about 50 g) of force in a 2-mm-diameter TSAD.[79] In a study of 51 patients who received 134 TSADs with three different diameters and 17 plates, there was no significant difference found between success rate and immediate loading, and the authors concluded that immediate loading is possible if the applied force is less than 2 N (about 200 g).[43] In a study in which TSADs were placed in cadavers at 90- and 45-degree angles on the palate and buccal alveolus, mechanical failure did not occur when up to 15 pounds of pressure was exerted on the TSAD.[80] Although this force was not sustained over a long period of time, this suggests that higher forces applied to the TSAD may be possible.

It has been demonstrated that immediate loading of an implant increases the cellular turnover and density of bone adjacent to the area of the implant compared with implants with no force applied, favoring the concept of immediate loading.[81] However, TSADs do not remain absolutely stationary and can have some mobility during loading in some patients with direct anchorage.[82,83] Therefore, to prevent TSADs from hitting any vital organs because of displacement, 2 mm of clearance must be provided between the TSAD and the root or major foramina, nerves, blood vessels, or pathways. Also, in a study by Motoyoshi et al,[74] adults demonstrated higher success rates versus adolescents with immediate loading, probably because of higher bone density. This suggests that it may be prudent to wait 2 weeks to begin loading a TSAD in adolescents.[57]

Angle of insertion

To avoid root injury, some clinicians have advised inserting TSADs at an angle of 30 to 45 degrees in the maxilla and 10 to 20 degrees in the mandible instead of perpendicular to the bone.[43,58,84] A more acute entry angle will result in increased stress because of the greater amount of cortical bone that the TSAD has to penetrate.[85] Increased stress may draw more cytokines, macrophages, and inflammatory mediators to the site, possibly resulting in a higher risk of TSAD failure through loss of primary stability. Most dental implant failures have been attributed to biomechanical stresses and strains at the bone-implant interface, resulting in peri-implant inflammation that can lead to bone loss.[86–90] Although there are no reported studies comparing angle of insertion to TSAD failure, a study that placed TSADs at different angulations in cadavers found that plain stress on bone was greater for the TSAD angled at 45 degrees to bone at both insertion and removal. This TSAD exerted greater stress on bone compared with TSADs that were placed perpendicular to the bone.[78] This increased stress may increase inflammation, which may influence success.

A finite element analysis and cadaver study by Woodall et al[79] demonstrated that TSADs placed at 90 degrees to bone provided greater anchorage resistance than 60- and 30-degree placements. This study refutes the concept that having more of the length of the TSAD in cortical bone increases resistance and stability and that angulation is not a factor in stability. The authors suggest that this is the result of an increase in the cantilever load arm for angles of 60 and 30 degrees versus 90 degrees. The increase in the distance of applied load at more acute angles of insertion would result in more force on the TSAD and a greater risk of failure.

Insertion torque is another potential factor in TSAD failure. Lim and colleagues[91] reported that increased torque can cause degeneration of bone at the implant-tissue interface. Also, increased torsional stress during placement can result in a TSAD bending, which can lead to TSAD fracture and small cracks in the peri-implant bone, further compromising implant stability.[92–96] The insertion torque increases with cortical bone thickness, which increases with the acuteness of the entry angle.[97]

Therefore, based on the available evidence and lack of clinical trials, it is difficult to recommend an angle at which to insert a TSAD. Clinical research in this area is needed.

TSAD Placement Technique

Each manufacturer promotes different placement techniques for its particular TSADs. There are no reported comparisons in the literature between different placement techniques on success or patient pain and comfort. The technique described here is used by the author.

1. The exact three-dimensional location of TSAD placement is determined using study casts, radiographs, and patient photographs.
2. A periapical radiograph or CBCT is preferred, particularly if the TSAD will be placed interdentally, to more accurately quantify the width of bone available. Because of rotation of teeth and patient positioning out of the focal trough, a panoramic radiograph is not an ideal tool to quantify the width of interdental bone.
3. Informed consent is obtained from the patient, who must understand the benefits and the risks of the procedure as well as the consequences of failure.
4. The patient is asked to rinse for 60 seconds with 0.12% or 0.2% chlorhexidine.
5. Surgical sterile gloves are recommended to avoid contamination and maintain proper infection control similar to that of a surgical extraction.
6. The author recommends a combination of topical and a small amount of local anesthesia for further patient comfort. An infiltration adjacent to a tooth, not a block, should be administered. If less than a quarter carpule of 2% lidocaine with 1:100,000 epinephrine is used, pulpal anesthesia should not be achieved, and the patient can warn the clinician if the TSAD is being inserted into a root. The advantage of using a local anesthetic with epinephrine is that it constricts the blood vessels, thereby decreasing the amount of hemorrhaging of the soft tissue and allowing for better visibility during insertion.
7. The area where the TSAD will be placed is scored with a periodontal probe, and the angle of entry is also marked. If the TSAD is being placed between roots, the roots are identified with the periodontal probe and scored to decrease the risk of insertion into a root.
8. A tissue punch is made if thick keratinized gingiva is present. If thick cortical bone is present, such as in the posterior palate, a 0.09-mm small round bur can score the bone. It is recommended that this be performed without air to avoid an air embolus and under saline irrigation to avoid overheating and infecting the bone.

9. If the TSAD system to be used requires pre-drilling, a pilot hole is made with saline irrigation and rotation at no more than 1,000 revolutions per minute.

10. The TSAD is inserted slowly with firm, consistent pressure. Once placed, it is important to carefully remove the driver to avoid torquing the TSAD. Torquing the TSAD with the driver may disturb the mechanical interlocking of the TSAD to the bone and prevent primary stability from being obtained.

11. Primary stability is then examined by attempting to move the TSAD; if the entire jaw or head moves with the TSAD, then primary stability has been obtained.

12. The procedure is concluded with another 60-second rinse of 0.12% or 0.2% chlorhexidine.

13. A follow-up radiograph is taken if the clinician is concerned that the TSAD is close to an anatomical structure.

14. Oral hygiene and postoperative instructions are given to the patient regarding proper care of the TSAD.

15. The patient is then instructed to take over-the-counter analgesics only if needed (eg, 500 mg of acetaminophen every 4 to 6 hours [4,000 mg max per day] and/or 600 mg of ibuprofen every 8 hours [2,400 mg max per day]).

16. A care call is then made to the patient the following day to ensure that the TSAD is in place and that the patient is not experiencing discomfort.

TSAD removal

TSAD removal is usually an uneventful, simple procedure, and local anesthesia is often not needed, provided there is no soft tissue overgrowth. The same manufacturer driver used to screw the TSAD should be used to unscrew it. If the TSAD cannot be removed, Melsen and Verna[98] advise to wait 3 to 7 days after the initial removal attempt because microfractures and bone remodeling may assist with loosening the TSAD.

Risks and Complications

Root damage

One of the risks of TSAD placement is root contact and damage. This can potentially result in devitalization, osteosclerosis, or ankylosis of the tooth. Enough clearance should be present when placing TSADs between roots, and it is recommended that a radiograph be taken following placement. If a root is contacted, the clinician should remove the TSAD from the bone and find another location for placement. Another risk is moving a tooth into a TSAD. Kadioglu et al[99] conducted a histologic investigation of roots in 10 patients in whom the roots of 20 maxillary premolars to be extracted were tipped into TSADs with tipping springs. The roots that were damaged demonstrated

repair and healing of cementum within a few weeks after removal of the TSADs.

It is important to be mindful that a TSAD does not necessarily remain stationary during treatment. Wang and Liou[100] undertook a prospective clinical study of 32 women who had TSADs placed in the infrazygomatic crest for en-masse retraction and intrusion with nickel-titanium closed-coil springs, half of which were pre-drilled and half of which were self-drilling, to quantify mobility with loading. The TSADs were loaded 2 weeks after placement, and movement of the TSAD was assessed with cephalometric superimposition at the time of initial force loading and at least 5 months later. The authors found that both types of TSADs displayed similar amounts and types of displacement. All TSADs remained stable without mobility or loosening, and the amount of displacement was significant in the direction of the force applied and correlated to the length of loading period. The amount of displacement was 0 to 1.6 mm with extrusion, 1.5 mm with forward or backward tipping at the screw tail, and 1.5 mm with forward tipping at the screw head. This study only assessed displacement in the infrazygomatic crest of the maxilla. The density of bone interdentally in the maxilla is lower, and displacement may be more significant. The authors therefore recommended that TSADs placed between roots in this area should have a clearance of 2 mm between the TSAD and the tooth root when forces are applied on the TSAD toward a root. Radiographs to monitor the proximity of the TSAD to the root during movement are valuable. Periapical radiographs at 90 degrees to the tooth are more clinically useful than a panoramic radiograph because the true proximity between the TSAD and the root would not be possible to assess on a panoramic radiograph.

Slippage

In areas where the bone may slope, there is a risk for the TSAD to slip and damage the periosteum and soft tissue. This can increase the overall postoperative pain. These high-risk areas include the infrazygomatic buttress, the bony place of the alveolar ridge, the retromolar pad, the buccal cortical shelf, and exostosis if present.[49] To avoid slippage, it may be prudent to place the TSAD at a 90-degree angle to bone in these areas.

Nerve injury

Careful planning and knowledge of facial anatomy is critical to prevent insertion into a nerve. The nerves at risk include the inferior alveolar nerve, the mental nerve, the greater palatine nerve, the long buccal nerve, and the lingual nerve. Because peripheral nerves have the capacity to regenerate, minor nerve damage is usually transient and manifests as paresthesia with recovery in 6 months, and treatment may involve corticosteroids, microneurosurgery, nerve grafting, or laser therapy.[49]

TSAD fracture

Because TSADs have the potential to partially osseointegrate, fracture can occur, most likely during removal. Fracture occurs if the torque applied upon removal exceeds the force the TSAD can withstand. This typically occurs in TSADs of smaller diameter and is a major reason for the recommendation not to use TSADs smaller than 1 mm in diameter.[43] If the TSAD fractures during removal, the clinician must decide if there is a risk of infection or potential harm from leaving it in the bone. If a fractured TSAD deep in bone requires removal, an additional surgical procedure with a trephine drill is required to remove it. This results in substantial bone loss as well as increased associated surgical morbidity.[49] The TSAD also must not be inserted beyond its neck because this can add torsional stress to the TSAD neck, which can cause TSAD loosening and potential fracture.

Air embolus/emphysema

If air enters the submucosa, soft tissue distension can occur, resulting in an air embolus or emphysema. The word *emphysema* comes from the Greek word meaning "to blow in." This is rare but can occur when a high-speed handpiece or air-water syringe is used on bone or under the soft tissue. It can manifest itself almost immediately as a crackling sound with associated pain from the distension of the tissues. It can lead to severe consequences, such as mucosal swelling, cervicofacial swelling, orbital swelling, otalgia, hearing loss, mild discomfort, airway obstruction, and possibly interseptal and interproximal alveolar necrosis.[101–103] Risks for an air embolus forming during TSAD placement exist when drilling a pilot hole, when scoring dense cortical bone with a round bur, and during TSAD insertion into loose alveolar tissue. An air-water syringe should therefore be avoided, and bleeding should be managed with gauze or cotton.

The clinician should be mindful of the risk of subcutaneous emphysema during TSAD placement through the loose alveolar tissue of the retromolar pad, on the buccal alveolar bone in the mandibular posterior area, and in the maxillary zygomatic regions. If a pilot hole is to be drilled through the mucosa, the clinician should use slow speed under low rotary pressure. If either a pilot hole or a mucosal punch is placed, an air-water syringe should never be used. Air from the syringe can enter the submucosal space through the small tissue opening, even in attached tissue. Bleeding and saliva should be controlled with suction, cotton, and gauze rather than an air-water syringe. If an air embolus occurs, the TSAD insertion should be stopped, and an ice pack should be applied to decrease the swelling. Once the swelling has stopped, the patient should be sent to a physician or to the emergency room to rule out an infection. The swelling typically resolves after 1 week.

Overheating of bone

TSADs should be placed with a controlled force and speed to prevent overheating of bone and potential infection. Saline irrigation should be applied if a pilot hole is placed or if dense cortical bone is scored with a round bur, and it should be undertaken with controlled torque on the driver.

Perforation into a sinus

Care must be taken to ensure that TSADs do not perforate the maxillary or nasal sinuses. If the risk does exist, a shorter TSAD of 6 mm should be utilized. If less than 2 mm of the TSAD perforates the sinus, healing usually occurs without complications and there is no impact on primary stability.[49]

Soft tissue pathology

TSADs that are placed in loose alveolar tissue have a greater risk of soft tissue coverage (Fig 8-9). This can occur within 1 day of placement from the distension of loose tissue during mastication, resulting in tissue growth around and sometimes over the TSAD. If the entire TSAD is covered with soft tissue, the patient may think that it has dislodged and perhaps that it has been swallowed. During TSAD insertion, loose alveolar tissue may be loose enough to twist around the TSAD. Therefore, it is recommended that the clinician push the soft tissue away from the TSAD with finger pressure during insertion. This will likely decrease the amount of inflammation. The clinician should also consider using a longer TSAD or a TSAD with a longer neck and not completely inserting the TSAD. Further measures to prevent failure such as prescribing an antimicrobial rinse or antibiotics as well as delaying loading should also be considered.

Contraindications

Absolute contraindications for using TSADs include patients with:

- Serious systemic diseases
- Use of bisphosphonate medications
- Uncontrolled hemorrhagic disorders
- Bone metabolism disorders
- Psychotic diseases
- Weakened immunoresistance and leukocyte dysfunctions
- Illnesses requiring the periodic use of steroids
- Uncontrollable endocrine disorders
- Nickel or titanium allergy

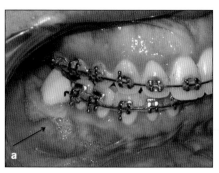 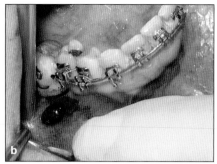 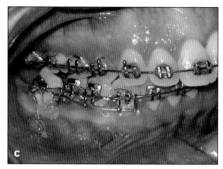

Fig 8-9 *(a) Arrow* pointing to soft tissue covering a TSAD. *(b)* The TSAD is uncovered by removing soft tissue. *(c)* The TSAD is then used clinically.

Relative contraindications for using TSADs include uncooperative patients, pregnant women, smokers, and patients with:

- Previously irradiated bone
- Diabetes mellitus
- Anticoagulant medication/hemorrhagic diathesis
- Poor oral hygiene
- Periodontal disease
- Drug, alcohol, or tobacco abuse
- Xerostomia
- High dental anxiety

Bayat and Bauss[104] assessed failure in 88 patients receiving 110 TSADs based on whether they were heavy smokers (10 or more cigarettes per day), light smokers (less then 10 cigarettes per day), or nonsmokers. *Failure* was defined as either a loosening of the TSAD that prevented its use for anchorage or peri-implant inflammation. They found a significant difference in failure between heavy smokers and light smokers/nonsmokers in the first 4 months following initial TSAD placement. There was no significant difference in failure between nonsmokers and light smokers. The effect of smoking on TSADs is consistent with the evidence in the dental implantology literature, which demonstrates the detrimental effect of smoking on dental implant success.[105]

Clinical Uses

The clinical use of TSADs has provided more treatment options for patients and innovative approaches for clinicians to manage malocclusions and mild skeletal maxillomandibular discrepancies. Applications for anchorage and the use of appliances in concert with TSADs are limited only by the limits of tooth movement within bone and the clinician's imagination.

Examples of dental corrections in which TSADs can be used include closure of extraction spaces, en-masse retraction of anterior teeth, alignment of the dental midline, extrusion of an impacted canine, extrusion and uprighting of impacted molars, molar intrusion, distalization, mesialization, uprighting, intrusion, and extrusion. Skeletal discrepancies that can be managed with TSADs include the correction of Class II and Class III sagittal relationships,[106–109] palatal expansion to avoid tipping of teeth,[110] the correction of skeletal cants, and the correction of anterior open bites.[111–113] The concern with using TSADs to correct skeletal discrepancies is relapse of the correction as a result of soft tissue. This issue is particularly relevant when discussing the correction of anterior open bites with TSADs because it is an attractive alternative to orthognathic surgery, and there are numerous case reports demonstrating excellent correction with short-term follow-up.[73,114,115]

Treatment options for anterior open bite include orthognathic surgery, extrusion of the incisors, extractions or interproximal reduction to retrocline the anterior teeth, growth modification in growing patients, intrusion of the posterior segment, or mere acceptance of the open bite. The first step in treatment is to determine the etiology of the anterior open bite. Numerous case reports describe the use of TSADs to treat anterior open bites with intrusion of maxillary molars.[73,114,115] These reports describe that molar intrusion results in a closure of the anterior open bite, counterclockwise rotation of the mandible and decreased mandibular plane angle, decreased overall facial height with an improved anteroposterior relationship of the mandible and maxilla, and an improved profile and overall facial esthetics with lip closure. This mode of treatment is likely more favorable in patients with anterior open bites as a result of long lower facial heights and who have associated Class I or mild Class II skeletal relationships.[114] In

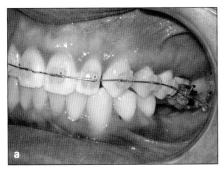 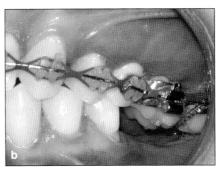 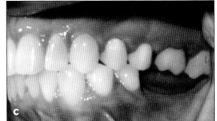

Fig 8-10 *(a)* Unopposed maxillary left molars have extruded, and the patient is unable to obtain implants in the mandibular left quadrant. *(b)* Intrusion of molars with a coil tied to buccal and palatal TSADs to create intrusive force. *(c)* Clearance for implant crowns in the mandibular left quadrant is achieved.

patients with anterior open bites with associated Class III skeletal relationships, counterclockwise mandibular auto-rotation would worsen the Class III relationship, resulting in a negative overjet and more concave profile. In these patients, orthognathic surgery is the preferred option. To correct this nonsurgically, TSADs could be placed in the retromolar pad to retract the mandibular arch, but this would overretrocline the mandibular incisors.

The biomechanics of molar intrusion can be achieved in different ways. TSADs can be placed on the buccal and lingual with a coil or elastic crossing the occlusion (Fig 8-10). Alternatively, a transpalatal appliance could receive a force from TSADs placed in the palate. It is beneficial to use a full-dimension stainless steel continuous archwire during intrusion to maintain the three-dimensional position of the posterior dentition because intrusive forces could result in uncontrolled tipping. A transpalatal appliance or force on both the buccal and lingual allows for more pure intrusion. As the molars intrude, there is a potential for periodontal pseudopockets to develop. Pocket reduction surgery may be necessary. Therefore, this type of treatment should not be undertaken in patients who have a compromised periodontium. The literature also suggests a relapse of 30% with molar intrusion, so overcorrection is therefore indicated.[116] Relapse would likely be greater if the etiology of the open bite is neuromuscular.

Degeshi et al[117] studied 30 adults with anterior open bites and similar skeletal cephalometric characteristics treated with either molar intrusion using TSADs or extrusion of incisors using conventional edgewise treatment and vertical anterior elastics. Patients treated with molar intrusion had more favorable soft tissue changes with counterclockwise rotation of the mandible, improved facial convexity, and an increase in the inferior labial sulcus angle, while those with incisor extrusion had clockwise rotation. Both groups demonstrated improvement in upper and lower lip protrusion. Patients were assessed 2 years after treatment.

Less stability was observed in patients treated by molar intrusion with TSADs. To prevent relapse, the authors recommended overcorrection, considering myofunctional therapy to correct a possible neuromuscular etiology, and a retainer with occlusal stops for the mandibular molars or TSADs in the mandible to prevent mandibular extrusion.

Summary Points

- Orthodontists are the ideal clinicians to place TSADs because of their understanding of the biomechanics of tooth movement.
- TSADs should be placed in keratinized gingiva and cortical bone when possible.
- Obtaining bicortical anchorage increases primary stability.
- The success rate of TSADs is approximately 85%, and proper treatment planning and site selection can increase success rates.
- TSADs can be immediately loaded because stability is based on primary stability.
- TSADs with a diameter less than 1.3 mm should not be utilized because of the risk of fracture.
- Indirect anchorage is a powerful clinical tool that allows for stabilization of a tooth or group of teeth to allow movement of another tooth or group of teeth.
- A protocol should be in place when placing TSADs to increase success rates.
- TSADs should be avoided in patients with compromised medical histories.
- Correcting a skeletal anterior open bite with TSADs should be undertaken in patients with a Class I or mild Class II skeletal relationship, but not a Class III skeletal relationship.

References

1. Kanomi R. Mini-implant for orthodontic anchorage. J Clin Orthod 1997;31:763–767.
2. Costa A, Raffaini M, Melsen B. Miniscrews as orthodontic anchorage: A preliminary report. Int J Adult Orthodon Orthognath Surg 1998;13:201–209.
3. Kyung HM, Park HS, Bae SM, Sung JH, Kim IB. Development of orthodontic micro-implants for intraoral anchorage. J Clin Orthod 2003;37:321–328.
4. Melsen B. Mini-implants: Where are we? J Clin Orthod 2005;39: 539–547.
5. Gainsforth BL, Higley LB. A study of orthodontic anchorage possibilities in basal bone. Am J Orthod Oral Surg 1945;31:406–416.
6. Linkow LI. The endosseous blade implant and its use in orthodontics. Int J Orthod 1969;7:149–154.
7. Creekmore TD, Eklund MK. The possibility of skeletal anchorage. J Clin Orthod 1983;17:266–269.
8. Block MS, Hoffman DR. A new device for absolute anchorage for orthodontics. Am J Orthod Dentofacial Orthop 1995;107:251–258.
9. Armbruster PC, Block MS. Onplant-supported orthodontic anchorage. Atlas Oral Maxillofac Surg Clin North Am 2001;9:53–74.
10. Wehrbein H, Merz BR, Diedrich P, Glatzmaier J. The use of palatal implants for orthodontic anchorage. Design and clinical application of the orthosystem. Clin Oral Implants Res 1996;7:410–416.
11. Wehrbein H, Feifel H, Diedrich P. Palatal implant anchorage reinforcement of posterior teeth: A prospective study. Am J Orthod Dentofacial Orthop 1999;116:678–686.
12. Arcuri C, Muzzi F, Santini F, Barlattani A, Giancotti A. Five years of experience using palatal mini-implants for orthodontic anchorage. J Oral Maxillofac Surg 2007;65:2492–2497.
13. Benson PE, Tinsley D, O'Dwyer JJ, Majumdar A, Doyle P, Sandler PJ. Midpalatal implants vs headgear for orthodontic anchorage—A randomized clinical trial: Cephalometric results. Am J Orthod Dentofacial Orthop 2007;132:606–615.
14. Douglass JB, Killiany DM. Dental implants used as orthodontic anchorage. J Oral Implantol 1987;13:28–38.
15. Roberts WE, Helm FR, Marshall KJ, Gongloff RK. Rigid endosseous implants for orthodontic and orthopedic anchorage. Angle Orthod 1989;59:247–256.
16. Roberts WE, Marshall KJ, Mozsary PG. Rigid endosseous implant utilized as anchorage to protract molars and close an atrophic extraction site. Angle Orthod 1990;60:134–152.
17. Kokich VG. Managing complex orthodontic problems: The use of implants for anchorage. Semin Orthod 1996;2:153–160.
18. Huang LH, Shotwell JL, Wang HL. Dental implants for orthodontic anchorage. Am J Orthod Dentofacial Orthop 2005;127:713–722.
19. Rozencweig G, Rozencweig S. Use of implants and ankylosed teeth in orthodontics. Review of the literature [in French]. J Parodontol 1989;8:179–184.
20. Jung BA, Kunkel M, Göllner P, Liechti T, Wehrbein H. Success rate of second-generation palatal implants. Angle Orthod 2009;79:85–90.
21. De Clerck HJ, Cornelis MA, Cevidanes LH, Heymann GC, Tulloch CJ. Orthopedic traction of the maxilla with miniplates: A new perspective for treatment of midface deficiency. J Oral Maxillofac Surg 2009;67:2123–2129.
22. Wilmes B, Drescher D, Nienkemper M. A miniplate system for improved stability of skeletal anchorage. J Clin Orthod 2009;43:494–501.
23. Chung KR, Kim SH, Kang YG, Nelson G. Orthodontic miniplate with tube as an efficient tool for borderline cases. Am J Orthod Dentofacial Orthop 2011;139:551–562.
24. Cha BK, Choi DS, Ngan P, Jost-Brinkmann PG, Kim SM, Jang IS. Maxillary protraction with miniplates providing skeletal anchorage in a growing Class III patient. Am J Orthod Dentofacial Orthop 2011;139:99–112.
25. Melsen B, Petersen JK, Costa A. Zygoma ligatures: An alternative form of maxillary anchorage. J Clin Orthod 1998;32:154–158.
26. Umemori M, Sugawara J, Mitani H, Nagasaka H, Kawamura H. Skeletal anchorage system for open-bite correction. Am J Orthod Dentofacial Orthop 1999;115:166–174.
27. Bae SM, Park HS, Kyung HM, Kwon OW, Sung JH. Clinical application of micro-implant anchorage. J Clin Orthod 2002;36:298–302.
28. Bantleon HP, Bernhart T, Crismani AG, Zachrisson BU. Stable orthodontic anchorage with palatal osseointegrated implants. World J Orthod 2002;3:109–116.
29. Erverdi N, Tosun T, Keles A. A new anchorage site for the treatment of anterior open bite: Zygomatic anchorage—Case report. J Clin Orthod 2002;3:147–153.
30. Chung K, Kim SH, Kook YC. Orthodontic microimplant for distalization of mandibular dentition in Class III correction. Angle Orthod 2004;75:119–128.
31. Mah J, Bergstrand F. Temporary anchorage devices: A status report. J Clin Orthod 2005;39:132–136.
32. Cope JB. Temporary anchorage devices in orthodontics: A paradigm shift. Semin Orthod 2005;11:3–9.
33. Choo H, Kim SH, Huang JC. TAD, a misnomer? Am J Orthod Dentofacial Orthop 2009;136:145–146.
34. Reddy KB, Kumar MP, Kumar MN. A grid for guiding miniscrew placement. J Clin Orthod 2008;42:531–532.
35. Noble J, Hechter FJ, Karaiskos NE, Lekic N, Wiltshire WA. Future practice plans of orthodontic residents in the United States. Am J Orthod Dentofacial Orthop 2009;135:357–360.
36. Buschang PH, Carrillo R, Ozenbaugh B, Rossouw PE. 2008 survey of AAO members on miniscrew usage. J Clin Orthod 2008;42: 513–518.
37. Hyde JD, King GJ, Greenlee GM, Spiekerman C, Huang GJ. Survey of orthodontists' attitudes and experiences regarding miniscrew implants. J Clin Orthod 2010;44:481–486.
38. Crismani AG, Bertl MH, Celar AG, Bantleon HP, Burstone CJ. Miniscrews in orthodontic treatment: Review and analysis of published clinical trials. Am J Orthod Dentofacial Orthop 2010;137: 108–113.
39. Schätzle M, Männchen R, Zwahlen M, Lang NP. Survival and failure rates of orthodontic temporary anchorage devices: A systematic review. Clin Oral Implants Res 2009;20:1351–1359.
40. Kim YH, Yang SM, Kim S, et al. Midpalatal miniscrews for orthodontic anchorage: Factors affecting clinical success. Am J Orthod Dentofacial Orthop 2010;137:66–72.
41. Brettin BT, Grosland NM, Qian F. Bicortical vs monocortical orthodontic skeletal anchorage. Am J Orthod Dentofacial Orthop 2008;134:625–635.
42. Carano A, Lonardo P, Velo S, Incorvati C. Mechanical properties of three different commercially available miniscrews for skeletal anchorage. Prog Orthod 2005;6:82–97.
43. Miyawaki S, Koyama I, Inoue M, Mishima K, Sugahara T, Takano-Yamamoto T. Factors associated with the stability of titanium screws placed in the posterior region for orthodontic anchorage. Am J Orthod Dentofacial Orthop 2003;124:373–378.
44. Chen CH, Chang CS, Hsieh CH, et al. The use of microimplants in orthodontic anchorage. J Oral Maxillofac Surg 2006;64:1209–1213.
45. Brunski JB. Biomaterials and biomechanics in dental implant design. Int J Oral Maxillofac Implants 1988;3:85–97.
46. Brinley CL, Behrents R, Kim KB, Condoor S, Kyung HM, Buschang PH. Pitch and longitudinal fluting effects on the primary stability of miniscrew implants Angle Orthod 2009;79:1156–1161.
47. Uhl RL. The biomechanics of screws. Orthop Rev 1989;18:1302–1307.
48. Suzuki EY, Suzuki B. Placement and removal torque values of orthodontic miniscrew implants. Am J Orthod Dentofacial Orthop 2011;139:669–678.
49. Kravitz ND, Kusnoto B. Risks and complications of orthodontic miniscrews. Am J Orthod Dentofacial Orthop 2007;131(4 suppl): S43–S51.
50. Maino BG, Mura P, Bednar J. Miniscrew implants: The spider screw anchorage system. Semin Orthod 2005;11:40–46.

51. Wehrbein H, Merz BR, Diedrich P. Palatal bone support for orthodontic implant anchorage —A clinical and radiological study. Eur J Orthod 1999;21:65–70.

52. Gracco A, Lombardo L, Cozzani M, Siciliani G. Quantitative cone-beam computed tomography evaluation of palatal bone thickness for orthodontic miniscrew placement. Am J Orthod Dentofacial Orthop 2008;134:361–369.

53. Kuroda S, Katayama A, Takano-Yamamoto T. Severe anterior open-bite case treated using titanium screw anchorage. Angle Orthod 2004;74:558–567.

54. Santiago RC, de Paula FO, Fraga MR, Picorelli Assis NM, Vitral RW. Correlation between miniscrew stability and bone mineral density in orthodontic patients. Am J Orthod Dentofacial Orthop 2009;136:243–250.

55. Lee KJ, Joo E, Kim KD, Lee JS, Park YC, Yu HS. Computed tomographic analysis of tooth-bearing alveolar bone for orthodontic miniscrew placement. Am J Orthod Dentofacial Orthop 2009;135:486–494.

56. Noble J, Cassolato S. Pre-prosthetic distalization using temporary skeletal anchorage. Ont Dent 2011;88(10):20–23.

57. Reynders R, Ronchi L, Bipat S. Mini-implants in orthodontics: A systematic review of the literature. Am J Orthod Dentofacial Orthop 2009;135:564.e1–564.e19.

58. Cheng SJ, Tseng IY, Lee JJ, Kok SH. A prospective study of the risk factors associated with failure of mini-implants used for orthodontic anchorage. Int J Oral Maxillofac Implants 2004;19:100–106.

59. Baek SH, Kim BM, Kyung SH, Lim JK, Kim YH. Success rate and risk factors associated with mini-implants reinstalled in the maxilla. Angle Orthod 2008;78:895–901.

60. Antoszewska J, Papadopoulos MA, Park HS, Ludwig B. Five-year experience with orthodontic miniscrew implants: A retrospective investigation of factors influencing success rates. Am J Orthod Dentofacial Orthop 2009;136:158.e1–158.e10.

61. Chen YJ, Chang HH, Huang CY, Hung HC, Lai EH, Yao CC. A retrospective analysis of the failure rate of three different orthodontic skeletal anchorage systems. Clin Oral Implants Res 2007;18:768–775.

62. Meredith N. Assessment of implant stability as a prognostic determinant. Int J Prosthodont 1998;11:491–501.

63. Park HS, Jeong SH, Kwon OW. Factors affecting the clinical success of screw implants used as orthodontic anchorage. Am J Orthod Dentofacial Orthop 2006;130:18–25.

64. Tseng YC, Hsieh CH, Chen CH, Shen YS, Huang IY, Chen CM. The application of mini-implants for orthodontic anchorage. Int J Oral Maxillofac Surg 2006;35:704–707.

65. Luzi C, Verna C, Melsen B. A prospective clinical investigation of the failure rate of immediately loaded mini-implants used for orthodontic anchorage. Prog Orthod 2007;8:192–201.

66. Kuroda S, Sugawara Y, Deguchi T, Kyung HM, Takano-Yamamoto T. Clinical use of miniscrew implants as orthodontic anchorage: Success rates and postoperative discomfort. Am J Orthod Dentofacial Orthop 2007;131:9–15.

67. Yerby S, Scott CC, Evans NJ, Messing KL, Carter DR. Effect of cutting flute design on cortical bone screw insertion torque and pullout strength. J Orthop Trauma 2001;15:216–221.

68. O'Sullivan D, Sennerby L, Meredith N. Influence of implant taper on the primary and secondary stability of osseointegrated titanium implants. Clin Oral Implants Res 2004;15:474–480.

69. Oktenoglu BT, Ferrara LA, Andalkar N, Ozer AF, Sarioglu AC, Benzel EC. Effects of hole preparation on screw pullout resistance and insertional torque: A biomechanical study. J Neurosurg 2001;94:91–96.

70. Motoyoshi M, Matsuoka M, Shimizu N. Application of orthodontic mini-implants in adolescents. Int J Oral Maxillofac Surg 2007;36:695–699.

71. Moon CH, Lee DG, Lee HS, Im JS, Baek SH. Factors associated with the success rate of orthodontic miniscrews placed in the upper and lower posterior buccal region. Angle Orthod 2008;78:101–106.

72. Wiechmann D, Meyer U, Büchter A. Success rate of mini- and micro-implants used for orthodontic anchorage: A prospective clinical study. Clin Oral Implants Res 2007;18:263–267.

73. Kuroda S, Yamada K, Deguchi T, Hashimoto T, Kyung HM, Takano-Yamamoto T. Root proximity is a major factor for screw failure in orthodontic anchorage. Am J Orthod Dentofacial Orthop 2007;131(4 suppl):S68–S73.

74. Motoyoshi M, Yoshida T, Ono A, Shimizu N. Effect of cortical bone thickness and implant placement torque on stability of orthodontic mini-implants. Int J Oral Maxillofac Implants 2007;22:779–784.

75. Hedayati Z, Hashemi SM, Zamiri B, Fattahi HR. Anchorage value of surgical titanium screws in orthodontic tooth movement. Int J Oral Maxillofac Surg 2007;36:588–592.

76. Chaddad K, Ferreira AF, Geurs N, Reddy MS. Influence of surface characteristics on survival rates of mini-implants. Angle Orthod 2008;78:107–113.

77. Berens A, Wiechmann D, Dempf R. Mini- and micro-screws for temporary skeletal anchorage in orthodontic therapy. J Orofac Orthop 2006;67:450–458.

78. Kinzinger G, Gulden N, Yildizhan F, Hermanns-Sachweh B, Diedrich P. Anchorage efficacy of palatally-inserted miniscrews in molar distalization with a periodontally/miniscrew-anchored distal jet. J Orofac Orthop 2008;69:110–120.

79. Woodall N, Tadepalli SC, Qian F, Grosland NM, Marshall SD, Southard TE. Effect of miniscrew angulation on anchorage resistance. Am J Orthod Dentofacial Orthop 2011;139:e147–e152.

80. Noble J, Karaiskos NE, Hassard TH, Hechter FJ, Wiltshire WA. Stress on bone from placement and removal of orthodontic miniscrews at different angulations. J Clin Orthod 2009;43:332–334.

81. Melsen B, Lang NP. Biological reactions of alveolar bone to orthodontic loading of oral implants. Clin Oral Implants Res 2001;12:223-230.

82. Liou EJ, Pai BC, Lin JC. Do miniscrews remain stationary under orthodontic forces? Am J Orthod Dentofacial Orthop 2004;126:42–47.

83. El-Beialy AR, Abou-El-Ezz AM, Attia KH, El-Bialy AM, Mostafa YA. Loss of anchorage of miniscrews: A 3-dimensional assessment. Am J Orthod Dentofacial Orthop 2009;136:700–707.

84. Park HS, Lee SK, Kwon OW. Group distal movement of teeth using microscrew implant anchorage. Angle Orthod 2005;75:602–609.

85. Ottoni JM, Oliveria ZF, Mansini R, Cabral AM. Correlation between placement torque and survival of single-tooth implants. Int J Oral Maxillofac Implants 2005;20:769–776.

86. Carano A, Velo S, Leone P, Siciliani G. Clinical applications of the Miniscrew Anchorage System. J Clin Orthod 2005;39:9–24.

87. Kyung HM, Park HS, Bae SM, Sung JH, Kim IB. Development of orthodontic micro-implants for intraoral anchorage. J Clin Orthod 2003;37:321–328.

88. Heckmann SM, Linke JJ, Graef F, Foitzik C, Wichmann MG, Weber HP. Stress and inflammation as a detrimental combination for peri-implant bone loss. J Dent Res 2006;85:711–716.

89. Yun HS, Kim HJ, Park YC. The thickness of the maxillary soft tissue and cortical bone related with an orthodontic implantation (thesis). Seoul, South Korea: Yonsei University, 2001.

90. Lee JS, Kim DH, Park YC, Kyung SH, Kim TK. The efficient use of midpalatal miniscrew implants. Angle Orthod 2004;74:711–714.

91. Lim SA, Cha JY, Hwang CJ. Insertion torque of orthodontic mini-screws according to changes in shape, diameter and length. Angle Orthod 2008;78:234–240.

92. Heidemann W, Gerlach KL, Gröbel KH, Köllner HG. Influence of different pilot hole sizes on torque measurements and pullout analysis of osteosynthesis screws. J Craniomaxillofac Surg 1998;26:50–55.

93. Trisi P, Rebaudi A. Progressive bone adaptation of titanium implants during and after orthodontic load in humans. Int J Periodontics Restorative Dent 2002;22:31–43.

94. Büchter A, Wiechmann D, Koerdt S, Wiesmann HP, Piffko J, Meyer U. Load-related implant reaction of mini-implants used for orthodontic anchorage. Clin Oral Implants Res 2005;16:473–479.

95. Jolley TH, Chung CH. Peak torque values at fracture of orthodontic miniscrews, J Clin Orthod 2007;41:326–328.

96. Freudenthaler JW, Haas R, Bantleon HP. Bicortical titanium screws for critical orthodontic anchorage in the mandible: A preliminary report on clinical applications. Clin Oral Implants Res 2001;12:358–363.

97. Phillips JH, Rahn BA. Comparison of compression and torque measurements of self-tapping and pretapped screws. Plast Reconstr Surg1989;83:447–458.

98. Melsen B, Verna C. Miniscrew implants: Ahe Aarhus Anchorage System. Semin Orthod 2005;11:24–31.

99. Kadioglu O, Büyükyilmaz T, Zachrisson BU, Maino BG. Contact damage to root surfaces of premolars touching miniscrews during orthodontic treatment. Am J Orthod Dentofacial Orthop 2008;134:353–360.

100. Wang YC, Liou EJ. Comparison of the loading behavior of self-drilling and predrilled miniscrews throughout orthodontic loading. Am J Orthod Dentofacial Orthop 2008;133:38–43.

101. McKenzie WS, Rosenberg M. Iatrogenic subcutaneous emphysema of dental and surgical origin: A literature review. J Oral Maxillofac Surg 2009;67:1265–1268.

102. Gamboa Vidal CA, Vega Pizarro CA, Almeida Arriagada A. Subcutaneous emphysema secondary to dental treatment: Case report. Med Oral Patol Oral Cir Bucal 2007;12:E76–E78.

103. Yang SC, Chiu TH, Lin TJ, Chan HM. Subcutaneous emphysema and pneumomediastinum secondary to dental extraction: A case report and literature review. Kaohsiung J Med Sci 2006;22:641–645.

104. Bayat E, Bauss O. Effect of smoking on the failure rates of orthodontic miniscrews. J Orofac Orthop 2010;71:117–124.

105. Bain CA, Moy PK. The association between the failure of dental implants and cigarette smoking. Int J Oral Maxillofac Implants 1993;8:609–615.

106. Choi NC, Park YC, Lee HA, Lee KJ. Treatment of Class II protrusion with severe crowding using indirect miniscrew anchorage. Angle Orthod 2007;77:1109–1118.

107. Maino BG, Gianelly AA, Bednar J, Mura P, Maino G. MGBM system: New protocol for Class II non extraction treatment without cooperation. Prog Orthod 2007;8:130–143.

108. Jamilian A, Showkatbakhsh R. Treatment of maxillary deficiency by miniscrew implants—A case report. J Orthod 2010;37:56–61.

109. Breuning KH. Correction of a Class III malocclusion with over 20 mm of space to close in the maxilla by using miniscrews for extra anchorage. Am J Orthod Dentofacial Orthop 2008;133:459–469.

110. Lee KJ, Park YC, Park JY, Hwang WS. Miniscrew-assisted nonsurgical palatal expansion before orthognathic surgery for a patient with severe mandibular prognathism. Am J Orthod Dentofacial Orthop 2010;137:830–839.

111. Kang YG, Nam JH, Park YG. Use of rhythmic wire system with miniscrews to correct occlusal-plane canting. Am J Orthod Dentofacial Orthop 2010;137:540–547.

112. Hashimoto T, Fukunaga T, Kuroda S, Sakai Y, Yamashiro T, Takano-Yamamoto T. Mandibular deviation and canted maxillary occlusal plane treated with miniscrews and intraoral vertical ramus osteotomy: Functional and morphologic changes. Am J Orthod Dentofacial Orthop 2009;136:868–877.

113. Jeon YJ, Kim YH, Son WS, Hans MG. Correction of a canted occlusal plane with miniscrews in a patient with facial asymmetry. Am J Orthod Dentofacial Orthop 2006;130:244–252.

114. Park YC, Lee HA, Choi NC, Kim DH. Open bite correction by intrusion of posterior teeth with miniscrews. Angle Orthod 2008;78:699–710.

115. Park HS, Kwon OW, Sung JH. Nonextraction treatment of an open bite with microscrew implant anchorage. Am J Orthod Dentofacial Orthop 2006;130:391–402.

116. Sugawara J, Baik UB, Umemori M, et al. Treatment and posttreatment dentoalveolar changes following intrusion of mandibular molars with application of a skeletal anchorage system (SAS) for open bite correction. Int J Adult Orthodon Orthognath Surg 2002;17:243–253.

117. Deguchi T, Kurosaka H, Oikawa H, et al. Comparison of orthodontic treatment outcomes in adults with skeletal open bite between conventional edgewise treatment and implant-anchored orthodontics. Am J Orthod Dentofacial Orthop 2011;139(4 suppl):S60–S68.

Tiziano Baccetti
DDS, PhD

CHAPTER

9

The Effectiveness of Treatment Procedures for Displaced and Impacted Maxillary Canines

Displacement and Impaction of the Maxillary Permanent Canine

Natural history studies on the prevalence of impacted maxillary canine teeth have estimated that 0.2% to 2.3% of the orthodontic population has at least one impacted maxillary canine.[1] In white populations, approximately 85% of maxillary canine impactions are oriented palatally.[1,2] Palatal maxillary canine impaction is thought to have a genetic etiology.[3] The pathogenesis of palatal canine impaction is characterized by an early developmental stage that can be reversed with treatment. During this stage, the canine is considered a *palatally displaced canine (PDC)* because it presents with an intraosseous palatal displacement prior to the expected time of eruption. If left untreated, PDCs generally progress into *palatally impacted canines (PICs)* after the pubertal growth spurt and require surgical intervention.[4–6] Recent studies reported prevalence rates for impaction of PDCs ranging from 75% to 85%.[7,8] Failure to recognize and treat maxillary canine displacement may result in root resorption of adjacent teeth[9–11] and/or the formation of cysts.[12–14] Furthermore, patients with PDCs that progress to impaction will incur higher treatment costs, more complex treatment plans, and delayed treatment timetables. Palatal impaction of the maxillary permanent canine is the final outcome of a PDC.

While in the past the expected time for canine eruption was correlated to chronologic age (12 years, 3 months in girls; 13 years, 1 month in boys),[2] attention has recently been given to the skeletal maturation of the patient. The maxillary permanent canine can erupt at any prepubertal or pubertal stage of skeletal development until CS5 in cervical vertebral maturation (CVM)[6] (Figs 9-1 and 9-2). Beyond this stage, which occurs on average 1 year after the end of the adolescent growth spurt, a PDC can be defined as a PIC. When the development of the dentition is used to determine the time of emergence of the maxillary permanent canine, delayed dental age is found in association with PDCs.[4]

Buccal displacement of the maxillary permanent canine is less frequent than palatal displacement. It is not associated with a positive family history, and it is mainly the result of a tooth size/arch length discrepancy and/or crowding in the maxillary arch. The identification of risk factors and the treatment planning to intercept the buccal displacement of the canine therefore involve assessment of these tendencies.

This chapter focuses on the evaluation and identification of risk indicators and interceptive treatment options for PDCs, which have been studied extensively with adequate research quality in recent years.

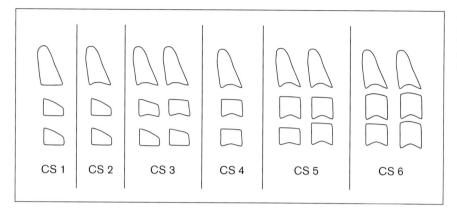

CS 1   CS 2   CS 3   CS 4   CS 5   CS 6

Fig 9-1 Schematic representation of the CVM method. Stages CS1 and CS2 are prepubertal, the pubertal growth spurt occurs between stages CS3 and CS4, and stages CS5 and CS6 are postpubertal.

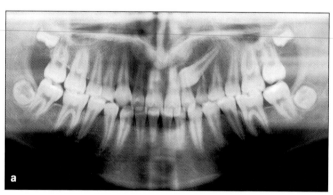
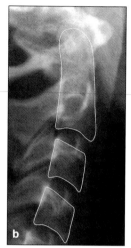

Fig 9-2 *(a)* Panoramic radiograph of a boy aged 12½ years. The maxillary left canine is impacted. *(b)* Diagnosis of impaction is corroborated by the presence of a mature CS5 stage (postpubertal) in the assessment of skeletal maturation by means of the CVM method.

Risk indicators for PDCs in the early mixed dentition

The early diagnosis of dental abnormalities that share a common genetic origin with PDCs (and PICs) can lead to the identification of risk indicators for PDCs. The etiology of PDCs, and subsequent PICs, is associated with a multifactorial genetic complex that controls the expression of other, possibly concurrent, tooth anomalies.[1,15–19] While the gene loci that dictate these anomalies are not yet known, Peck and collaborators[1] have indicated multiple evidential categories for the genetic origin of PDCs, ie, familial occurrence, bilateral occurrence (17% to 45%), sex differences, differences in prevalence rates among different populations, and increased occurrence of other concomitant dental anomalies. Box 9-1 reports the list of dental anomalies that present with a significant association with PDCs and that can be used as risk indicators for the eruption anomaly of the maxillary canine[20] (Fig 9-3).

Once a patient is diagnosed with a PDC (in most instances during the late mixed dentition phase), interceptive measures can be implemented to avoid the final establishment of a PIC. These interceptive measures classically tend to facilitate eruption of the canine by acting on local/mechanical factors that may affect the evolution from PDC to PIC.

The aim of the following sections is to review the effectiveness of alternative interceptive therapies to avoid canine impaction in the presence of a PDC.

Dental anomalies that are significantly associated with PDCs

Small size of maxillary permanent incisors (unilateral or bilateral)

Agenesis of maxillary lateral incisors

Agenesis of maxillary second premolars

Infraocclusion of primary molars

Distal angulation of mandibular second premolars (before their eruption)

Enamel hypoplasia (maxillary central incisors and permanent first molars)

Dental anomalies that are not significantly associated with PDCs

Supernumerary teeth

Ectopic eruption of permanent first molars

Agenesis of permanent third molars

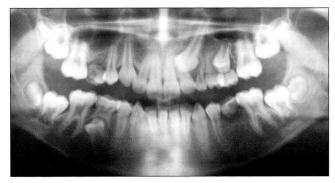

Fig 9-3 Panoramic radiograph of a girl aged 11 years, 3 months reveals several dental anomalies associated with a palatally displaced maxillary left canine: agenesis of the maxillary right second premolar, agenesis of the mandibular left second premolar, and a distally angulated unerupted mandibular right second premolar.

Alternative Treatment Options to Intercept PDCs

As mentioned above, while etiology of PDCs (and subsequent PICs) has been linked to a genetic component, the evolution from PDC to PIC can be affected by local/mechanical factors, which have become the targets of "interceptive treatment" of PDCs in order to prevent the final occurrence of PICs as well as allow the canines to erupt without surgical intervention.

Extraction of the primary canine

The procedure of extracting the corresponding primary canine in order to reduce the prevalence of a PDC from becoming impacted has been present in the dental literature since 1936.[9] The outcomes in several individual cases during the subsequent 50 years corroborated the clinical recommendation for this interceptive measure, as reviewed by Jacobs.[21] The prospective study by Ericson and Kurol[22] in 1988 analyzed the effects of the extraction of the primary canine on PDCs in terms of rate and time of "spontaneous" eruption.[22] A total of 36 out of 46 PDCs (78%) presented with an improvement in the eruption pathway 6 to 12 months after removal of the primary canines. In 1993, after conducting a longitudinal 2-year investigation, Power and Short[23] described the achievement of a normal eruptive position of a PDC in 62% of the cases following the extraction of the primary canine. It should be emphasized

that both the studies by Ericson and Kurol[22] and by Power and Short[23] were conducted before the establishment of a genetic basis for PDCs. Both studies calculated prevalence rates of canine eruption by using the number of erupting individual teeth, which is not recommended because of the genetic etiology of the tooth developmental disorder. In fact, patients with bilateral PDCs should not count as two independent statistical units because the same etiologic factors act on both sides of the maxillary arch. Therefore, individual *subjects* and not individual *teeth* are indicated as statistical units when analyzing data pertaining to PDCs or PICs, in order to avoid inflated prevalence rates. Also, the prevalence rate for successful outcomes indicated by Ericson and Kurol[22] included both PDCs that improved their pathway and PDCs that actually erupted.

A study by Leonardi and associates[24] failed to find extraction of the primary canine to be an effective treatment for PDCs. However, the power of this study was limited, as stated in a more recent study that was represented by a randomized prospective approach to interceptive treatment of PDC with the incorporation of untreated controls and a statistically appropriate number of subjects.[25] In this recent personal investigation, the removal of the primary canine as an isolated measure to intercept palatal displacement of maxillary canines showed a 65.2% prevalence rate of success, which was significantly greater (almost double) than the success rate in untreated controls (36%). The prevalence rate of canine eruption here was calculated on individual subjects, and *eruption* was defined as the time at which a bracket could be placed on the crown of the canine.

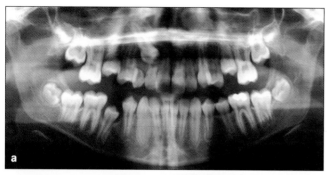

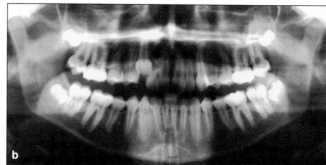

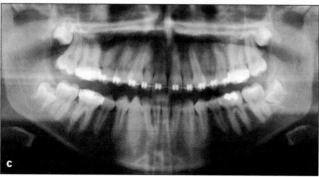

Fig 9-4 *(a)* Panoramic radiograph of a girl aged 11 years, 5 months shows severe displacement of the maxillary right canine in the late mixed dentition. The patient has a Class II tendency and a tendency to a hypodivergent facial pattern. *(b)* Interceptive treatment of canine displacement by means of a maxillary headgear worn at nighttime only for 10 months with light forces (150 g) to avoid the mesial advancement of the maxillary posterior teeth. Note the dramatic change in tooth angulation and favorable eruption pathway achieved after 10 months of interceptive therapy. *(c)* Alignment of the maxillary right canine within the maxillary dental arch during orthodontic finalization with fixed appliances.

Interceptive therapies

In recent years, two randomized controlled trials (RCTs) and one prospective controlled clinical study have evaluated the role of alternative interceptive approaches to PDCs that consisted of extraction of the primary canine in association with the use of either a headgear appliance[24] or a rapid maxillary expander.[7,8,26]

The RCT by Baccetti and associates[25] in 2008 evaluated the effectiveness of primary canine extraction in combination with the nighttime-only use of a cervical headgear (Fig 9-4). The randomized prospective design of the investigation comprised 75 patients with PDCs (92 maxillary canines) who were randomly assigned to three groups: *(1)* extraction of the primary canine only, *(2)* extraction of the primary canine and use of the cervical headgear, and *(3)* the untreated control group. Panoramic radiographs were evaluated at the time of initial observation at an average age of 11.7 years old (T1) and after an average time period of 18 months (T2). At T2, an evaluation of the relative success of canine eruption was performed, with a statistical comparison between the groups. A superimposition study on lateral cephalometric radiographs at T1 and T2 evaluated the changes in the sagittal position of the maxillary molars in the three groups. As previously mentioned, the extraction of the primary canine as an isolated measure to intercept palatal displacement of maxillary canines showed a 65.2% prevalence rate of success, which was significantly greater than the success rate in untreated controls (36%). The nighttime use of a headgear in addition to the extraction of the primary canine was able to induce

successful eruption in 87.5% of the cases, with a significant improvement in the measures for intraosseous canine position. There was no significant difference between the two interceptive approaches regarding the time it took for canine eruption.

The cephalometric superimposition study showed a significant mesial movement of the maxillary first molars in the control group and the extraction only group when compared with the extraction plus headgear group. It appears, therefore, that the main effect of the headgear is to prevent the mesial movement of the posterior segments of the maxillary arch, thus facilitating the maintenance of an eruption pathway for the canine (Fig 9-5). It should be remembered that a nonrandomized retrospective study by Olive[27] in 2002 had already reported the significantly favorable effects of a clinical protocol including the extraction of the primary canine followed by fixed appliance therapy to increase the maxillary arch perimeter.

A second prospective RCT aimed to assess the prevalence rate of eruption of PDCs when diagnosed at an early developmental stage by means of posteroanterior radiographs and consequently treated by rapid maxillary expansion (RME). The trial included 60 patients in the early mixed dentition with PDCs diagnosed on periapical radiographs according to the method by Sambataro and associates.[28] The age range of the patients at first observation (T1) was 7.6 to 9.6 years, with a prepubertal stage of skeletal maturity (CS1 or CS2). The diagnosis of PDCs was performed on posteroanterior lateral cephalometric radiographs because the assessment of PDCs on panoramic radiographs is not reliable at these early ages. The 60 pa-

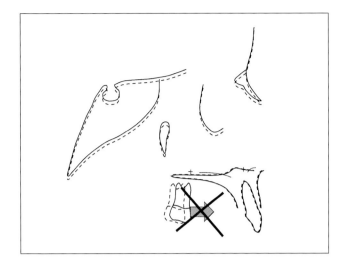

Fig 9-5 Cephalometric superimposition of the longitudinal changes in the average craniofacial configuration of control subjects with PDCs. Without interceptive treatment, the maxillary molars move physiologically in a mesial direction by 2.5 mm, thus jeopardizing space available for the maxillary canine on the maxillary dental arch. Interceptive treatment (headgear or transpalatal arch [TPA]) prevents the mesial movement of the maxillary molars.

tients were randomly allocated to either the treatment group (35 cases) or the control group (25 cases). The treatment group was treated with a banded rapid maxillary expander. At the end of expansion, all patients were retained with the expander in place for 6 months; thereafter the expander was removed, and patients wore a retention plate at night for 1 year. The control group did not receive any treatment. At T2 (early permanent dentition, postpubertal, CS5), all patients were reevaluated. No statistically significant differences were found for any variable at T1. It should be noted that patients with PDCs in the early mixed dentition did not exhibit transverse deficiency of the maxillary arch. Therefore, the transverse features of the maxilla were not related to the etiology of the eruption disorder of the canine, as indicated already by Langberg and Peck.[29] In fact, the indication for RME in the patients enrolled in the clinical study was the presence of a mild to moderate tooth size/arch length discrepancy and/or Class II or Class III tendency, not a transverse maxillary deficiency.

The use of the orthopedic device (rapid maxillary expander) assisted in preventing final impaction of the PDCs during the developmental stages from PDC to PIC. Once again, while a genetic etiology has been postulated for initial palatal displacement of maxillary canines, the pathogenesis of the displacement and of final impaction is related especially to the anatomical complexity of the eruption pathway of this tooth,[30] which can be affected by environmental alterations. The prevalence rate of successful eruption of the maxillary canines was 65.7% in the group treated with RME, while it was only 13.6% in the untreated control group. The comparison was obviously statistically significant and led to the conclusion that the use of a rapid maxillary expander as an early interceptive approach is an effective procedure to increase the rate of eruption of PDCs. The low prevalence rate for spontaneous eruption of canines in the control group is a result of the methodologic aspects of the study, which included patients with not only a diagnosis of PDCs but also a prognosis of PICs, as derived by the analysis of periapical radiographs according to the method by Sambataro et al.[28]

Finally, a prospective controlled clinical trial was aimed to investigate the effect of RME and transpalatal arch (TPA) therapy in combination with primary canine extraction on the eruption rate of PDCs in the late mixed dentition by means of a two-center prospective study. Seventy subjects with PDCs diagnosed on panoramic radiographs were enrolled.[8] The treatment group (40 subjects) underwent RME followed by TPA therapy plus extraction of primary canines. The control group (30 subjects) received no orthodontic treatment. At T2 (CVM stage CS5 or CS6), all patients were reevaluated, and eruption of permanent maxillary canines was assessed. At T1, panoramic radiographs and dental casts were compared between the two groups by means of the Mann-Whitney test ($P < .05$). The prevalence rates of successful cases in the treatment group were compared with those in the control group by means of chi-square tests ($P < .05$). The association of PDCs with other dental anomalies was assessed. The results showed that no statistically significant difference was found for any measurement at T1 between the two groups. The prevalence rate of eruption of the maxillary canines was 80% for the treatment group versus 28% in the control group, a statistically significant difference ($\chi^2 = 16.26$, $P < .001$). The prevalence rate at T1 for pubertal stages of CVM (63%) was significantly greater in unsuccessfully treated cases than in successfully treated cases (16%). In the controls, all successful cases presented PDCs that overlapped the corresponding primary canine or the distal aspect of the lateral incisor. Eruption of PDCs in both the treatment group and the control group was associated significantly with the presence of an open root apex. The conclusions of the study were that RME followed by a TPA combined with extraction of the primary canines is effective in treating patients with PDCs in the late mixed dentition. Predictive pretreatment variables for the success of treatment on the eruption of PDCs included less severe sectors of

Table 9-1 Comparison of the outcomes of studies on interceptive treatment of PDCs

Study	Interceptive treatment	Age at time of interceptive treatment	Prevalence rate of successful canine eruption in treated patients	Prevalence rate of successful canine eruption in untreated control patients
Ericson and Kurol[12] (1988)	Extraction of primary canine alone	10–13 y	78%* (including improvement in eruption pathway)	No controls
Power and Short[23] (1993)	Extraction of primary canine alone	11.2 y ± 1.4 y	62%*	No controls
Olive[27] (2002)	Extraction of primary canine and fixed appliances	11.4–16.1 y	75%*	No controls
Baccetti et al[25] (2008)	Extraction of primary canine alone	11.7 y ± 0.8 y	65.2%[†]	36%
Baccetti et al[25] (2008)	Extraction of primary canine and headgear on maxillary molars (at night)	11.9 y ± 0.9 y	87.5%[†]	36%
Baccetti et al[7] (2009)	RME	7–9 y	65.7%[†]	13.6% (severe PDCs with prediction of impaction)
Sigler et al[8] (2011)	RME and TPA ± extraction of primary canine	10.6 y ± 0.9 y (late mixed dentition)	80%[†]	28%
Baccetti et al[26] (2011)	TPA and extraction of primary canine	10.8 y ± 0.9 y (late mixed dentition)	79%[†]	28%

*Based on the number of teeth.
[†]Based on the number of patients.

displacement, prepubertal stages of skeletal maturity, and an open root apex of PDCs. Several dental anomalies were associated significantly with PDCs, thus confirming the genetic etiology of this eruption disturbance.

RME treatment shows a rate of effectiveness (65.7%) similar to those described for extraction of the primary canines alone (78% according to Ericson and Kurol,[22] including improvement of the eruption path; 62% according to Power and Short[23]; 65.2% according to Baccetti et al[25]) or in combination with fixed appliances (75% according to Olive[27]) but smaller than the prevalence rate for eruption of the canines following the nighttime use of a cervical headgear (87.5% according Baccetti et al[25]) or the use of RME and TPA therapy in the late mixed dentition (80%). Recent unpublished data suggest that the use of a TPA in combination with the extraction of the primary canine may provide very similar results (79% of canine eruption) in cases that do not require maxillary expansion[26] (Table 9-1).

Clinical considerations and critical approach

Several considerations need to be made when evaluating the outcomes of the alternative interceptive treatment approaches to PDCs. First of all, the extraction of the primary canine alone, though less effective than the same procedure in combination with headgear or RME appliances, presents also with a significantly smaller "burden of treatment" for the patient. The same can be affirmed for the use of a TPA in conjunction with the extraction of the primary canine. Also, the extraction of the primary canine alone presents with the same effectiveness in preventing a PIC as RME therapy performed in the early mixed dentition (when the diagnosis of PDCs is less reliable). Obviously, patients showing an indication for the use of orthodontic forces to distalize maxillary molars (patients with a Class II or end-to-end malocclusion or patients with a tendency to crowding of the maxillary arch) will benefit from the combined treatment (extraction of the primary canine and headgear) both in terms of correction of their malocclusions and improvement in the probability of canine eruption.

Secondly, when tested at an early developmental age (7 to 9 years old), the RME approach resulted in less favorable results compared with when it was used in the late mixed dentition. This dentitional stage in combination with a prepubertal stage of skeletal maturation and an open apex of the PDC appears to be the most effective time at which to perform either of these interceptive treatments. Moreover, once again, before 10 years of age (in the early mixed dentition), the diagnosis of PDCs on periapical radiographs can be effectively carried out only in cases with severe displacement of the canine toward the midfacial structures. PDCs can be diagnosed more accurately in the late mixed dentition.

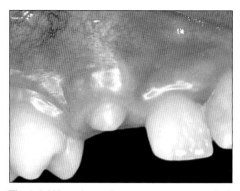

Fig 9-6 When the canine erupts spontaneously, it ideally erupts at the center of the alveolar ridge so that some attached gingiva is present on both the palatal and buccal sides of the tooth.

Orthodontic-Surgical Approach to Impacted Canines

When interceptive treatment of displaced canines, both buccal and palatal, is not successful, or when the patient comes under observation too late to attempt interceptive approaches to the displaced tooth or teeth, orthodontic-surgical repositioning of the impacted canine is required. The following sections review the factors predicting the outcomes of this type of therapy, with special regard to the use of a surgical procedure (the "tunnel technique") aimed to provide the repositioned canine with periodontal health in the long term by reproducing the physiologic eruption of the canine at the center of the alveolar ridge so that an adequate amount of attached gingiva is present on both the buccal and palatal sides of the tooth (Fig 9-6).

Factors predicting the outcomes of orthodontic-surgical repositioning

A specific study was conducted by Baccetti et al[30] to evaluate the influence of pretreatment radiographic features (angulation, distance from the occlusal plane, and sector of displacement) on the duration of active orthodontic traction of impacted maxillary canines treated by a combined surgical (flap approach) and orthodontic (direct traction to the center of the ridge) treatment. A study population of 168 patients (168 canines) was evaluated. Multiple regression analysis was used. Pretreatment radiographic variables were associated significantly with the duration of orthodontic traction, while the sex of the patient and the site of impaction did not affect the duration of traction significantly. Age (older than 20 years) may play negatively in terms of final outcomes of therapy.

Angulation, distance from the occlusal plane, and sector of displacement appeared as valid indicators for the duration of orthodontic traction. For every 5 degrees of initial angulation, 1 more week of traction can be expected; for every 1 mm of distance from the occlusal plane, 1 more week of traction can be expected; for canines impacted in a zone apparently overlapping the central incisor in the panoramic radiograph, 6 more weeks of traction can be expected with regard to a more favorable sector of displacement.

The "tunnel technique"

In 1994, Crescini et al[31] proposed in the international literature the very favorable orthodontic and periodontal results of the "tunnel technique" in repositioning impacted canines. A surgical-orthodontic procedure was used to treat deep infraosseous impacted canines (test teeth) associated with the persistence of the primary tooth in 15 patients who had the contralateral canine normally erupted (control teeth). The periodontal outcome was evaluated at the end of the orthodontic treatment and 3 years later. In the "tunnel technique" (Fig 9-7), after extraction of the primary canine, a mucoperiosteal flap was raised on the buccal (seven cases) or palatal (eight cases) aspect to expose the cusp of the impacted tooth. The empty socket of the primary tooth was extended to reach the impacted cusp and to form an osseous tunnel. A chain was passed through the tunnel and fixed to a bonded device on the impacted cusp. The flap was sutured back into its original position. The chain was used for traction to the impacted canine toward the center of the alveolar ridge. No attachment loss and no recession were observed at the end of the active therapy or 3 years later. No significant differences in keratinized tissue width were observed between test and control teeth at the follow-up examination.

The purpose of a further study by Crescini et al[32] was to evaluate the periodontal variables of impacted maxillary canines that were treated with a combined surgical and orthodontic approach aimed at reproducing the physiologic eruption pattern of a larger number of canines with re-

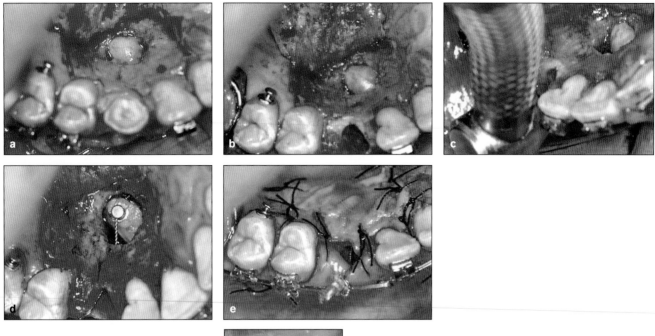

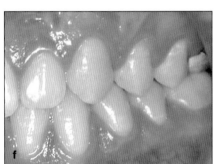

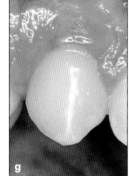

Fig 9-7 Surgical phases of the "tunnel technique" to reposition a palatally impacted canine and final outcomes. *(a)* The persistence of the primary canine can be very useful, allowing the option of the "tunnel technique." *(b)* Once the full-thickness flap is created and elevated, the primary canine is extracted and a bony tunnel is performed in order to reach the exposed crown of the impacted canine. *(c)* Creation of the tunnel. *(d)* Bonded attachment for orthodontic traction by means of a metal chain that passes through the tunnel. *(e)* The flap is sutured, and orthodontic traction is initiated with the final goal of "pulling" the canine to the center of the alveolar ridge, like pulling up a bucket in a well. *(f and g)* Final results with the canine well aligned and with a very natural-looking gingival tissue on the buccal side.

spect to the original report. Twenty-five patients who presented with unilateral impacted maxillary canines were consecutively enrolled (age range, 13.2 to 23.2 years). They were treated with a surgical flap and orthodontic traction directed to the center of the crest and were evaluated periodontally at the end of treatment and again at a follow-up visit (2 to 5 years posttreatment). Pocket depth, keratinized tissue width, and gingival recession were recorded. At the end of orthodontic treatment, all 25 treated canines presented with normal pocket depth (2.0 ± 0.3 mm) and a normal amount of keratinized tissue (5.0 ± 1.2 mm). No sites showed gingival recession. At the follow-up visit, both pocket depths and keratinized tissues were slightly reduced. The combined technique permits traction of the impacted canines to the center of the crest, simulating the physiologic eruption pattern and resulting in correct alignment and good periodontal status.

Summary Points

- Palatal displacement of the canine is the developmental antecedent of palatal impaction.
- Skeletal maturation (by means of the CVM method) can assist in the determination of the evolution from PDCs to PICs: The canine is impacted when it is still in an intraosseous position at CS5 or beyond this stage (2 or more years after the adolescent growth spurt). If not intercepted with early treatment modalities, PDCs develop into PICs in two out of three cases.
- Different interceptive approaches to PDCs (headgear, RME, RME/headgear, RME/TPA, TPA) are able to promote eruption of the displaced canine with a success rate that ranges from two to three times the rate shown by untreated controls (up to almost 90% of the cases), as assessed in several evidence-based investigations. In-

terceptive treatment of PDCs to avoid PICs is therefore clinically recommended.

- Interceptive treatment approaches are indicated in the late mixed dentition, before CS4, and before the apex of the displaced canine is completely formed.

- When the orthodontic-surgical repositioning of an impacted canine is required, the "tunnel technique" is an easy, predictable procedure to bring the impacted tooth to the center of the alveolar ridge, thus reproducing natural eruption and warranting an adequate amount of keratinized gingiva surrounding the repositioned canine. For this reason, the presence of the primary canine on the maxillary dental arch can be a valid option facilitating the tunnel procedure.

- Factors influencing the outcomes of orthodontic-surgical repositioning of the impacted canine include the age of the patient and especially the radiographic pretreatment characteristics that describe the canine malposition (angulation, distance from the occlusal plane, and sector of displacement).

References

1. Peck S, Peck L, Kataja M. The palatally displaced canine as a dental anomaly of genetic origin. Angle Orthod 1994;64:249–256.
2. Hurme V. Range of normalcy in the eruption of permanent teeth. J Dent Child 1949;16:11–15.
3. Pirinen S, Arte S, Apajalahti S. Palatal displacement of canine is genetic and related to congenital absence of teeth. J Dent Res 1996;75:1742–1746.
4. Becker A, Chaushu S. Dental age in maxillary canine ectopia. Am J Orthod Dentofacial Orthop 2000;117:657–662.
5. Baccetti T, Franchi L, McNamara JA Jr. The Cervical Vertebral Maturation Method for the assessment of optimal treatment timing in dentofacial orthopedics. Semin Orthod 2005;11:119–129.
6. Baccetti T, Franchi L, De Lisa S, Giuntini V. Eruption of the maxillary canines in relation to skeletal maturity. Am J Orthod Dentofacial Orthop 2008;133:748–751.
7. Baccetti T, Mucedero M, Leonardi M, Cozza P. Interceptive treatment of palatal impaction of maxillary canines with rapid maxillary expansion: A randomized clinical trial. Am J Orthod Dentofacial Orthop 2009;136:657–661.
8. Sigler LM, Baccetti T, McNamara JA Jr. Effect of rapid maxillary expansion and transpalatal arch treatment associated with deciduous canine extraction on the eruption of palatally displaced canines: A 2-center prospective study. Am J Orthod Dentofacial Orthop 2011;139:e235–e244.
9. Buchner HJ. Root resorption caused by ectopic eruption of maxillary cuspid. Int J Orthod 1936;22:1236–1237.
10. Hoffmeister H. Undermining resorption of the second deciduous molar by the permanent molars as a microsymptom of hereditary dentition disorders [in German]. Schweiz Monatsschr Zahnmed 1985;95:151–154.
11. Ericson S, Kurol J. Radiographic examination of ectopically erupting maxillary canines. Am J Orthod Dentofacial Orthop 1987;91:483–492.
12. Ericson S, Kurol J. Resorption of maxillary lateral incisors caused by ectopic eruption of the canines: A clinical and radiographic analysis of predisposing factors. Am J Orthod Dentofacial Orthop 1988;94:503–513.
13. Alling CC, Helfrick JF, Alling RD. Impacted maxillary teeth. In: Impacted Teeth. Philadelphia: WB Saunders, 1993:247–269.
14. Hyomoto M, Kawakami M, Inoue M, Kirita T. Clinical conditions for eruption of maxillary canines and mandibular premolars associated with dentigerous cysts. Am J Orthod Dentofacial Orthop 2003;124:515–520.
15. Bjerklin K, Kurol J, Valentin J. Ectopic eruption of maxillary first permanent molars and association with other tooth and developmental disturbances. Eur J Orthod 1992;14:369–375.
16. Baccetti T. An analysis of the prevalence of isolated dental anomalies and of those associated with hereditary syndromes: A model for evaluating the genetic control of the dentition characteristics [in Italian]. Minerva Stomatol 1993;42:281–294.
17. Sacerdoti R, Baccetti T. Dentoskeletal features associated with unilateral or bilateral palatal displacement of maxillary canines. Angle Orthod 2004;74:725–732.
18. Leifert S, Jonas IE. Dental anomalies as a microsymptom of palatal canine displacement. J Orofac Orthop 2003;64:108–120.
19. Shalish M, Chaushu S, Wasserstein A. Malposition of unerupted mandibular second premolar in children with palatally displaced canines. Angle Orthod 2009;79:796–799.
20. Baccetti T. A controlled study of associated dental anomalies. Angle Orthod 1998;68:267–274.
21. Jacobs SG. Reducing the incidence of unerupted palatally displaced canines by extraction of primary canines. The history and application of this procedure with some case reports. Aust Dent J 1998;43:20–27.
22. Ericson S, Kurol J. Early treatment of palatally erupting maxillary canines by extraction of the primary canines. Eur J Orthod 1988;10:283–295.
23. Power SM, Short MB. An investigation into the response of palatally displaced canines to the removal of primary canines and an assessment of factors contributing to favourable eruption. Br J Orthod 1993;20:215–223.
24. Leonardi M, Armi P, Franchi L, Baccetti T. Two interceptive approaches to palatally displaced canines: A prospective longitudinal study. Angle Orthod 2004;75:581–586.
25. Baccetti T, Leonardi M, Armi P. A randomized clinical study of two interceptive approaches to palatally displaced canines. Eur J Orthod 2008;30:381–385.
26. Baccetti T, Sigler LM, McNamara JA Jr. An RCT on treatment of palatally displaced canines with RME and/or a transpalatal arch. Eur J Orthod 2011;33:601–607.
27. Olive RJ. Orthodontic treatment of palatally impacted maxillary canines. Aust Orthod J 2002;18:64–70.
28. Sambataro S, Baccetti T, Franchi L, Antonini F. Early predictive variables for upper canine impaction as derived from posteroanterior cephalograms. Angle Orthod 2005;75:28–34.
29. Langberg BJ, Peck S. Adequacy of maxillary dental arch width in patients with palatally displaced canines. Am J Orthod Dentofacial Orthop 2000;118:220–223.
30. Baccetti T, Crescini A, Nieri M, Rotundo R, Pini Prato GP. Orthodontic treatment of impacted maxillary canines: An appraisal of prognostic factors. Prog Orthod 2007;8:6–15.
31. Crescini A, Clauser C, Giorgetti R, Cortellini P, Pini Prato GP. Tunnel traction of infraosseous impacted maxillary canines. A three-year periodontal follow-up. Am J Orthod Dentofacial Orthop 1994;105:61–72.
32. Crescini A, Nieri M, Rotundo R, Baccetti T, Cortellini P, Prato GP. Combined surgical and orthodontic approach to reproduce the physiologic eruption pattern in impacted canines: Report of 25 patients. Int J Periodontics Restorative Dent 2007;27:529–537.

M. Ali Darendeliler
BDS, PhD, Dip Orth, Certif Orth,
Priv Doc, MRACD (Ortho)

Lam L. Cheng
BDSc, MDSc, MOrth RCS (Ed),
MRACD (Ortho)

CHAPTER

10

Orthodontically Induced Inflammatory Root Resorption

Introduction

Orthodontically induced inflammatory root resorption (OIIRR) is an unavoidable side effect of orthodontic treatment. It is a pathologic process that is related to the local injury of the periodontal ligament (PDL) and resorption of cementum and dentin that occurs in association with the removal of hyalinized tissue during tooth movement.[1,2] The severity of OIIRR is unpredictable. It occurs in all orthodontic patients, but only about 1% to 5% of treated individuals have greater than 4 mm of root resorption.[3,4] Fortunately, there is a reparative process in the periodontium, which commences when the applied orthodontic force is discontinued or reduced below a certain level.[5,6] This healing process can occur as early as the first week of retention following orthodontic treatment and increases over time.[7–9] There are biologic and mechanical factors that influence the severity of OIIRR. Mechanical causative factors can be controlled by the clinician to minimize the adverse effects of OIIRR and allow initiation of repair. It is important to know these causative factors because in cases of severe OIIRR, the crown-to-root ratio of the affected dentition can be significantly altered. This will pose limitations to future dental treatment options, particularly in regard to coexisting periodontal disease or trauma. This chapter focuses on research evidence that shows how mechanical factors affect the severity of OIIRR and possible strategies to control these factors. In addition, clinical implications and preventive measures for OIIRR are evaluated.

Factors Affecting OIIRR

OIIRR can be influenced by biologic and/or mechanical factors (Box 10-1). However, biologic factors are not within the control of the clinician. Some of these factors are genetic, while others are environmental. Mechanical factors, on the other hand, are attributed to the nature of the orthodontic appliance and can be controlled by both the clinician and the patient.

Physical Properties of Cementum in OIIRR

Cementum at the cervical and middle thirds of the root has greater hardness and elastic modulus than that of the apical third[10,11] (Fig 10-1). This is because of the variable mineral content of cellular and acellular cementum. It has also been found that hardness is positively correlated to the amount of mineralization.[10,11] Hence, OIIRR is typically found to more severely affect the apical part of the tooth roots. Chutimanutskul et al[12] conducted a study that assessed the relationship between the magnitude of orthodontic forces and physical properties of the human cementum. This study revealed that the mean hardness and elastic modulus of cementum was greater in the light force group than the heavy force group. The mean hardness and

Box 10-1	Factors influencing the extent of OIIRR

Biologic factors

Genetic factors

Environmental factors

Systemic factors

- Asthma and allergy
- Endocrine and hormone imbalance
- Alcohol
- Nutrition
- Drugs
- Psychologic stress
- Chronologic age
- Dental age
- Sex

Local factors

- Habits
- History of trauma
- Density and turnover of alveolar bone
- Types of malocclusion
- Hypofunctional periodontium
- Occlusal trauma
- Missing teeth
- Tooth type
- Dental invagination
- Abnormal root morphology
- Root resorption prior to orthodontic treatment
- Previous endodontic treatment

Mechanical factors

Treatment duration

Distance of tooth movement

Magnitude of orthodontic force

Orthodontic appliance (removable versus fixed) and technique (different bracket systems)

Force direction (tip, rotation, torque, translation)

Duration of force application (continuous versus intermittent)

Extraction versus nonextraction therapy

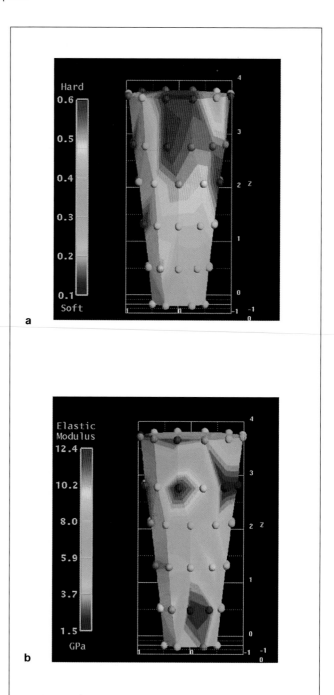

Fig 10-1 Color-coded three-dimensional maps of cementum hardness (a) and elasticity (b).

elastic modulus of cementum gradually decreased from the cervical to the apical regions. This study concluded that the hardness and elastic modulus of cementum were affected by the application of orthodontic forces.

Rex et al[13] studied the mineral composition (calcium, phosphorus, and fluoride) of human premolar cementum following the application of orthodontic forces. The results showed limited change in the mineral composition of cementum after the application of light force. There was a trend toward an increase in the calcium and phosphorus concentrations of cementum at various areas of PDL compression. The application of heavy force caused a significant decrease in the calcium concentration of cementum at certain areas of PDL tension. Although there was a trend toward a decreasing flouride content in cementum with the application of orthodontic forces, definitive conclusions could not be made because of the large interindividual variation in the flouride content.

Mechanical Factors

Orthodontic tooth movement and biomechanics have been found to account for approximately one-tenth to one-third of the total variation in OIIRR.[14,15] One study showed that up to 90% of variation can be attributed to the extent of tooth movement.[16]

Magnitude of applied force

Many animal studies[17–19] and human studies[20–24] have found that the force magnitude is directly proportional to the severity of OIIRR. Heavy force induces excessive hyalinization and interferes with the repair process of resorption craters.[5,18,24–27] Three-dimensional (3D) quantitative studies on human maxillary first premolars, one comparing 25 g to 225 g of buccal force in a scanning electron microscopy (SEM) stereoimaging study and one comparing 25 g to 225 g of intrusive force in a micro-computed tomography (micro-CT) study, found an increased amount of OIIRR with an increased force level.[28,29]

On the other hand, Owman-Moll et al[30,31] claimed that root resorption was not force dependent. They compared the effects of two controlled, continuous forces of 50 cN (1 cN = about 1 gram) and 100 cN on tooth movement and root resorption. The severity of root resorption, which was measured as the extension and depth of resorbed root contour and size of root area on histologic sections, did not differ significantly when the applied force was doubled to 100 cN or when the force was fourfold larger (200 cN). These studies have been criticized by Weltman et al[32] because the accuracy of the serial sectioning protocol to identify and measure the resorption craters on histologic slides was questionable. In addition, the selection criteria for the studies' premolars were not strict; therefore, other external factors may have predisposed the experimental teeth to OIIRR.

Treatment duration

Most studies support the finding that the severity of OIIRR is directly related to the duration of orthodontic treatment.[33–41] Only a limited number of studies do not support this finding.[42,43]

Paetyangkul et al[44] used micro-CT analysis to quantitatively compare the degree of OIIRR resulting from buccally directed force (both light [25 g] and heavy [225 g]) for 4, 8, and 12 weeks. The amounts of OIIRR from 4 and 8 weeks of light force were similar. However, when light force was applied for 12 weeks, there was a significant increase in the amount of OIIRR (Fig 10-2). There was also a statistically significant increase in the amount of OIIRR in the heavy force group between 4, 8, and 12 weeks. Therefore, the treatment duration is an important influence: The longer the force application, the more severe the OIIRR.

Artun et al[45] evaluated standardized periapical radiographs of the maxillary incisors taken before treatment (T1) and at about 6 and 12 months after bracket placement (T2 and T3, respectively) of 2,467 patients. The risk of one or more teeth undergoing more than 1.0 mm of resorption from T2 to T3 was 3.8 times higher than that from T1 to T2.

Smale et al[46] radiographically assessed the amount of apical root resorption on average 6 months after initiation of fixed orthodontic appliance therapy. The results showed that root resorption began in the early leveling stages of orthodontic treatment. About 4.1% of the patients studied had an average resorption of ≥ 1.5 mm in the maxillary incisors, and about 15.5% had one or more maxillary incisors with resorption of ≥ 2.0 mm from 3 to 9 months after initiation of fixed appliance therapy.

In a randomized clinical trial study, Brin et al[47] compared the amount of OIIRR in cases of Class II malocclusion treated with one phase or two phases of treatment. The results showed that 11% of central incisors and 14% of lateral incisors demonstrated moderate to severe OIIRR (ie, 2 mm). The proportion of incisors with moderate to severe OIIRR was slightly greater in the one phase treatment group. Significant associations existed among OIIRR, the magnitude of overjet reduction, and the fixed orthodontic appliance treatment time.

Distance of tooth movement

The severity of OIIRR has been shown to be positively related to the distance of tooth movement.[40,43,48–50] The maxillary incisors are commonly moved the greatest distance and are therefore at the highest risk of OIIRR.[40,48,49,51,52]

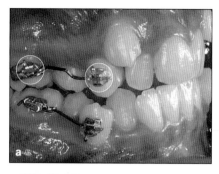
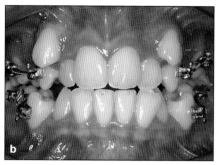
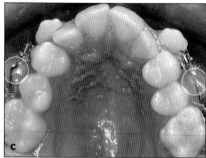
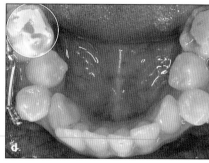

Fig 10-2 *(a to d)* Clinical experimental setup for evaluating the amount of root resorption following 4, 8, and 12 weeks of light and heavy orthodontic force. *(e)* Box-plot displaying a statistically significant difference in OIIRR between 4, 8, and 12 weeks of orthodontic force. A statistically significant difference was also found between 4 and 8 weeks of heavy orthodontic force. NS—not statistically significant. *(f)* Micro-CT image of a premolar root displaying resorption craters following 12 weeks of heavy force.

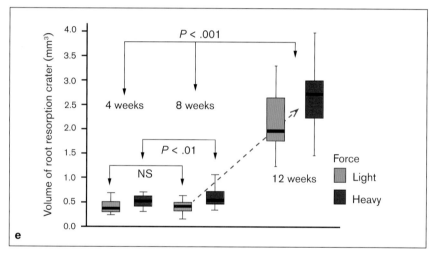

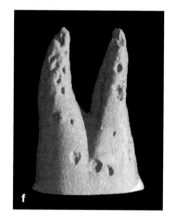

Different appliances and treatment techniques

Numerous studies have compared the extent of OIIRR following treatment with different types of orthodontic appliances. Most of the studies found no statistically significant difference among various orthodontic appliances (eg, Tweed, Begg, edgewise, and self-ligating systems).[16,33,53] This could be the result of individual variation. It is also difficult to utilize split-mouth designs in these comparative studies because malocclusion on one side differs from that on the other.

In contrast, some radiographic studies have shown significant differences between different orthodontic techniques. McNab et al[54] found more OIIRR in patients treated with Begg appliances compared with those treated with edgewise appliances, probably because of the excessive lingualization of the maxillary incisor root by torquing force at the end of the third stage of the Begg technique. This tipping style of mechanics followed by uprighting to obtain torque would result in round tripping of the apex. Janson et al[55] compared OIIRR after orthodontic treatment with three different fixed appliance techniques: the standard edgewise technique, the edgewise straight-wire system, and bioefficient therapy. The bioefficient therapy resulted in less root resorption compared with the other techniques. It was suggested that this is because of the use of heat-activated and superelastic wires, a different bracket design, and smaller rectangular stainless steel wires during incisor retraction and finishing.

Sequential aligners are becoming a more popular treatment alternative, especially in the adult population. Barbagallo et al[56] compared the amount of OIIRR associated with a buccally directed movement with clear sequential thermoplastic aligners and fixed orthodontic appliances for an 8-week period. The degree of OIIRR from clear sequential thermoplastic aligners was comparable to that of a light buccally directed force of 25 g. The heavy force of 225 g from fixed orthodontic appliances induced twice as much OIIRR as the light force of 25 g. Removable appliances are usually considered less detrimental in terms of creating OIIRR because of the intermittent force used.[57,58] However, frequent removal and replacement of the appliance in the mouth generates jiggling forces, which can increase the amount of OIIRR to the same extent as that of wearing elastics.[57]

Skeletal anchorage and miniscrews can be used as an adjunct to orthodontic treatment. Careful placement of the skeletal anchorage and miniscrew is necessary to avoid damage to the root structure and minimize discomfort for the patient. Several studies have investigated the tissue responses following intentional placement of miniscrews on root surfaces and have found that the cementum regenerated after miniscrews were removed.[59–62] Dao et al[61] also found that in cases of severe injury from miniscrews, ankylosis can occur with root fragmentation. Cementum repair was also found in cases in which the tooth had tipped in contact with the miniscrew.[63]

Intermittent versus continuous force

There are conflicting reports as to whether continuous or intermittent force produces a difference in the amount of OIIRR. A pause in tooth movement allows the resorbed cementum to heal, which may produce less root resorption.[64–69] A number of studies with varying durations and frequencies of interruption in the applied forces have led to varied results.

Reitan[6,70,71] advocated the use of intermittent forces to prevent the development of root resorption by allowing reparative processes to occur during periods with little or no force. Using this approach in an animal experiment, Rygh and Brudvik[72] showed an association between the duration of both the root resorptive process and force and the presence of necrotic tissue in the PDL.

Levander et al[65] radiographically evaluated the effect of a 2- to 3-month pause in treatment on teeth in which OIIRR was discovered after an initial treatment period of 6 months with fixed appliances. The amount of root resorption was significantly less in patients treated with a pause compared to those treated without interruption. The inter-

mission of the forces facilitated reorganization of damaged periodontal tissue and reduced root shortening. Maltha and Dijkman[66] compared the amount of root resorption after continuous (24 hours per day) and discontinuous (16 hours per day) force application in dogs and reported more resorption when continuous forces were used. Acar et al[64] also compared the effects of continuous and discontinuous force application on root resorption. The degree of root blunting was assessed by visual scoring on composite electron micrographs. It was discovered that the mean percentage of resorption-affected areas was smaller and apical blunting was less severe under the discontinuous force. Weiland[69] compared the amount of root resorption effected by constant and dissipating forces. Constant force was induced by a superelastic wire for 12 weeks, whereas dissipating forces were induced by stainless steel wire that was activated every 4 weeks. The volume of resorption craters was measured using 3D digital images made with a confocal laser-scanning microscope. The results showed that the resorption craters on the teeth receiving constant force were 140% greater than those on the teeth receiving dissipating forces. Kameyama et al[73] examined the effects of inactive periods of force on the amount of root resorption during experimental tooth movement in rats. The area of root resorption in the groups receiving 4 and 9 hours of inactivation per day was significantly less than that in the groups receiving 0 and 1 hour of inactivation per day. This was the result of a decrease in mechanical stress and hyalinized tissue, recovery of form and function of the blood vessels, reduction of cytokine production, and subsequent odontoclast formation. Kumasako-Haga et al[74] also found that intermittent forces (8 hours a day) are biologically better than continuous orthodontic forces.

On the other hand, Owman-Moll et al[75] compared the effects of continuous (24 hours per day) and interrupted continuous (interrupted 1 week every 4 weeks) forces in adolescents and reported no difference in the amount or severity of root resorption. Once again, Weltman et al[32] criticized this study because the springs used in the continuous force group showed force decay. Therefore, the results should be interpreted with caution.

If, in fact, intermittent forces result in less OIIRR than continuous force, how often should the force application be paused? The micro-CT studies carried out by Ballard et al[76] and Aras et al[77] utilized the same experimental design but different intermittent force application schemes (Table 10-1). In the study by Ballard et al,[76] continuous buccally directed forces were applied for 14 days followed by 6 weeks of continuous or intermittent force of 225 g. The intermittent force scheme entailed 3 days of rest followed by 4 days of force application. The results showed that the intermittent orthodontic forces caused less OIIRR than continuous forces. However, this intermittent scheme is not clinically practical and less efficient in orthodontic tooth movement. A more recent study by Aras et al[77] compared two different intermittent schemes with a continuous force. Group 1 compared the difference between continuous and intermittent force (150 g) of 11 days of

Table 10-1 Amount of OIIRR with intermittent and continuous forces of varying schemes

Force application scheme	Force level	Difference in OIIRR between intermittent and continuous forces
4 days on, 3 days off	225 cN	Less with intermittent force
11 days on, 3 days off	150 cN	No difference
18 days on, 3 days off	150 cN	Less with intermittent force

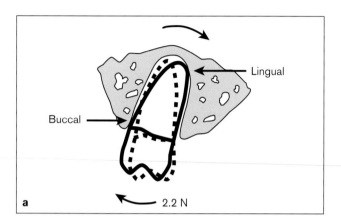

Fig 10-3 *(a)* Schematic tooth diagram showing the movement of a premolar subjected to buccally directed force. *(b)* Finite element mapping of the stressed area on a tooth root following buccally directed orthodontic force.

Lingual

Buccal

2.2 N

a

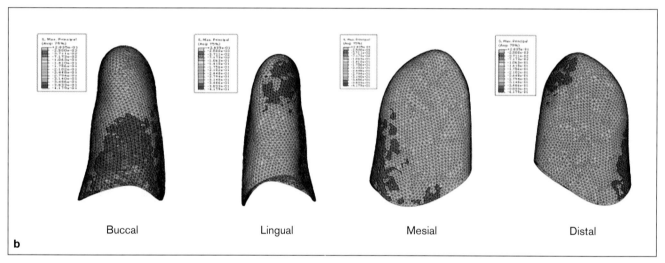

| Buccal | Lingual | Mesial | Distal |

b

force application and 3 days of rest. Group 2 compared the difference between continuous and intermittent force (150 g) of 18 days of force application and 3 days of rest. The results showed similar amounts of OIIRR between the continuous and intermittent force group for the 11/3–day scheme. The intermittent force group also produced less tooth movement. Therefore, this scheme is deemed clinically inefficient and not biologically beneficial. The 18/3–day scheme, on the other hand, produced statistically significantly less OIIRR compared with the continuous force. Even though the continuous force causes more resorptive effect, however, it is more effective at tooth movement than the intermittent force.

Direction of force

The type and direction of tooth movement have a considerable role in OIIRR. Generally, the distribution of root resorption is dictated by the pressure zone created by different types of tooth movement (Fig 10-3). However, OIIRR tends to occur preferentially in the apical region for the following reasons:

• The force concentrates at the root apex because orthodontic tooth movement is not entirely translatory and the fulcrum of force is usually occlusal to the apical half of the root.[78]

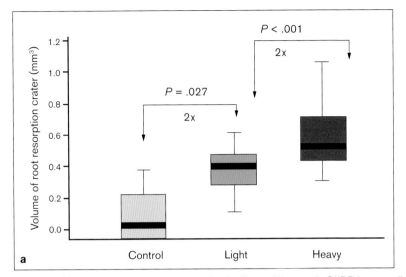
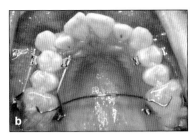
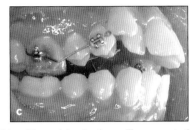

Fig 10-4 *(a)* Box-plot displaying a statistically significant difference in OIIRR between light and heavy intrusive force. The amount of root resorption resulting from heavy intrusive force was twice as much as that from light intrusive force. The control group also displayed some degree of physiologic root resorption. *(b)* Occlusal view of the experimental setup. *(c)* Buccal view of the experimental setup showing the intrusion spring.

- The orientation of the periodontal fibers in the apical end is different, which increases the stress in the region.[79]
- More friable acellular cementum covers the apical third of the root, which can be easily injured.[14,78,79]

It is expected that intrusion and torque have a higher force per unit area and thus cause more tissue necrosis and OIIRR.[6] Some authors suggest that less root resorption is associated with bodily movement than with tipping because of the different stress distribution.[6,68]

Intrusion

Harris et al[29] compared the amount of OIIRR between light (25 g) and heavy (225 g) intrusive forces for 4 weeks. The results showed that light intrusion induced a significantly higher degree of OIIRR than the control group of no force. The heavy intrusion force also induced significantly more root resorption than the light force and control group (almost two and four times as much, respectively) (Fig 10-4). Because of the nature of the intrusive force, with force concentration at the root tip, the apical part of the tooth should be more affected by OIIRR. This study found a trend toward greater root resorption in the apical third of the tooth, with the mesioapical and distoapical surfaces having significantly greater resorption volumes compared with the other regions of the tooth roots.

Clinically, McFadden et al[39] looked at retrospective data of 38 patients with deep bite who were treated with utility arches to intrude incisors, and they reported an average root shortening of 1.84 mm for maxillary incisors and 0.61 mm for mandibular incisors with no significant correlation between resorption and the amount of intrusion. Melsen et al[80] investigated the degree of root resorption after intrusion of incisors in adult patients with marginal bone loss. The results showed that root resorption varied from 1 to 3 mm.

Extrusion

Jiménez et al[81] investigated the impact of 4 weeks of light (25 g) and heavy (225 g) extrusive forces on OIIRR. The results showed that heavy extrusive forces caused significantly more root resorption than light extrusive forces (Fig 10-5). Han et al[82] compared the amount of root resorption in the same individual after application of continuous intrusive and extrusive forces using SEM. The study showed that intrusion of teeth caused about four times more root resorption than extrusion. In addition, Weekes and Wong[83] observed root resorption at the interproximal region of the cervical third of the root after extrusion, indicating that orthodontic extrusion is not without risk.

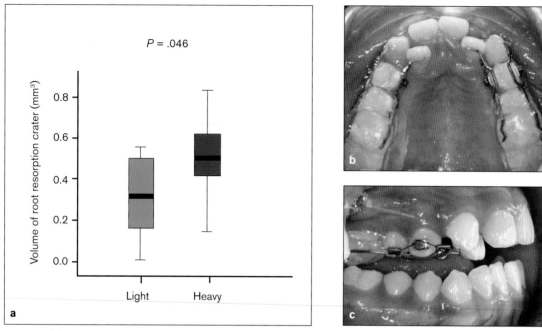

Fig 10-5 *(a)* Box-plot displaying a statistically significant difference in OIIRR between light and heavy extrusive force. *(b)* Occlusal view of the experimental setup. *(c)* Buccal view of the experimental setup showing the extrusion spring.

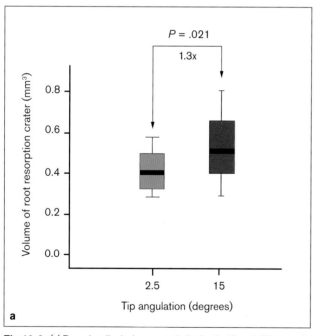

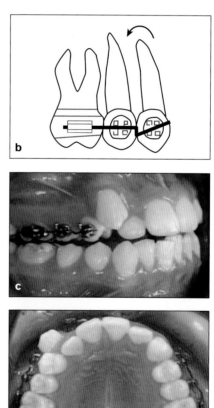

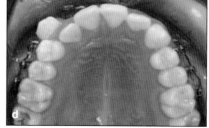

Fig 10-6 *(a)* Box-plot displaying no statistically significant difference in OIIRR between 2.5- and 15-degree distal tipping force. *(b)* Schematic diagram showing the distal tipping force exerted by the wire. *(c)* Buccal view of the experimental setup showing the tipping spring. *(d)* Occlusal view of the experimental setup.

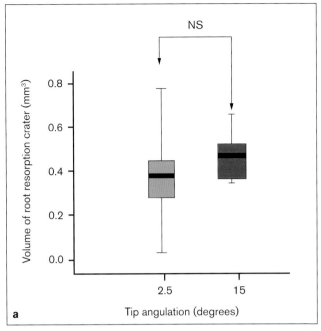
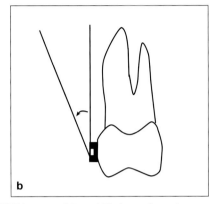

Fig 10-7 *(a)* Box-plot displaying no statistically significant difference in OIIRR between 2.5- and 15-degree buccal torque force. NS—not statistically significant. *(b)* Schematic diagram showing the buccal torque exerted by the wire.

Tip

Several micro-CT studies have compared the amount of root resorption between light and heavy buccally directed tipping force.[44,56,84] All experiments have shown that heavy forces create more severe root resorption craters. The crater distribution was usually at the buccal cervical region and also the lingual apical region. This indicates the location of the pressure zones on the periodontium when buccally directed force was induced.

King et al[85] explored the amount of root resorption in the mesiodistal tipping direction. The study compared the severity of root resorption quantitatively by inducing 2.5 degrees of distal tip in one experimental group and 15 degrees of distal tip in the other experimental group. The larger angulation of tipping caused 1.3-fold more root resorption than the smaller angulation (Fig 10-6).

Torque

Torque movement has always been considered the main culprit of root resorption because of the proximity of the root surface to the cortical bone plate. Bartley et al[86] compared the amount of root resorption between 2.5- and 15-degree buccal root torque in premolars. There was no statistically significant difference in total root resorption between the two groups (Fig 10-7). However, in the apical third region, the larger degree of torquing resulted in more severe root resorption than the smaller degree of torquing. More root resorption was seen in the buccoapical, midbuccal, and palatocervical regions compared with the palatoapical, midpalatal, and buccocervical regions, respectively. Once again, the distribution of root resorption craters indicated the location of the pressure zones.

Casa et al[20] investigated the occurrence, localization, and extension of root resorption after fixed appliance treatment with a continuous torque force. The SEM analysis showed many resorption craters on the lingual side in the apical third of the roots. Resorption processes were also observed on the buccal root surface in the cervical third of the roots. Goldin[37] investigated the effect of labial root torque on the maxillary incisor root apex. The overall amount of apical root resorption was 12.7% per year.

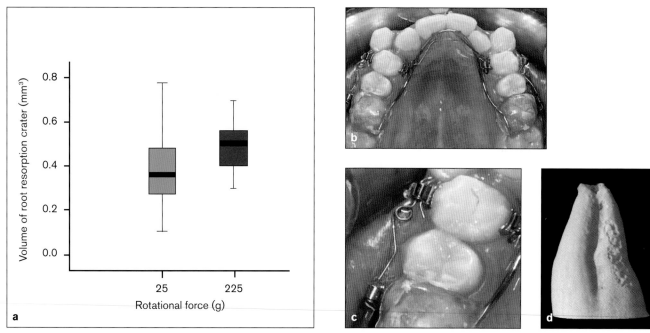

Fig 10-8 (a) Box-plot displaying a statistically significant difference in OIIRR between light and heavy rotational force. NS—not statistically significant. (b) Occlusal view of the experimental setup showing the rotation springs. (c) Close-up view of the rotation spring. (d) A micro-CT photograph shows the resorption craters concentrated at the lingual distal surface.

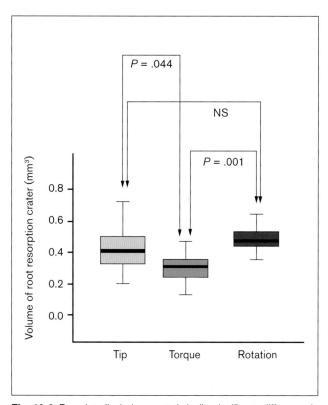

Fig 10-9 Box-plot displaying a statistically significant difference in OIIRR between tip and torque movement. A highly statistically significant difference in OIIRR was found between torque and rotational movement. NS—not statistically significant.

Rotation

Wu et al[87] quantitatively measured and compared the locations and volumes of root resorption craters following light (25 g) and heavy (225 g) rotational forces. Heavy rotational forces resulted in significantly more root resorption than light rotational forces (Fig 10-8). The compression areas (ie, buccodistal and linguomesial surfaces) showed significantly higher root resorption than other areas of the root.

Jimenez-Pellegrin and Arana-Chavez[88] investigated the presence, location, and severity of root resorption after orthodontic rotation for different lengths of time. SEM revealed many root resorption craters on all rotated teeth. The resorption areas were located mainly at the mesial root third and in regions that corresponded to the prominent zones of the roots.

All movements

A recent systematic review by Weltman et al[32] comparing the amount of OIIRR with different types of movement revealed that intrusion causes the greatest damage because the pressure is concentrated at the tooth apex. Lingual root torque movements in the maxillary central incisors also strongly correlated with OIIRR.

Neizert et al[89] evaluated the amount of root resorption on premolars following the application of buccal root torque of 15 degrees, distal root tipping of 15 degrees, and axial rotation with a force of 225 g for 4 weeks and concluded that 225 g of rotating forces caused more root resorption than 15-degree buccal root torquing force. Fifteen degrees of distal tipping force induced greater amounts of root resorption than 15-degree buccal root torquing force. Similar amounts of root resorption were induced by 225 g of rotating force and 15-degree distal root tipping force (Fig 10-9).

Extraction versus nonextraction treatment protocol

There are studies that have looked at the amount of OIIRR associated with extraction treatment.[39,40,54] The approach of comparing extraction with nonextraction treatment and its association with OIIRR is overly simplistic. Attention should be drawn to the distance the teeth are moved. Extractions for severe crowding do not have as much impact on movement of the maxillary incisors as the displacement following extractions for overjet reduction.

In a radiologic study by Sameshima and Sinclair[40] involving 868 patients from six fixed edgewise practices, extractions and the extraction pattern were among the variables assessed and related to the severity of OIIRR. The authors found that patients who had four first premolars extracted had more root resorption than those patients who were treated with a nonextraction protocol. In addition, patients with other types of extractions, including four second premolars, a mandibular incisor, and asymmetric extractions, also had more OIIRR than nonextraction patients. In contrast, cases that involved only extraction of the maxillary first premolars did not result in more resorption than the nonextraction cases. The authors acknowledged that this contradicted their own conclusions that overjet and horizontal distance of movement of root apices are significant contributing factors to OIIRR.

Root Resorption Repair

Repair of root resorption craters begins when the applied orthodontic force is discontinued or reduced below a certain threshold.[5,6] According to Schwartz,[90] when the pressure in the PDL is 20 to 26 g/cm^2, root resorption stops. The reparative process may be seen simultaneously with the resorption process.[7,24,25,91] Many studies have demonstrated that the resorptive defects are repaired by deposition of new cementum and reestablishment of new PDL.[7,8,92–94] Therefore, the risk of tooth loss following orthodontic therapy is not high.[43,95,96]

Numerous studies have documented the time of onset of root resorption repair. Root resorption repair was recorded as early as the first week of retention.[9] Filho et al[97] suggested that cementum repair following root resorption was likely to occur within 2 to 3 weeks if the affected surface was not very large.

The amount of root resorption repair increases with time.[7–9,30] Owman-Moll and Kurol[98] demonstrated more reparative cementum in the resorption cavities after 6 and 7 weeks of retention when compared with 2 and 3 weeks of

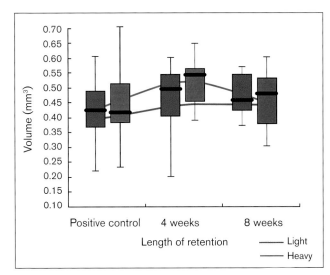

Fig 10-10 Temporal pattern of repair for heavy and light force groups. Volume indicates the average amount of root resorption.

retention. The reparative process increased during the first 4 weeks of retention, and after 5 to 6 weeks, the process slowed down and reached a steady phase.[9]

Cheng et al[99] utilized the micro-CT technique to quantitatively compare the volumes of the root resorption craters after 4 and 8 weeks of retention following 4 weeks of continuous light and heavy orthodontic force application. The study concluded that root resorption continued for another 4 weeks after the orthodontic force had stopped and was more pronounced in the heavy orthodontic force group. Following a retention period of 8 weeks, cementum repair of this continued resorption resulted in its complete repair. Eight weeks of retention following 4 weeks of light orthodontic force application showed the least amount of root resorption (Fig 10-10). Therefore, light orthodontic forces are once again recommended to encourage better recovery of the resorbed cementum.

Owman-Moll et al[9] documented the amount of root resorption cavities repaired at different retention periods following 6 weeks of light buccally directed orthodontic force of 50 cN. After the first week of retention, 28% of the resorption craters showed some degree of repair. The repair rose to 75% after 8 weeks of retention. In a later study, Owman-Moll and Kurol[98] found 38%, 44%, and 82% of resorption craters repaired after 2, 3, and 6 to 7 weeks of retention, respectively.

Brudvik and Rygh[100] found that the reparative process started in the periphery of the root resorption craters while active resorption was still occurring beneath the centrally located overcompressed hyalinized zone. An SEM study on the postmortem orthodontically treated tooth material showed that the resorption area was characterized by the coexistence of centrally located active resorption processes and reparative activity in the marginal zones.[101] On the

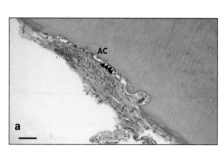
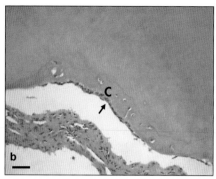
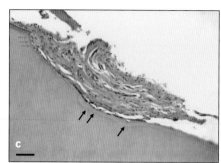

Fig 10-11 *(a)* Histologic section of a root resorption crater showing active cementum repair with acellular cementum (AC) lining the base of the resorption cavity and cementocytes trapped in the superficial layer of newly formed cementum *(arrows)*. Bar = 1 mm. *(b)* Histologic section of a root resorption crater showing cellular cementum (C) overlaid by a layer of mononuclear cells *(arrow)*. Bar = 1 mm. *(c)* Histologic section of a root resorption crater showing reparative cementum that is thicker in the central part *(black arrows)* than the peripheral part *(green arrows)* of the resorption cavity. Bar = 1 mm.

contrary, Owman-Moll and Kurol[98] revealed in their study that healing cementum only occurred centrally in the bottom of the cavity and the central periphery on one of the lateral walls of the cavity. Cheng et al[102] also found in their study that reparative cementum was a mixture of acellular and cellular cementum and that repair seems to commence at the central part of the resorption cavity and expand to the periphery (Fig 10-11).

Clinical consequences of OIIRR

The clinical significance of OIIRR lies in the fact that there is shortening of the root length, which could potentially compromise the long-term prognosis of the affected teeth, especially in periodontally affected cases. This would also make dental treatment planning difficult because these teeth are not favorable for ideal restorations.

A long-term radiographic evaluation of root resorption after active orthodontic therapy revealed progressive remodeling of the root surface.[95] The jagged resorbed edges were smoothed, and the sharply pointed root ends were rounded with time. However, the original root contours and lengths were never reestablished. Severely resorbed teeth were scarce and were found to be functioning in a reasonable manner. Out of the 100 patients that were studied, the worst outcome was hypermobility, which was observed in only two patients.[95] Similarly, VonderAhe[43] examined 57 patients who had suffered from mild, moderate, or severe amounts of OIIRR, and only one case of hypermobility or other detrimental consequences was detected 6.5 years postretention.

A study involving a long-term evaluation of maxillary incisors with severe apical resorption 5 to 15 years after orthodontic treatment showed a significant correlation between tooth mobility, total root length, and intra-alveolar root length.[103] The authors found a significant risk of tooth mobility if a maxillary incisor had OIIRR resulting in a root length of 9 mm or less. Thus, they recommended regular follow-up assessments of teeth with severe OIIRR.[103] Similarly, Jonsson et al[104] found that for teeth with extremely resorbed roots (< 10 mm root length), mobility is expected to increase with age. Teeth with longer root lengths (≥ 10 mm) and a healthy periodontium remain stable.

A reduction in root length as a result of apical resorption has been described as less detrimental than an equivalent loss of periodontal attachment at the alveolar crest, especially in cases with less than 3 mm of early root resorption.[3] Kalkwarf et al,[105] with the aid of a computer graphics system, showed a nearly linear relationship between root length and percentage of periodontal attachment. Results indicated that 4 mm of root resorption translated into 20% of total attachment loss and 3 mm of apical root loss equaled only 1 mm of crestal bone loss. Calculations revealed that after the initial 2-mm apical root loss, every additional 2 mm of root loss equaled only 1 mm of crestal bone loss. Therefore, patients who are susceptible to marginal periodontal breakdown may have a higher risk of losing severely resorbed teeth prematurely. This emphasizes the importance of periodontal disease control in patients with severely resorbed teeth. In addition, teeth with abnormally short roots and loss of periodontal attachment may not be suitable as future fixed partial denture abutments.

Lee et al[106] investigated the perceptions of different dental professionals (eg, general practitioners, orthodontists, periodontists, prosthodontists) toward the significance of root resorption and found that general dental practitioners were the most concerned about root resorption. However, none of the groups thought that a resorption level of over 50% was a good enough reason to extract and prosthetically replace the tooth.

Prevention and Management of OIIRR

Although little to no documentation shows that OIIRR could result in tooth loss, other minor clinical consequences such as mobility, pulpal changes, periodontal attachment loss, and future difficulty in restorations may occur. This could become a potential medicolegal issue; therefore, patient education, identification of at-risk patients, and preventive measures must be considered prior to orthodontic treatment.

Clinically, a number of approaches have been suggested in the literature to minimize OIIRR. These approaches have been summarized by Vlaskalic et al[41] and Ghafari.[107] Together with the recent research findings from micro-CT studies, these are the recommendations for clinically reducing the risk of OIIRR:

- A thorough assessment of familial tendency and medical history[39,108–110]
- Habit control[111]
- Treatment of moderate to severe malocclusions when most of the incisors have open apices because incomplete root formation has been found to be significantly associated with a lower severity of OIIRR[57,112,113]
- Decreased treatment duration by careful treatment planning and efficient mechanics
- Use of light orthodontic forces especially for intrusion, lingual torque of maxillary incisors, and rotation of premolars
- Assessment of the use of intermittent forces where possible to allow resorption repair
- Progress radiographs after 6 to 12 months of treatment[114] and assessment for a rest period from orthodontic force if rapid root resorption is found[65] or reassessment of the treatment plan
- Avoidance of sustained jiggling intermaxillary elastics[58]
- Limiting of tooth movement for OIIRR-prone teeth

It has been strongly suggested that periapical radiographs should be taken at least every year to determine the presence of root resorption.[107] In a study by Levander and Malmgren,[38] minor resorption or an irregular contour of the root that was seen 6 to 9 months after the last radiograph indicated an increased risk of further root resorption.[38] If further root resorption occurs, the original treatment goals must be reassessed depending on the extent of root resorption detected, and a compromised orthodontic result may need to be accepted. The force levels should at least be modified, or a 2- to 3-month pause in treatment with passive archwires should be implemented.[65] Additional radiographs should be taken every 3 months in at-risk patients to monitor the progress of root resorption.[107,115] The amount of additional tooth movement required should be considered against the amount of root resorption acceptable, that is, no more than one-third of the root length. It is

mandatory to take final radiographs at the time of removal of fixed appliances.[116] In the case of teeth with severe OIIRR, follow-up radiographs are recommended until additional root loss is no longer detected.[103] If OIIRR continues to worsen, sequential root canal therapy with calcium hydroxide might be considered.[117] Retention of teeth with severely resorbed roots should be considered carefully to avoid occlusal trauma, which can cause further root resorption.[116]

Can we prevent OIIRR?

Numerous animal studies have been conducted to investigate the possibility of reducing the risk of OIIRR by applying drugs that modulate the activity of osteoblasts, osteoclasts, and odontoclasts. Arginine-glycine-aspartic acid–containing peptides that inhibit the resorptive activity of isolated clast cells by targeting the integrin receptor expressed by odontoclasts have shown to be effective in reducing root resorption during tooth movement.[118] Low-dose systemic administration of doxycycline in rats may have an inhibitory effect on OIIRR via reduction of odontoclasts, osteoclasts, mononuclear cells, and tartrate-resistant acid phosphatase (TRAP)–positive cells on the root.[119] Low doses of thyroid hormone have also played a protective role on the root surface against OIIRR.[120] Steroid-treated rats also displayed significantly less root resorption on the compression side and fewer TRAP-positive cells within the PDL space on the same side compared to controls.[121] Clodronate (a first-generation bisphosphonate) controls the formation and dissolution of calcium phosphate and has also been found to decrease OIIRR.[122] However, many of the above-mentioned drugs also alter the activity of osteoblasts and osteoclasts in alveolar bone, which may decrease the rate of tooth movement.[123,124]

Fluoride has been used in preventive dentistry to strengthen the enamel and protect against caries attack. Can fluoride then protect against OIIRR by strengthening the root cementum? Foo et al[125] investigated the amount of root resorption in Wistar rats' molars after exposing them to systemic fluoride and orthodontic force. The study concluded that fluoride reduced the size of resorption craters, but the effect was variable and not statistically significant. Lim et al[126] examined the elemental composition of OIIRR craters of rat molar cementum that was exposed to fluoride utilizing proton-induced x-ray and gamma-ray emission. The results showed that there was less calcium in the resorption craters in the nonfluoridated group and higher concentrations of fluorine and zinc in the fluoridated group. Does this mean that there is a link between exposure of fluoride and preservation of more calcium that increases resistance to resorption? Gonzales et al[127] evaluated the effect on OIIRR of fluoride administered via drinking water in rats prior to and during orthodontic tooth movement. When fluoride was administered from birth, it suppressed OIIRR and tooth movement. The duration of fluoride administration affected the severity of OIIRR, ie, the longer the fluo-

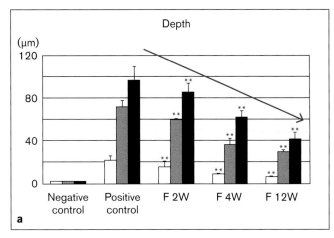

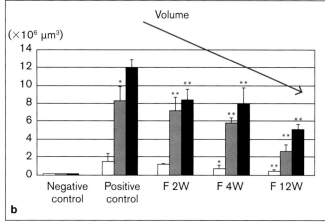

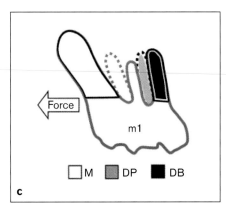

Fig 10-12 *(a and b)* Bar graphs showing that depth and volume of root resorption craters decreased as the duration of fluoride treatment increased. F—fluoride; W—weeks. *(c)* Schematic diagram of a rat molar tooth (m1). M—mesial; DP—distopalatal; DB—distobuccal.

ride was administered, the smaller the amount of OIIRR (Fig 10-12). Based on the results of this research, the effect of systemic fluoride in preventing OIIRR was investigated in humans with a micro-CT technique. Karadeniz et al[128] studied the effect of systemic fluoride intake on OIIRR and its repair when 4 weeks of light and heavy buccal tipping forces were applied to maxillary premolars. Forty-nine patients were recruited in the study and separated into two groups based on the demographics in Turkey: Group 1 was exposed to high water fluoridation (> 2 ppm), and Group 2 was exposed to low water fluoridation (< 0.05 ppm). Each group was subdivided further into two groups, with each exposed to either light (25 g) or heavy orthodontic force (225 g). After 4 weeks of force application, the high fluoride intake group showed significantly less OIIRR when heavy forces were used compared to the low fluoride intake group. After a further 8 weeks of retention, the same group continued to show significantly less OIIRR. Therefore, perhaps fluoride can lessen the effect of OIIRR when heavy force is used. However, the exact dosage of fluoride necessary to be effective is yet to be determined.

Blood and saliva test

Several studies have identified an association of polymorphism of the interleukin 1β (IL-1β) gene with OIIRR.[129,130] However, it might not be cost-effective or clinically effi-

cient to perform genetic tests on all patients. Recent research has focused on identifying biologic markers in the gingival crevicular fluid (GCF) and relating them to the risk of OIIRR. If successful, this technique could be easily implemented in identifying the patients at risk of OIIRR prior to orthodontic treatment, and treatment planning could be modified accordingly. Mah and Prasad[131] showed elevated levels of dentin phosphoproteins in the GCF in resorbing primary teeth and active orthodontically treated teeth compared with untreated permanent teeth. In addition, Balducci et al[132] identified an increase in dentin phosphophoryn and dentin sialoprotein concentration in the GCF of the severe root resorption group. Therefore, dentin phosphophoryn and dentin sialoprotein could be suitable biologic markers for identifying at-risk patients and monitoring root resorption during orthodontic treatment. Ramos et al[133] analyzed serum immunoglobulin G (IgG) levels and salivary secretory immunoglobulin A (sIgA) levels in human dentin extract before and after orthodontic treatment and discovered that elevated levels of salivary sIgA before treatment were associated with more severe root resorption. This could also be another salivary marker to identify patients at risk of OIIRR.

Recent studies have shown the role of osteoprotegerin (OPG) and receptor activator of nuclear factor kappa B ligand (RANKL) in osteoclastogenesis[134] and hence the possibility of their role in root resorption.[135] These studies

Fig 10-13 *(a to c)* Initial panoramic radiograph and clinical photographs of case study. *Circles* highlight the root resorption sites.

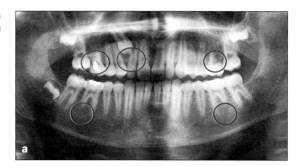

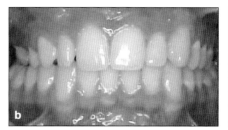
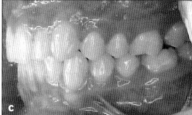

found an increase in RANKL and a decrease in the level of OPG expression in physiologic root resorption in primary human teeth. It was then postulated that the expression of RANKL regulated by the decoy receptor OPG had direct involvement in osteoclastogenesis and therefore the activation of physiologic root resorption. Low et al[136] investigated the role of OPG and RANKL in artificially induced root resorption in a rat model. Tooth movement was induced by heavy forces, and an increased level of both RANKL and OPG was reported at sites adjacent to resorption zones compared with the control teeth with no resorption. Yamaguchi et al[137] investigated the effect of compressive force on the production of RANKL and OPG. The findings revealed an increase of RANKL and a decrease of OPG in the severe root resorption group. George and Evans[138] confirmed the presence of matrix proteins and cytokines in GCF of patients with root resorption. This identification is not specific to severe and mild resorption cases, but when compared with control teeth with no orthodontic force, there was an increased RANKL/OPG ratio, which indicated an increase in bone resorption activity.

Vibration and repair

El-Bialy et al[139] investigated the effect of low-intensity pulsed ultrasound (LIPUS) on root resorption. SEM showed a statistically significant reduction in resorption area and the number of resorption craters in LIPUS-exposed premolars. Histology showed healing of some resorbed roots by hypercementosis. All lesions repaired anatomically (ie, original root contour was established with repaired cementum). Results suggested that the use of LIPUS during orthodontic treatment enhanced repair of root resorption with continuous orthodontic force. The increased formation of reparative cementum that covers most resorption

craters suggested the direct stimulatory effect of LIPUS as cementogenesis.

Grove[140] applied 150 g of buccally directed force to the bilateral maxillary first premolars in 14 patients for a period of 28 days. In a split-mouth procedure, buccally directed vibration of 113 Hz was applied to the maxillary first premolar on the "vibration" side for 10 minutes a day for the entire experimental period. The maxillary first premolars were then extracted and analyzed with micro-CT scan. There was a significant difference in the total root resorption volume between vibration and nonvibration sides ($P = 0.003$), with vibration reducing the amount of OIIRR by 33% on average. Vibration as applied in this study shows its potential in preventing or reducing OIIRR. However, the clinical significance of such application should be evaluated on a sample undergoing a complete course of orthodontic treatment.

Case report

A 15½-year-old boy who had a Class II, division 1 malocclusion had severe root resorption of the maxillary right lateral incisor because of an impacted maxillary right canine (Figs 10-13a to 10-13c). There was also severe root resorption of the maxillary right first molar and mild root resorption of the other first molars. This indicates that the patient had a high risk of OIIRR. When treatment planning this case, the following had to be considered:

- Can the maxillary right canine be left, or should it be extracted? If the maxillary right canine is to be brought down into the arch, how should space be opened for it?
- The maxillary right first molar is severely resorbed and needs to be extracted. How will the space be handled?
- Can the Class II molar relationship be corrected?

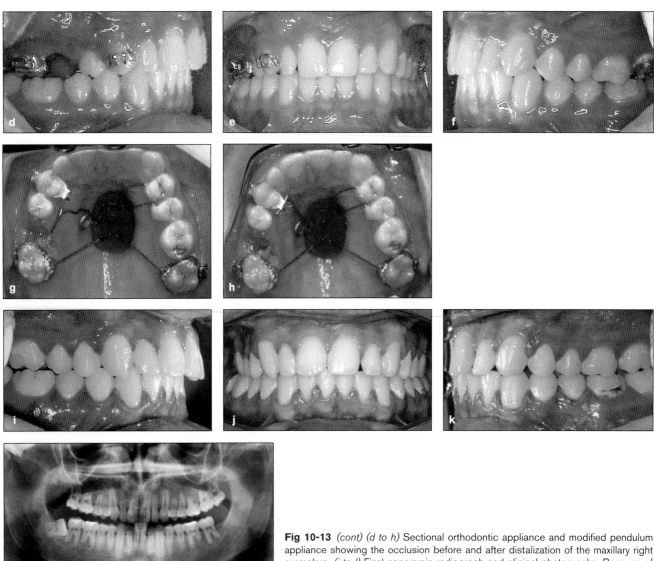

Fig 10-13 *(cont) (d to h)* Sectional orthodontic appliance and modified pendulum appliance showing the occlusion before and after distalization of the maxillary right premolars. *(i to l)* Final panoramic radiograph and clinical photographs. Because of the extent of root resorption and lack of patient compliance with oral hygiene, treatment was terminated early, and the buccal segment of the left side remained Class II.

Because of the severity of the root resorption, the treatment plan was to extract the maxillary right first molar and distalize the maxillary right first and second premolars to provide space for the impacted maxillary right canine. The correction of the Class II relationship on the left side was dependent on the degree of OIIRR present during treatment. First, sectional mechanics with a modified pendulum device were used to distalize the maxillary right first and second premolars (Figs 10-13d to 10-13h). The sectional mechanics were used in an attempt to localize the orthodontic movement that was needed to distalize the maxillary right first and second premolars and reduce the risk of any unwanted pressure on the rest of the dentition. The modified pendulum device provided intermittent force, which allowed for a rest period for resorption repair. Once adequate space was achieved for alignment of the impacted maxillary right canine, full fixed orthodontic appliances were placed. Because of the amount of root resorption present during treatment, the treatment plan was modified, and a Class I molar relationship on the left side was not achieved. The end result was an acceptable occlusion with good esthetics and teeth that had adequate root length (Figs 10-13i to 10-13l). This case illustrates that even in the presence of severe root resorption, orthodontic treatment can be carried out safely with careful planning of treatment objectives and mechanics.

Conclusion

In order to minimize the risk of root resorption related to orthodontic treatment, the following should be considered first:

- Careful treatment planning, taking into consideration family, medical, and social history.
- Use of light forces especially for intrusion, lingual torque of maxillary incisors, and rotation of premolars. This could be achieved with slow progression of archwire sequence.
- For at-risk patients, regular radiographs (6- to 12-month intervals) should be taken and the treatment plan reassessed if required.
- Even though continuous force causes more resorption, it is more effective on tooth movement than intermittent force.
- Periodontal disease control in patients with severely resorbed teeth is prudent.
- The most important consideration of all is to obtain informed consent prior to orthodontic treatment by explaining the risks and benefits of the orthodontic treatment and the potential for root resorption associated with orthodontic treatment.

References

1. Brudvik P, Rygh P. Root resorption after local injection of prostaglandin E_2 during experimental tooth movement. Eur J Orthod 1991;13:255–263.
2. Brudvik P, Rygh P. Root resorption beneath the main hyalinized zone. Eur J Orthod 1994;16:249–263.
3. Lupi JE, Handelman CS, Sadowsky C. Prevalence and severity of apical root resorption and alveolar bone loss in orthodontically treated adults. Am J Orthod Dentofacial Orthop 1996;109:28–37.
4. Killiany DM. Root resorption caused by orthodontic treatment: An evidence-based review of literature. Semin Orthod 1999;5:128–133.
5. Rygh P. Orthodontic root resorption studied by electron microscopy. Angle Orthod 1977;47:1–16.
6. Reitan K. Biomechanical principles and reactions. In: Graber TM, Swain BF (eds). Orthodontics: Current Principles and Techniques. St Louis: Mosby, 1985:101–192.
7. Barber AF, Sims MR. Rapid maxillary expansion and external root resorption in man: A scanning electron microscope study. Am J Orthod 1981;79:630–652.
8. Langford SR, Sims MR. Root surface resorption, repair, and periodontal attachment following rapid maxillary expansion in man. Am J Orthod 1982;81:108–115.
9. Owman-Moll P, Kurol J, Lundgren D. Repair of orthodontically induced root resorption in adolescents. Angle Orthod 1995;65:403–408.
10. Malek S, Darendeliler MA, Swain MV. Physical properties of root cementum: Part I. A new method for 3-dimensional evaluation. Am J Orthod Dentofacial Orthop 2001;120:198–208.
11. Poolthong S. Determination of the Mechanical Properties of Enamel, Dentine and Cementum by an Ultra Micro-Indentation System [thesis]. Sydney: University of Sydney, 1998.
12. Chutimanutskul W, Ali Darendeliler M, Shen G, Petocz P, Swain M. Changes in the physical properties of human premolar cementum after application of 4 weeks of controlled orthodontic forces. Eur J Orthod 2006;28:313–318.
13. Rex T, Kharbanda OP, Petocz P, Darendeliler MA. Physical properties of root cementum: Part 6. A comparative quantitative analysis of the mineral composition of human premolar cementum after the application of orthodontic forces. Am J Orthod Dentofacial Orthop 2006;129:358–367.
14. Baumrind S, Korn EL, Boyd RL. Apical root resorption in orthodontically treated adults. Am J Orthod Dentofacial Orthop 1996;110:311–320.
15. Horiuchi A, Hotokezaka H, Kobayashi K. Correlation between cortical plate proximity and apical root resorption. Am J Orthod Dentofacial Orthop 1998;114:311–318.
16. Parker RJ, Harris EF. Directions of orthodontic tooth movements associated with external apical root resorption of the maxillary central incisor. Am J Orthod Dentofacial Orthop 1998;114:677–683.
17. Dellinger EL. A histologic and cephalometric investigation of premolar intrusion in the *Macaca speciosa* monkey. Am J Orthod 1967;53:325–355.
18. King GJ, Fischlschweiger W. The effect of force magnitude on extractable bone resorptive activity and cemental cratering in orthodontic tooth movement. J Dent Res 1982;61:775–779.
19. Vardimon AD, Graber TM, Voss LR, Lenke J. Determinants controlling iatrogenic external root resorption and repair during and after palatal expansion. Angle Orthod 1991;61:113–122.
20. Casa MA, Faltin RM, Faltin K, Sander FG, Arana-Chavez VE. Root resorptions in upper first premolars after application of continuous torque moment. Intra-individual study. J Orofac Orthop 2001;62:285–295.
21. Darendeliler MA, Kharbanda OP, Chan EK, et al. Root resorption and its association with alterations in physical properties, mineral contents and resorption craters in human premolars following application of light and heavy controlled orthodontic forces. Orthod Craniofac Res 2004;7:79–97.
22. Faltin RM, Arana-Chavez VE, Faltin K, Sander FG, Wichelhaus A. Root resorptions in upper first premolars after application of continuous intrusive forces. Intra-individual study. J Orofac Orthop 1998;59:208–219.
23. Faltin RM, Faltin K, Sander FG, Arana-Chavez VE. Ultrastructure of cementum and periodontal ligament after continuous intrusion in humans: A transmission electron microscopy study. Eur J Orthod 2001;23:35–49.
24. Harry MR, Sims MR. Root resorption in bicuspid intrusion. A scanning electron microscope study. Angle Orthod 1982;52:235–258.
25. Stenvik A, Mjör IA. Pulp and dentine reactions to experimental tooth intrusion. A histologic study of the initial changes. Am J Orthod 1970;57:370–385.
26. Reitan K. Initial tissue behavior during apical root resorption. Angle Orthod 1974;44:68–82.
27. Bondevik O. Tissue changes in the rat molar periodontium following application of intrusive forces. Eur J Orthod 1980;2:41–49.
28. Chan EK, Darendeliler MA, Petocz P, Jones AS. A new method for volumetric measurement of orthodontically induced root resorption craters. Eur J Oral Sci 2004;112:134–139.
29. Harris DA, Jones AS, Darendeliler MA. Physical properties of root cementum: Part 8. Volumetric analysis of root resorption craters after application of controlled intrusive light and heavy orthodontic forces: A microcomputed tomography scan study. Am J Orthod Dentofacial Orthop 2006;130:639–647.
30. Owman-Moll P, Kurol J, Lundgren D. The effects of a four-fold increased orthodontic force magnitude on tooth movement and root resorptions. An intra-individual study in adolescents. Eur J Orthod 1996;18:287–294.
31. Owman-Moll P, Kurol J, Lundgren D. Effects of a doubled orthodontic force magnitude on tooth movement and root resorptions. An inter-individual study in adolescents. Eur J Orthod 1996;18:141–150.

32. Weltman B, Vig KW, Fields HW, Shanker S, Kaizar EE. Root resorption associated with orthodontic tooth movement: A systematic review. Am J Orthod Dentofacial Orthop 2010;137:462–476.

33. Beck BW, Harris EF. Apical root resorption in orthodontically treated subjects: Analysis of edgewise and light wire mechanics. Am J Orthod Dentofacial Orthop 1994;105:350–361.

34. Taner T, Ciger S, Sencift Y. Evaluation of apical root resorption following extraction therapy in subjects with Class I and Class II malocclusions. Eur J Orthod 1999;21:491–496.

35. Brezniak N, Wasserstein A. Root resorption after orthodontic treatment: Part 2. Literature review. Am J Orthod Dentofacial Orthop 1993;103:138–146.

36. Brezniak N, Wasserstein A. Root resorption after orthodontic treatment: Part 1. Literature review. Am J Orthod Dentofacial Orthop 1993;103:62–66.

37. Goldin B. Labial root torque: Effect on the maxilla and incisor root apex. Am J Orthod Dentofacial Orthop 1989;95:208–219.

38. Levander E, Malmgren O. Evaluation of the risk of root resorption during orthodontic treatment: A study of upper incisors. Eur J Orthod 1988;10:30–38.

39. McFadden WM, Engstrom C, Engstrom H, Anholm JM. A study of the relationship between incisor intrusion and root shortening. Am J Orthod Dentofacial Orthop 1989;96:390–396.

40. Sameshima GT, Sinclair PM. Predicting and preventing root resorption: Part II. Treatment factors. Am J Orthod Dentofacial Orthop 2001;119:511–515.

41. Vlaskalic V, Boyd RL, Baumrind S. Etiology and sequelae of root resorption. Semin Orthod 1998;4:124–131.

42. Phillips JR. Apical root resorption under orthodontic therapy. Angle Orthod 1955;25:1–12.

43. VonderAhe G. Postretention status of maxillary incisors with root-end resorption. Angle Orthod 1973;43:247–255.

44. Paetyangkul A, Türk T, Elekdağ-Türk S, et al. Physical properties of root cementum: Part 16. Comparisons of root resorption and resorption craters after the application of light and heavy continuous and controlled orthodontic forces for 4, 8, and 12 weeks. Am J Orthod Dentofacial Orthop 2011;139:e279–e284.

45. Artun J, Smale I, Behbehani F, Doppel D, van't Hof M, Kuijpers-Jagtman AM. Apical root resorption six and 12 months after initiation of fixed orthodontic appliance therapy. Angle Orthod 2005;75:919–926.

46. Smale I, Artun J, Behbehani F, Doppel D, van't Hof M, Kuijpers-Jagtman AM. Apical root resorption 6 months after initiation of fixed orthodontic appliance therapy. Am J Orthod Dentofacial Orthop 2005;128:57–67.

47. Brin I, Tulloch JF, Koroluk L, Philips C. External apical root resorption in Class II malocclusion: A retrospective review of 1- versus 2-phase treatment. Am J Orthod Dentofacial Orthop 2003;124:151–156.

48. Hollender L, Ronnerman A, Thilander B. Root resorption, marginal bone support and clinical crown length in orthodontically treated patients. Eur J Orthod 1980;2:197–205.

49. Sharpe W, Reed B, Subtelny JD, Polson A. Orthodontic relapse, apical root resorption, and crestal alveolar bone levels. Am J Orthod Dentofacial Orthop 1987;91:252–258.

50. Dermaut LR, De Munck A. Apical root resorption of upper incisors caused by intrusive tooth movement: A radiographic study. Am J Orthod Dentofacial Orthop 1986;90:321–326.

51. DeShields RW. A study of root resorption in treated Class II, Division I malocclusions. Angle Orthod 1969;39:231–245.

52. Goldson L, Henrikson CO. Root resorption during Begg treatment: A longitudinal roentgenologic study. Am J Orthod 1975;68:55–66.

53. Blake M, Woodside DG, Pharoah MJ. A radiographic comparison of apical root resorption after orthodontic treatment with the edgewise and Speed appliances. Am J Orthod Dentofacial Orthop 1995;108:76–84.

54. McNab S, Battistutta D, Taverne A, Symons AL. External apical root resorption following orthodontic treatment. Angle Orthod 2000;70:227–232.

55. Janson GR, De Luca Canto G, Martins DR, Henriques JF, De Freitas MR. A radiographic comparison of apical root resorption after orthodontic treatment with 3 different fixed appliance techniques. Am J Orthod Dentofacial Orthop 2000;118:262–273.

56. Barbagallo LJ, Jones AS, Petocz P, Darendeliler MA. Physical properties of root cementum: Part 10. Comparison of the effects of invisible removable thermoplastic appliances with light and heavy orthodontic forces on premolar cementum. A microcomputed-tomography study. Am J Orthod Dentofacial Orthop 2008;133:218–227.

57. Linge BO, Linge L. Apical root resorption in upper anterior teeth. Eur J Orthod 1983;5:173–183.

58. Linge L, Linge BO. Patient characteristics and treatment variables associated with apical root resorption during orthodontic treatment. Am J Orthod Dentofacial Orthop 1991;99:35–43.

59. Asscherickx K, Vannet BV, Wehrbein H, Sabzevar MM. Root repair after injury from mini-screw. Clin Oral Implants Res 2005;16:575–578.

60. Chen Y, Shin HI, Kyung HM. Biomechanical and histological comparison of self-drilling and self-tapping orthodontic microimplants in dogs. Am J Orthod Dentofacial Orthop 2008;133:44–50.

61. Dao V, Renjen R, Prasad HS, Rohrer MD, Maganzini AL, Kraut RA. Cementum, pulp, periodontal ligament, and bone response after direct injury with orthodontic anchorage screws: A histomorphologic study in an animal model. J Oral Maxillofac Surg 2009;67:2440–2445.

62. Renjen R, Maganzini AL, Rohrer MD, Prasad HS, Kraut RA. Root and pulp response after intentional injury from miniscrew placement. Am J Orthod Dentofacial Orthop 2009;136:708–714.

63. Kadioglu O, Büyükyilmaz T, Zachrisson BU, Maino BG. Contact damage to root surfaces of premolars touching miniscrews during orthodontic treatment. Am J Orthod Dentofacial Orthop 2008;134:353–360.

64. Acar A, Canyurek U, Kocaaga M, Erverdi N. Continuous vs. discontinuous force application and root resorption. Angle Orthod 1999;69:159–163.

65. Levander E, Malmgren O, Eliasson S. Evaluation of root resorption in relation to two orthodontic treatment regimes. A clinical experimental study. Eur J Orthod 1994;16:223–228.

66. Maltha JC, Dijkman GE. Discontinous forces cause less extensive root resoprtiion than continuous forces. Eur J Orthod 1996;20:420.

67. Oppenheim A. Human tissue response to orthodontic intervention of short and long duration. Am J Orthod Oral Surg 1942;28:263–301.

68. Reitan K. Effects of force magnitude and direction of tooth movement on different alveolar bone types. Angle Orthod 1964;34:244–255.

69. Weiland F. Constant versus dissipating forces in orthodontics: The effect on initial tooth movement and root resorption. Eur J Orthod 2003;25:335–342.

70. Reitan K. Some factors determining the evaluation of forces in orthodontics. Am J Orthod 1957;43:32–45.

71. Reitan K. Evaluation of orthodontic forces as related to histologic and mechanical factors. SSO Schweiz Monatsschr Zahnheilkd 1970;80:579–596.

72. Rygh P, Brudvik P. Root resorption and new wire qualities. Eur J Orthod 1993;15:343.

73. Kameyama T, Matsumoto Y, Warita H, Soma K. Inactivated periods of constant orthodontic forces related to desirable tooth movement in rats. J Orthod 2003;30:31–37.

74. Kumasako-Haga T, Konoo T, Yamaguchi K, Hayashi H. Effect of 8-hour intermittent orthodontic force on osteoclasts and root resorption. Am J Orthod Dentofacial Orthop 2009;135:278.e1–278.e8.

75. Owman-Moll P, Kurol J, Lundgren D. Continuous versus interrupted continuous orthodontic force related to early tooth movement and root resorption. Angle Orthod 1995;65:395–401.

76. Ballard DJ, Jones AS, Petocz P, Darendeliler MA. Physical properties of root cementum: Part 11. Continuous vs intermittent controlled orthodontic forces on root resorption. A microcomputed-tomography study. Am J Orthod Dentofacial Orthop 2009;136:8.e1–8.e8.

77. Aras B, Cheng LL, Turk T, Elekdag-Turk S, Jones AS, Darendeliler MA. Physical properties of root cementum: Part 23. Effects of 2 or 3 weekly reactivated continuous or intermittent orthodontics forces on root resorption and tooth movement: A microcomputed tomography study. Am J Orthod Dentofacial Orthop 2012;141:e29–e37.

78. Harris EF, Boggan BW, Wheeler DA. Apical root resorption in patients treated with comprehensive orthodontics. J Tenn Dent Assoc 2001;81:30–33.

79. Henry JL, Weinmann JP. The pattern of resorption and repair of human cementum. J Am Dent Assoc 1951;42:270–290.

80. Melsen B, Agerbaek N, Markenstam G. Intrusion of incisors in adult patients with marginal bone loss. Am J Orthod Dentofacial Orthop 1989;96:232–241.

81. Montenegro VC, Jones A, Petocz P, Gonzales C, Darendeliler MA. Physical properties of root cementum: Part 22. Root resorption after the application of light and heavy extrusive orthodontic forces: A microcomputed tomography study. Am J Orthod Dentofacial Orthop 2012;141:e1–e9.

82. Han G, Huang S, Von den Hoff JW, Zeng X, Kuijpers-Jagtman AM. Root resorption after orthodontic intrusion and extrusion: An intra-individual study. Angle Orthod 2005;75:912–918.

83. Weekes WT, Wong PD. Extrusion of root-filled incisors in beagles—A light microscope and scanning electron microscope investigation. Aust Dent J 1995;40:115–120.

84. Paetyangkul A, Türk T, Elekdağ-Türk S, Jones AS, Petocz P, Darendeliler MA. Physical properties of root cementum: Part 14. The amount of root resorption after force application for 12 weeks on maxillary and mandibular premolars: A microcomputed-tomography study. Am J Orthod Dentofacial Orthop 2009;136:492.e1–492.e9.

85. King A, Türk T, Colak C, et al. Physical properties of root cementum: Part 21. The extent of root resorption after the application of 2.5° and 15° tips for four weeks: A microcomputed tomography study. Am J Orthod Dentofacial Orthop 2011;140:e299–e305.

86. Bartley N, Türk T, Colak C, et al. Physical properties of root cementum: Part 17. Root resorption after the application of 2.5° and 15° of buccal root torque for 4 weeks: A microcomputed tomography study. Am J Orthod Dentofacial Orthop 2011;139:e353–e360.

87. Wu AT, Türk T, Colak C, et al. Physical properties of root cementum: Part 18. The extent of root resorption after the application of light and heavy controlled rotational orthodontic forces for 4 weeks: A microcomputed tomography study. Am J Orthod Dentofacial Orthop 2011;139:e495–e503.

88. Jimenez-Pellegrin C, Arana-Chavez VE. Root resorption in human mandibular first premolars after rotation as detected by scanning electron microscopy. Am J Orthod Dentofacial Orthop 2004;126:178–184.

89. Neizert S, Turk T, Kara C, et al. Comparison of the Amount of Root Resorption When Heavy Tip, Torque and Rotational Forces were Applied for 4 Weeks [thesis]. Sydney: University of Sydney, 2009.

90. Schwartz AM. Tissue changes incidental to tooth movement. Int J Orthod 1932;18:331–352.

91. Kurol J, Owman-Moll P, Lundgren D. Time-related root resorption after application of a controlled continuous orthodontic force. Am J Orthod Dentofacial Orthop 1996;110:303–310.

92. Listgarten MA. Electron microscopic study of the junction between surgically denuded root surfaces and regenerated periodontal tissues. J Periodontal Res 1972;7:68–90.

93. Andreasen JO. Cementum repair after apicoectomy in humans. Acta Odontol Scand 1973;31:211–221.

94. Brice GL, Sampson WJ, Sims MR. An ultrastructural evaluation of the relationship between epithelial rests of Malassez and orthodontic root resorption and repair in man. Aust Orthod J 1991;12:90–94.

95. Remington DN, Joondeph DR, Artun J, Riedel RA, Chapko MK. Long-term evaluation of root resorption occurring during orthodontic treatment. Am J Orthod Dentofacial Orthop 1989;96:43–46.

96. Parker WS. Root resorption—Long-term outcome. Am J Orthod Dentofacial Orthop 1997;112:119–123.

97. Filho PF, Letra A, Carvalhal JC, Menezes R. Orthodontically induced inflammatory root resorptions: A case report. Dent Traumatol 2006;22:350–353.

98. Owman-Moll P, Kurol J. The early reparative process of orthodontically induced root resorption in adolescents—Location and type of tissue. Eur J Orthod 1998;20:727–732.

99. Cheng LL, Türk T, Elekdağ-Türk S, Jones AS, Petocz P, Darendeliler MA. Physical properties of root cementum: Part 13. Repair of root resorption 4 and 8 weeks after the application of continuous light and heavy forces for 4 weeks: A microcomputed-tomography study. Am J Orthod Dentofacial Orthop 2009;136:320.e1–320.e10.

100. Brudvik P, Rygh P. Transition and determinants of orthodontic root resorption-repair sequence. Eur J Orthod 1995;17:177–188.

101. Fritz U, Rudzki-Janson I, Paschos E, Diedrich P. Light microscopic and SEM findings after orthodontic treatment—Analysis of a human specimen. J Orofac Orthop 2005;66:39–53.

102. Cheng LL, Türk T, Elekdağ-Türk S, Jones AS, Yu Y, Darendeliler MA. Repair of root resorption 4 and 8 weeks after application of continuous light and heavy forces on premolars for 4 weeks: A histology study. Am J Orthod Dentofacial Orthop 2010;138:727–734.

103. Levander E, Malmgren O. Long-term follow-up of maxillary incisors with severe apical root resorption. Eur J Orthod 2000;22:85–92.

104. Jonsson A, Malmgren O, Levander E. Long-term follow-up of tooth mobility in maxillary incisors with orthodontically induced apical root resorption. Eur J Orthod 2007;29:482–487.

105. Kalkwarf KL, Krejci RF, Pao YC. Effect of apical root resorption on periodontal support. J Prosthet Dent 1986;56:317–319.

106. Lee KS, Straja SR, Tuncay OC. Perceived long-term prognosis of teeth with orthodontically resorbed roots. Orthod Craniofac Res 2003;6:177–191.

107. Ghafari JG. Root resorption associated with combined orthodontic treatment and orthognathic surgery: Modified definitions of the resorptive process sugested. In: Davidovitch Z (ed). Biological Mechanisms of Tooth Eruption, Resorption and Replacement by Implants. Birmingham: EBSCO Media, 1994:545–556.

108. Newman WG. Possible etiologic factors in external root resorption. Am J Orthod 1975;67:522–539.

109. Jacobson O. Clinical significance of root resorption. Am J Orthod 1952;38:687–696.

110. Sameshima GT, Sinclair PM. Predicting and preventing root resorption: Part I. Diagnostic factors. Am J Orthod Dentofacial Orthop 2001;119:505–510.

111. Odenrick L, Brattström V. Nailbiting: Frequency and association with root resorption during orthodontic treatment. Br J Orthod 1985;12:78–81.

112. Rosenberg HN. An evaluation of the incidence and amount of apical root resorption and dilaceration occurring in orthodontically treated teeth having incompletely formed roots at the beginning of Begg treatment. Am J Orthod 1972;61:524–525.

113. Rudolph CE. An evaluation of root resorption occuring during orthodontic treatment. J Dent Res 1940;19:367.

114. Artun J, Van 't Hullenaar R, Doppel D, Kuijpers-Jagtman AM. Identification of orthodontic patients at risk of severe apical root resorption. Am J Orthod Dentofacial Orthop 2009;135:448–455.

115. Levander E, Bajka R, Malmgren O. Early radiographic diagnosis of apical root resorption during orthodontic treatment: A study of maxillary incisors. Eur J Orthod 1998;20:57–63.

116. Brezniak N, Wasserstein A. Orthodontically induced inflammatory root resorption. Part II: The clinical aspects. Angle Orthod 2002;72:180–184.

117. Pizzo G, Licata ME, Guiglia R, Giuliana G. Root resorption and orthodontic treatment. Review of the literature. Minerva Stomatol 2007;56:31–44.

118. Talic NF, Evans C, Zaki AM. Inhibition of orthodontically induced root resorption with echistatin, an RGD-containing peptide. Am J Orthod Dentofacial Orthop 2006;129:252–260.

119. Mavragani M, Brudvik P, Selvig KA. Orthodontically induced root and alveolar bone resorption: Inhibitory effect of systemic doxycycline administration in rats. Eur J Orthod 2005;27:215–225.

120. Vazquez-Landaverde LA, Rojas-Huidobro R, Alonso Gallegos-Corona M, Aceves C. Periodontal 5'-deiodination on forced-induced root resorption—The protective effect of thyroid hormone administration. Eur J Orthod 2002;24:363–369.

121. Ong CK, Walsh LJ, Harbrow D, Taverne AA, Symons AL. Orthodontic tooth movement in the prednisolone-treated rat. Angle Orthod 2000;70:118–125.

122. Choi J, Baek SH, Lee JI, Chang YI. Effects of clodronate on early alveolar bone remodeling and root resorption related to orthodontic forces: A histomorphometric analysis. Am J Orthod Dentofacial Orthop 2010;138:548.e1–548.e8.

123. Fujimura Y, Kitaura H, Yoshimatsu M, et al. Influence of bisphosphonates on orthodontic tooth movement in mice. Eur J Orthod 2009;31:572–577.

124. Iglesias-Linares A, Yanez-Vico RM, Solano-Reina E, Torres-Lagares D, Gonzalez Moles MA. Influence of bisphosphonates in orthodontic therapy: Systematic review. J Dent 2010;38:603–611.

125. Foo M, Jones A, Darendeliler MA. Physical properties of root cementum: Part 9. Effect of systemic fluoride intake on root resorption in rats. Am J Orthod Dentofacial Orthop 2007;131:34–43.

126. Lim E, Belton D, Petocz P, Arora M, Cheng LL, Darendeliler MA. Physical properties of root cementum: Part 15. Analysis of elemental composition by using proton-induced x-ray and gamma-ray emissions in orthodontically induced root resorption craters of rat molar cementum after exposure to systemic fluoride. Am J Orthod Dentofacial Orthop 2011;139:e193–e202.

127. Gonzales C, Hotokezaka H, Karadeniz EI, et al. Effects of fluoride intake on orthodontic tooth movement and orthodontically induced root resorption. Am J Orthod Dentofacial Orthop 2011;139:196–205.

128. Karadeniz EI, Gonzales C, Nebioglu-Dalci O, et al. Effect of Systemic Fluoride Intake on Orthodontic Root Resorption and Its Repair when 4 Weeks Light and Heavy Buccal Tipping Forces Applied on Maxillary Premolars [thesis]. Sydney: University of Sydney, 2010.

129. Bastos Lages EM, Drummond AF, Pretti H, et al. Association of functional gene polymorphism IL-1β in patients with external apical root resorption. Am J Orthod Dentofacial Orthop 2009;136:542–546.

130. Al-Qawasmi RA, Hartsfield JK, Hartsfield JK Jr, et al. Root resorption associated with orthodontic force in IL-1β knockout mouse. J Musculoskelet Neuronal Interact 2004;4:383–385.

131. Mah J, Prasad N. Dentine phosphoproteins in gingival crevicular fluid during root resorption. Eur J Orthod 2004;26:25–30.

132. Balducci L, Ramachandran A, Hao J, Narayanan K, Evans C, George A. Biological markers for evaluation of root resorption. Arch Oral Biol 2007;52:203–208.

133. Ramos Sde P, Ortolan GO, Dos Santos LM, et al. Anti-dentine antibodies with root resorption during orthodontic treatment. Eur J Orthod 2011;33:584–591.

134. Kong YY, Yoshida H, Sarosi I, et al. OPGL is a key regulator of osteoclastogenesis, lymphocyte development and lymph-node organogenesis. Nature 1999;397:315–323.

135. Fukushima H, Kajiya H, Takada K, Okamoto F, Okabe K. Expression and role of RANKL in periodontal ligament cells during physiological root-resorption in human deciduous teeth. Eur J Oral Sci 2003;111:346–352.

136. Low E, Zoellner H, Kharbanda OP, Darendeliler MA. Expression of mRNA for osteoprotegerin and receptor activator of nuclear factor kappa beta ligand (RANKL) during root resorption induced by the application of heavy orthodontic forces on rat molars. Am J Orthod Dentofacial Orthop 2005;128:497–503.

137. Yamaguchi M, Aihara N, Kojima T, Kasai K. RANKL increase in compressed periodontal ligament cells from root resorption. J Dent Res 2006;85:751–756.

138. George A, Evans CA. Detection of root resorption using dentin and bone markers. Orthod Craniofac Res 2009;12:229–235.

139. El-Bialy T, El-Shamy I, Graber TM. Repair of orthodontically induced root resorption by ultrasound in humans. Am J Orthod Dentofacial Orthop 2004;126:186–193.

140. Grove J. The Effects of Mechanical Vibration on Orthodontic Root Resorption [thesis]. Sydney: University of Sydney, 2011.

Donald J. Rinchuse
DMD, MS, MDS, PhD

Sanjivan Kandasamy
BDSc, BSc Dent, Doc Clin Dent,
MOrth RCS, MRACDS

11 | Orthodontics and TMD

The natural history of temporomandibular disorder (TMD) is one that has certainly taken on a life of its own, with debates muddled with differences of opinion on definition, etiology, diagnosis, and treatment. From early on many fallacious notions have been derived from empirical clinical observations. Gradually over the decades, false beliefs on the topics of occlusion, condyle position, and TMD have been nurtured and disseminated through the generations as gospel truths.[1,2] Unfortunately, the acceptance of these beliefs has almost always been based more on faith than on science. In this respect, some professionals in dentistry and orthodontics have acquired their views on occlusion, condyle position, and TMD based on some combination of authority, rationalism, tenacity, and empiricism, with little attention spent on objectively analyzing and evaluating the science and evidence.[2] This chapter provides a contemporary and evidence-based evaluation of the topics of occlusion, condyle position, and TMD as they relate to orthodontics, as well as a general discussion of the management of TMD for orthodontists. Much of the evidence-based information pertinent to these topics is derived from systematic reviews and/or randomized controlled trials (RCTs) (Table 11-1).

Does Orthodontics Cause TMD?

Although the functional aspects of occlusion were recognized by orthodontists in the 1930s, it was not until the early 1970s that the "gnathologic-prosthodontic view" of occlusion and TMD made its way into mainstream orthodontics through the influence of the late Ronald H. Roth.[3–5] It was argued by Roth and other orthodontic gnathologists that although orthodontists do not "cut" or modify the natural dentition, orthodontics is analogous to prosthodontic full-mouth occlusal rehabilitation. Therefore, as argued by Roth, orthodontists should have the same knowledge as prosthodontists and should be charged with attaining a prosthodontic "gnathologic occlusal" functional occlusion finish as well as attaining traditional orthodontic static occlusal goals. The general gnathologic requisites were to[3–6]:

- Attain canine-protected (mutually protected) functional occlusion
- Attain a centric occlusion (CO), also known as *maximal intercuspation* (MI), position that is coincident with the condyles in anterior-superior centric relation (CR)
- Advocate the use of articulators as an aid to orthodontic diagnostics and treatment planning

Orthodontic gnathologists were of the opinion that if these goals were not achieved, patients would be predisposed to develop TMDs. In addition, they believed that TMDs could be mitigated or cured by applying the principles of orthodontic gnathology to patient treatments.[3–6]

However, there was no hard scientific data or evidence in the 1970s to support orthodontic gnathology. That is, the basis for the principles of gnathology was empirical rather than scientific. Nonetheless, the landmark US court case in 1987 of Brimm v Malloy reinvigorated research and debate among orthodontic communities worldwide on whether or not orthodontic treatment, occlusion, and condyle position caused TMD.[7] In the Brimm case, a Michigan orthodontist allegedly caused a TMD in a 16-year-old girl who presented with an Angle Class II, division 1 malocclusion.[7] The orthodontic treatment carried out involved the extraction of the maxillary first premolars and the use of a headgear. The defendant orthodontist was purported to have caused a TMD (temporomandibular joint [TMJ] internal derangement) by distal displacement of the mandible as a result of the overretraction of the maxillary incisors.

Table 11-1 Evidence-based view on the relationship of various factors and TMD*

Variable	Cause of TMD (Y/N)	Diagnosis/ treatment of TMD (Y/N)	Comments
Dental-based model			
Occlusion	N	N	No longer considered the primary cause of TMD
Condyle position (CR)	N	N	No longer considered the primary cause of TMD
Centric slides > 4 mm	N	N	Believed to be the result rather than the cause of TMD
Orthodontics	—	N	Does not cause or correct/mitigate TMD
Articulator (diagnostic aid in orthodontics)	—	—	No evidence-based data supporting the use of articulators to enhance orthodontic diagnostics
Biopsychosocial model			
Behavioral risk-conferring factors	Y	Y	Current evidence-based view on the cause of and treatment for TMD
Psychosocial traits/states	Y	Y	Current evidence-based view on the diagnosis of and treatment for TMD
Cognitive-behavioral therapy	—	Y	Current evidence-based approach for the treatment of TMD
Biofeedback	—	Y	Current evidence-based approach for the treatment of TMD
Conservative and reversible treatment (at least initially)	—	Y	Current evidence-based approach for the treatment of TMD
Oral occlusal appliances			
Repositioning splints	—	N	No evidence supporting their use; cannot "recapture" displaced TMJs
Stabilizing (flat-plane) splints	—	Y	Preferred type of oral occlusal appliance; recent evidence demonstrating that occlusal splints are no more effective than other TMD therapies
Future/research			
Genetics	Y	Y	Exciting future of TMD research and possible treatment
Endocrinology	Y	Y	TMD diagnostics and possible treatment
Central-brain processing	—	Y	TMD diagnostics
Imaging of the pain-involved brain	—	Y	TMD diagnostics

*Based on population data.
—, not applicable.

However, many studies carried out immediately following the Brimm case rejected all of the allegations made in that case.[8–14] The contemporary evidenced-based view on the relationship between orthodontics and TMD is that orthodontic treatment does not generally cause, mitigate, or cure TMD and does not prevent the future development of TMD.[8] This is irrespective of the type of appliance used or treatment carried out (ie, chin cup, headgear, extractions). Hence, orthodontics is considered neutral[8–17] in regard to its relationship with TMD.

TMD, once considered a single disease/dysfunction with a single cause, is now considered a collection of disorders embracing many clinical problems that involve the masticatory muscles, joints, and associated structures[18,19] (Fig 11-1). Occlusion and/or specific locations of the condyles in the glenoid fossae are no longer considered primary factors in the multifactorial nature of TMD. The multifactorial nature of TMD is complicated in that the multifactorial etiology previously mentioned is for each of the half-dozen or so subclasses of TMD and not for the general, single category of TMD. The current view of the etiology, diagnosis, and treatment of TMD is based on a biopsychosocial model that integrates the host of biologic, behavioral, and social factors to the onset, maintenance, and mitigation of TMD.[6,20–26] A medical orthopedic approach for TMD treatment is advocated that focuses on the biomedical sciences and musculoskeletal therapies similar to those for most chronic pain. Cognitive-behavioral therapies (CBTs) and biofeedback (BFB) are contemporary TMD treatment modalities.

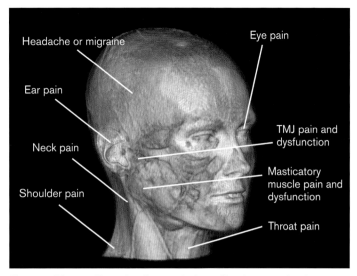

Fig 11-1 Diagram illustrating the complexity and involvement of various structures that contribute to TMD: the masticatory muscles, TMJs, and associated craniofacial structures.

It should be mentioned, however, that the evidence-based view related to occlusion, condyle position (CR), orthodontics, and TMD does not imply that occlusion has no relevance to the etiology of TMD. A gross examination of the occlusion is still important in the diagnosis and treatment of TMD to identify and eliminate major occlusal discrepancies.[27] In addition, the data and evidence for the passive role of occlusion, condyle position, and orthodontics related to TMD is based on population rather than the individual patient. This implies that, at the individual patient level and for a select few patients, there is the rare possibility that orthodontic treatment, occlusion, and/or condyle position may precipitate (and cause) TMD in a susceptible or vulnerable individual.

Functional Occlusion, Centric Relation, and Orthodontics

Functional occlusion

The optimal functional occlusal scheme has been debated for over a century. This is in spite of the fact that the criteria that denote an ideal functional occlusion have not been elucidated. Based more on anecdotal data than on science and evidence, it is conjectured that the optimal functional occlusion for orthodontic and other patient groups is canine-protected occlusion (CPO), also known as *mutually protected occlusion*.[28] The concept of CPO was developed based on the tenet that during laterotrusive movements of the mandible, only the canines contact and hence protect

the remaining dentition from adverse occlusal torsion forces as the mandible moves side-to-side from CO (MI).[28–30] When CPO is not established in orthodontic patients, it is argued that patients would be predisposed to TMD as well as orthodontic tooth relapse.[4,5]

However, the literature as a whole does not indicate the predominance of CPO in nature. Namely, it appears that balanced occlusion (with very light nonworking contacts, not inferences, on the posterior teeth) seems to be the most prevalent functional occlusion type in individuals with Class I and/or optimal static occlusions.[28] In addition, in a literature review published in the *Journal of Prosthodontics* that dates back to the late 1970s, Woda and coworkers[31] argued that CPO and group function rarely exist in their pure form and that current populations show balancing contacts to be the general rule.

CPO as the optimal functional occlusal scheme in orthodontics is equivocal and unsupported by the available evidence. To be clear, there is nothing inherently wrong with CPO, but it may only be one of several acceptable functional occlusal schemes. McNamara et al[32] pointed out that although the goal in orthodontic treatment is to achieve a stable occlusion, the failure to achieve a specific gnathologic ideal does not result in TMD signs and symptoms. In other words, not achieving a CPO does not necessarily lead to TMD. Incidentally, a benign balancing occlusal *contact* is very light and not pathologic, whereas a balancing occlusal *interference* is pathologic in the sense that it can cause tooth mobility, fremitus, and deviated and deflective mandibular movement. Occlusal contacts can be considered normal and do not need to be addressed, whereas occlusal interferences can be harmful and are in need of intervention. In studies finding the predominance of balanced occlusion in orthodontic patients as well as other population groups, patients typically possessed balancing side contacts and not interferences.[28] Hence, irrespective of the type of laterotrusive functional occlusal patterns on the working side, the nonworking side should not possess balancing side interferences.

Furthermore, if a particular functional occlusal scheme (eg, CPO) is advocated and achieved for orthodontic patients, it will not necessarily be stable over the lifetime of the patient. A patient's occlusal environment is dynamic in nature, constantly changing with time based on myriad factors, including tooth attrition, occlusal settling, and changes in the oral environment. Craniofacial morphology, chewing kinematics, static occlusion type, current oral health condition (periodontal and other), and especially parafunctional habits must be assessed prior to deciding on a particular functional occlusal scheme for each individual. Many patients possess more vertical chewing patterns (as gleaned from a frontal plane evaluation) and function laterally close to CR, not making the extremely lateral side-to-side movements governed by the "test" position of the philosophy of the current functional occlusion paradigm involving CPO. Clearly, traditional functional occlusal schemes including CPO do not adequately evaluate the above-cited variables. Given the complex interrelationships of the previously mentioned factors, prescribing one functional occlusal scheme over another makes no sense and fails to take into consideration individual patient variability.[28]

Centric relation

The definition of *centric relation* and the location of the condyles has "migrated" from a retruded, posterior, and, for the most part, superior condyle position (in the glenoid fossa) to an anterior-superior position.[33] Whether CO or MI should be coincident with the condyles in CR is controversial. The gnathologists have consistently argued that they should be coincident, but there is little to no hard data or evidence to support this viewpoint.[34] Interestingly, the intraoral telemetry studies that date back to the 1960s did not support the notion of retruded CR that originally captivated the attention of the early orthodontic gnathologists. In these early intraoral telemetry studies, when research patients' entire dentitions were restored to retruded CR, these patients were found to still function some 2 mm anterior to retruded CR.[35-37] Further, centric slides of 4 mm or greater that have been found in studies to be associated with TMJ arthropathies are most likely the consequence rather than the cause of the TMD.[32,38]

Even though by contemporary definition CR is considered an anterior-superior position, this is not supported by scientific evidence.[6] The change of definition from a posterior-superior condyle position in the 1970s to an anterior-superior condyle position in the 1980s was arbitrarily determined and motivated by magnetic resonance imaging (MRI) findings of TMJ internal derangements in selected patients. Namely, the preponderance of the population-based evidence supports the view that there is a range of clinically appropriate CR positions and not one particular CR position that is universally optimal for all persons. The range of acceptable CR positions from a population perspective does not mean that each individual typically functions in a wide range of CR positions but rather that there is probably one unique condyle position ("seated position" within a small range) that is optimal for each person (eg, mid-CR or somewhere anterior and superior). It is worth mentioning that CR may change locations very slightly during the day for each individual based on several factors such as fatigue of the masticatory and facial muscles, posture, tongue position, and the slight changes in the size, shape, and position of the disc based on the level and extent of loading. As previously discussed, the notion that certain orthodontic appliances and procedures (eg, extraction treatment, interarch elastics, chin cups) cause a posterior displacement (or position) of the mandibular condyles, which then leads to TMD, is not supported by the evidence.[8-12,15-17,39]

Deprogramming appliances

It is believed that mandibular movements are governed by preprogrammed muscle engrams, or habitual muscular patterns. *Muscle engrams* are the memorized patterns of muscle activity developed from the habitual repetition of proprioceptive sensory information. Gnathologists hypothesize that these memorized patterns of the masticatory muscles may adversely change the position of the mandible in the presence of occlusal interferences. They therefore recommend the use of a deprogramming splint or other type of apparatus before obtaining centric bite registrations. It is believed that using various deprogramming splints to disocclude the posterior teeth would remove any occlusal interferences or proprioceptive errors and permit the muscles of mastication to establish a more physiologic engram.[4-6,40,41]

Nonetheless, the evidence for using deprogrammers is equivocal and lacks a true physiologic basis. In 1999, following the use of a "Lucia type anterior deprogramming jig" (ie, anterior tooth contact without posterior tooth contact) in TMD subjects, Karl and Foley[42] found small differences in articulator condyle position indicator (CPI) centric recordings before and after using the deprogrammer for 6 hours. Compared with traditional centric bite registrations, the differences were very minor. The most prevalent type of centric slide on average resulted in a posterior and inferior distraction of the articulator condyles from CR-CO (condyles) of 0.37 mm horizontally and 0.57 mm vertically.[42] Interestingly, Kulbersh et al[43] in 2003 did not find a difference in MI-CR measurements between 34 postorthodontic patients who wore gnathologic full-coverage splints for 3 weeks (24 hours/day) and 14 postorthodontic patients who did not wear splints.

It appears that the use of various deprogramming appliances for either short or long periods to establish a more accurate CR is neither evidence-based nor justified. It seems that deprogramming splints simply serve to complicate and introduce more error and procedures into a gnathologic treatment modality that already struggles for recognition.[6] Another consideration is the question of how one knows that the deprogrammed CR position is healthier or more physiologic in comparison to the original position.

Do Articulators Improve Orthodontic Diagnostics?

There are many different articulator types: arcon, nonarcon, fully adjustable, semiadjustable, polycentric hinge, etc. There is no doubt that articulators can have utility for gross fixed and removable prosthodontic and orthognathic surgical procedures to at least maintain a certain vertical dimension while laboratory procedures are performed. The use of articulators as a diagnostic aid in orthodontics is a topic that has been debated since the early 1970s when the late Dr Ronald Roth introduced the historic prosthodontics-gnathology philosophy to the orthodontic profession.[3–5] Roth believed that by "mounting" orthodontic patient dental casts on articulators, orthodontists would then be able to deduce three-dimensional centric discrepancies. Early on, Dr Roth focused on being able to identify discrepancies in a sagittal plane such as "Sunday Bites" (patient can bite both forward and backward), but later his focus shifted to the orthodontic diagnoses of hidden transverse and vertical discrepancies. The orthodontic gnathologic camp contends that for a certain percentage of orthodontic patients (ranging from 18.7% to 40.9% according to Utt et al[44] and Cordray,[41] respectively), the diagnosis of Angle's classification of malocclusion will be affected and different for those who have had articulator mountings. Not all gnathologists, however, believe that all cases need to be mounted. Some believe that only certain cases require mounting, such as patients requiring orthognathic surgery, TMD patients, most adult patients, those with many missing permanent teeth, those with functional crossbites and midline discrepancies, and those with deviations on opening and/or closing. Frank Cordray, a contemporary Roth advocate, believes that all cases need to be mounted based on the assertion that no practitioner can determine beforehand which cases are or will turn out to be the troublesome ones.[40] It seems that although much is written and discussed concerning articulators, the critical issue is not so much about the articulator mountings per se but rather about the reliability, validity, and transferability of the bite registrations used to "set" or mount the casts on the articulator. Nonetheless, orthodontic gnathologists contend that the best way to evaluate CR is with the use of the Roth power bite registration followed by an articulator mounting.[40,45]

More than a half-century ago, Posselt developed the concept of the "terminal hinge axis."[46] He proposed that in the initial 20 mm or so of opening and closing, the mandible (condyles) rotates similar to a door hinge (and does not simultaneously translate). Articulators were essentially based on this concept of Posselt's. However, Posselt's theory was made in the era when CR was considered a retruded, posterior position of the condyles in the glenoid fossa and was recorded with distal guided pressure applied to the chin.[6] In 1995, Lindauer et al[47] demonstrated that during opening and closing, the condyles not only rotated but also simultaneously translated (moved downward and forward). Their findings supported the notion of an "instantaneous center of rotation" (simultaneous rotation and translation) that is different in every patient and cannot be simulated on an articulator, demonstrating that the terminal hinge axis does not exist.

The scientific data supports the view that clinicians are not able to estimate where patient condyles are located based on their particular bite registration.[48] This makes it imperative that clinicians furnish data from TMJ images such as MRIs that substantiate that patients' condyles are actually located in the CR positions that they claim. Furthermore, it appears that the difference between gnathologic and non-gnathologic diagnostic records is on average as little as 1 mm or less, and this is typically in the vertical dimension.[45,49] The question here, then, is: Are such small differences between gnathologic and non-gnathologic records a real health concern? Incidentally, it is not really known which of the centric records is more valid (ie, the gnathologic or non-gnathologic); the gnathologists assume that their record is superior just because it is applied after non-gnathologic recording in research protocols.

A summary of the shortcomings of the use of articulators to enhance orthodontic diagnostics are as follows[9]:

- Although the centric bite registrations are reliable, orthodontic gnathologists have not furnished any evidence (MRI data) to demonstrate that the condyles are actually in the positions they have described them to be in.
- It has been shown that condyles are not actually located in the assumed positions as advocated and produced by several gnathologic centric bite registrations.
- The difference between gnathologic and non-gnathologic findings is generally as little as 1 mm or less, and this is mostly in the vertical dimension. Is such a difference actually a health concern? When one takes into consideration the errors associated with the entire registration and mounting process, this further reduces the significance of these differences and the gnathologists' claims.
- In children, the TMJ condyle–glenoid fossa complex changes location with growth; the fossae are generally displaced posteriorly and inferiorly.[50] Gnathologists would therefore need to perform new mountings throughout treatment in order to maintain an ideal CR.
- Articulators (and their bite registrations) cannot discern patients' chewing kinematics.

In conclusion, the bottom line is that there is no valid evidence to support the routine mounting of dental casts to enhance orthodontic diagnoses and facilitate treatment planning that would lead to improved stomatognathic health.[49,51] Articulator mountings are not a cost-effective exercise and provide no additional biologic information about the presence of disease in orthodontic patients. Diseases of the TMJ such as disc displacement and osteoarthrosis are best diagnosed with TMJ imaging (MRI) and a thorough clinical examination and not through the use of articulators. Interestingly, the most destructive occlusal forces of all are those produced during parafunction (bruxing and clenching), and articulators have never been and cannot be used to capture and analyze these types of movements and forces.[49] The evidence-based opinion is that use of articulators in orthodontics is perfunctory, with no valid support for their efficacy.

Internal Derangements and Recapturing TMJ Discs

Internal derangements

Internal derangements (IDs) are defined as any interference with smooth joint movement. The term is used interchangeably with *disc displacements* in this chapter, but it also encompasses disc adherences, adhesions, subluxations, and dislocations of the disc-condyle complex.[52] It appears that as many as 30% or more of TMD asymptomatic subjects have TMJ IDs, most commonly disc displacements.[53-55] A current controversy is whether or not TMD asymptomatic patients with TMJ ID need some form of dental or orthodontic treatment to reduce or prevent the risk of developing TMD symptoms in the future.

The relationship of disc displacement to pain, mandibular dysfunction, osteoarthrosis, and growth disturbances remains unclear, and, given the fact that each patient adapts differently to variations in disc-condyle relationships, the presence of asymptomatic IDs should be discussed with the patient, though in general they are best left untreated. With regards to ID and growth, not all growing patients with disc displacement grow abnormally, nor do all patients with growth deficiencies have disc displacement.[56-58] It seems that if disc displacement were a significant cause of mandibular growth deficiency, the signs and symptoms of disc displacement would be more common and/or more dramatically displayed in this population than in the normal population.

TMD asymptomatic patients who are characterized as having a disc displacement commonly have atypical TMJ disc locations in relation to the condyle–glenoid fossa complex. In the long term, it has been demonstrated that patients with moderate to severe TMJ dysfunction with associated disc displacement without reduction will improve with minimal or no treatment. On average, the nat-

ural course for patients with nonreducing disc displacements without treatment tends to be a lessening in clinical signs and symptoms over time, with improvements in jaw movement and masticatory efficiency.[52,58-60] TMJ imaging may help to confirm a particular diagnosis, but this does not axiomatically lead to a particular treatment like in orthopedic medicine. Namely, TMD asymptomatic patients can have discernable TMJ IDs that arguably may not require treatment.

Recapturing TMJ displaced discs

In the 1970s, Farrar[61] introduced the concept of "recapturing the disc." Some professionals in dentistry and orthodontics still believe that anteriorly displaced discs, even in asymptomatic patients, need to be treated in order to avoid progression to TMD, such as degenerative disease or painful dysfunction.[61-63] Some in dentistry and orthodontics have advocated treating anteriorly displaced TMJ discs with anterior repositioning splints. The rationalization for this treatment is that by anteriorly positioning the mandible with a so-called anterior positioning appliance or device, the disc would be "recaptured" in a forward position, and then the appliance could be adjusted or remade to facilitate the gradual "walking back" of the disc-condyle relationship to a normal position. By positioning the mandible in a forward position, the retrodiscal tissues are allowed to recover, facilitating adaptive and reparative changes. The retrodiscal tissues become avascular and fibrotic, allowing the condyles to eventually function "off the disc" or articulate on the newly adapted retrodiscal tissues with no pain.[18,56,64-67] After the use of the anterior repositioning splint, there is the added consideration by "recapture" advocates for stabilizing the mandible in this anterior position with the help of orthodontic treatment, prosthodontics, orthognathic surgery, or a combination of these treatments. Unfortunately, these practices are not evidence-based, and the validity for the use of repositioning splints is based on anecdotal reports rather than hard scientific data; the use of such splints may actually lead to adverse occlusal changes.[18,27,56] Furthermore, there is no known anatomical mechanism that accounts for the retraction of an anteriorly displaced disc to its normal position.[68] It appears that the TMJ disc always remains anteriorly displaced. The bottom line is that displaced TMJ discs cannot be "recaptured." Incidentally, flat-planed, stabilizing splints are preferred over repositioning splints for treatment of TMD, including disc displacements when TMJ surgery is not advised.

Management of TMD

TMD treatment/management philosophy has migrated away from the historic dental-based model to a biopsychosocial model that focuses on the integration of biologic,

Fig 11-2 *(a and b)* Maxillary stabilizing (flat-plane) splint. *(c and d)* Mandibular stabilizing (flat-plane) splint. Mandibular splints are generally preferred over maxillary splints when at all possible because patients are able to function better (eg, speech).

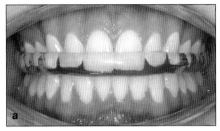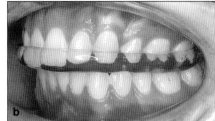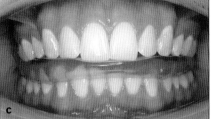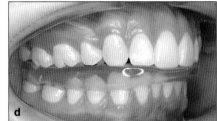

genetic, social, psychologic, and behavioral variables that account for the onset, maintenance, and remission of TMD (see Table 11-1). Factors that have received the most attention recently include genetics (vulnerabilities related to pain), central-brain processing of thinking and emotions, imaging of the pain-involved brain, behavioral risk-conferring factors, endocrinology, sexual dimorphism, and psychosocial traits and states. Nonetheless, some orthodontists still tell TMD patients that certain features of their occlusions are the cause of their complaint.

A first step in TMD diagnosis is to classify the patient's TMD as arthrogenous (originating from a joint) or myogenous (originating from a muscle), realizing that both conditions could be present concomitantly. It is recommended from both clinical and medicolegal perspectives that for arthrogenous TMD conditions, the orthodontist should make a referral to an oral surgeon before intervening. Myogenous conditions can be initially managed by the orthodontist without prior referral to an oral surgeon. Concomitant arthrogenous and myogenous conditions should be handled as per the recommendation for arthrogenous conditions. In addition, classification of TMD pain should involve two levels or axes of consideration. Axis I is the physical side and axis II the emotional or psychologic side of an ailment. The two axes must be evaluated individually and together because they are usually interrelated. Acute pain is typically more related to axis I factors and chronic pain to axis II factors, but this is not totally true in all cases.

The orthodontist should have an understanding of the contemporary evidence-based information on TMD management. Typically, TMD treatments are symptomatic and palliative and generally do not address cause. In medicine, for certain illnesses such as fibromyalgia, the symptoms are managed rather than treatment directed toward a cause (ie, the cause is illusive and not really known). TMD therapies should be conservative, reversible (at least initially), symptomatic, and, when possible, have a scientific basis.[18,27] Irreversible and invasive TMD treatments

are rarely indicated, with the exception of when patients' TMD symptoms cannot be managed in a conservative way. This does not imply that irreversible and definitive TMD treatment is the best option when conservative treatments fail. In summary, the orthodontist is obliged to provide orthodontic TMD patients with what they most need and desire—relief from pain and the ability to get on with their normal daily activities.[68,69]

Evidence-based treatment options

Orthodontists should be capable of providing scientifically based palliative, conservative, and reversible TMD treatments. The majority of TMD patients can be managed (at least initially) with simple treatments such as counseling/reassurance, medications, physical therapies, and occlusal splints, even though part of the therapeutic success observed for many TMD treatments may be the result of placebo or a patient's cognitive awareness.[18,27,66,70,71]

Regarding oral occlusal appliances, a recent systematic review based on 12 RCTs concluded that not enough evidence exists either to support or deny the efficacy of stabilization splint therapy compared with other active interventions for the treatment of TMD[72] (Fig 11-2). Nonetheless, it appears that occlusal splints (stabilizing rather than repositioning) work best initially, and CBT and BFB work better later in treatment.[24–26,73]

There are essentially four main categories for the treatment of muscle-generated TMD[66]:

1. Patient self-directed therapy
2. Office-based physical medicine
3. Pharmacologic treatment
4. Behavioral therapies

Patient self-directed therapies usually involve avoidance therapies, local ice-cold therapy, stretch therapy, and exercise therapy. Stretching should be performed multiple times a day to suppress muscle tension levels (not to strengthen or condition the muscles). As a holistic approach to better well-being, efforts aimed at reducing stress, such as somatic physical exercise (aerobic and anaerobic), may be beneficial. Depending on whether the pain is influenced by physical or psychologic factors, pharmacologic agents can be used. These may involve analgesic and anti-inflammatory agents as well as anti-anxiety agents, tranquilizers, and antidepressant medications. Behavior therapies include mind-body therapies (MBTs) such as autogenic training, relaxation exercises, meditation, CBT, hypnosis, guided imagery, BFB, education on a specific disorder, or coping skills training.[66]

Conclusion

TMD is a collective term embracing a number of clinical problems that involve the masticatory musculature and the TMJs and are of a multifactorial etiology. The historic dental-based model has been gradually replaced by a biologic-medical model used in the treatments of other chronic musculoskeletal disorders. The contemporary biopsychosocial approach to TMD management focuses on the integration of biologic, clinical, and behavioral factors that may ultimately account for the onset, maintenance, and remission of TMD.[20–26,57,74,75] Genetics (vulnerabilities related to pain), endocrinology, behavioral risk-conferring factors, and psychosocial traits and states appear to be the variables currently being researched and receiving the most attention. However, some professionals in orthodontics are reluctant to change and still embrace past unscientific notions that lead to the use of empirically based treatments. It is critical that orthodontists pay attention to the new research developments so that they can ultimately provide their patients with the best possible care.[69]

Summary points

- The biopsychosocial model has replaced the historic dental-based model.
- Orthodontics does not cause or "cure" TMD.
- One particular functional occlusion scheme (eg, CPO) has not been demonstrated to be optimal for all patients.
- *Centric relation* has become a nebulous term, and there does not appear to be one optimal CR position for all patients.
- TMD treatments should be conservative, reversible (at least initially), palliative, and when possible have a scientific basis.

References

1. Rinchuse DJ, Rinchuse DJ. The impact of the American Dental Association's guidelines for the management of temporomandibular disorders on orthodontic practice. Am J Orthod 1983;83:518–522.
2. Rinchuse DJ, Rinchuse DJ, Kandasamy S. Evidence-based versus experience-based views on occlusion and TMD. Am J Orthod Dentofacial Orthop 2005;127:249–254.
3. Roth RH. Temporomandibular pain-dysfunction and occlusal relationships. Angle Orthod 1973;43:136–153.
4. Roth RH. The maintenance system and occlusal dynamics. Dent Clin North Am 1976;20:761–788.
5. Roth RH. Functional occlusion for the orthodontist. II. J Clin Orthod 1981;25:100–123.
6. Rinchuse DJ, Kandasamy S. Centric relation: A historical and contemporary orthodontic perspective. J Am Dent Assoc 2006;137:494–501.
7. Pollack B. Cases of note: Michigan jury awards $850,000 in ortho case: A tempest in a teapot. Am J Orthod Dentofacial Orthop 1988;94:358–360.
8. Gianelly AA. Orthodontics, condylar position and TMJ status. Am J Orthod Dentofacial Orthop 1989;95:521–523.
9. Gianelly AA, Hughes HM, Wohlgemuth P, Gildea C. Condylar position and extraction treatment. Am J Orthod Dentofacial Orthop 1988;93:201–205.
10. Gianelly AA. Condylar position and class II deep bite, no-overjet malocclusion. Am J Orthod Dentofacial Orthop 1989;96:428–432.
11. Gianelly AA, Cozzanic M, Boffa J. Condylar position and maxillary first premolar extraction. Am J Orthod Dentofacial Orthop 1991;99:473–476.
12. Gianelly AA, Anderson CK, Boffa J. Longitudinal evaluation of condylar position in extraction and nonextraction treatment. Am J Orthod Dentofacial Orthop 1991;100:416–420.
13. Reynders RM. Orthodontics and temporomandibular disorders: A review of the literature (1966–1988). Am J Orthod Dentofacial Orthop 1990;97:463–471.
14. Kim MR, Graber TM, Vianna MA. Orthodontics and temporomandibular disorders: A meta-analysis. Am J Orthod Dentofacial Orthop 2002;121:438–446.
15. Arat ZM, Akcam MO, Gökalp H. Long-term effects of chin-cup therapy on the temporomandibular joints. Eur J Orthod 2003,25:471–475.
16. Beattie JR, Paquette DE, Johnston LE Jr. The functional impact of extraction and nonextraction treatment: A long-term comparison in patients with "borderline," equally susceptible Class II malocclusions. Am J Orthod Dentofacial Orthop 1994;105:444–449.
17. Luppanapornlap S, Johnston LE Jr. The effects of premolar extraction: A long-term comparison of outcomes in "clear-cut" extraction and nonextraction Class II patients. Angle Orthod 1993;63:257–272.
18. McNeill C, Mohl ND, Rugh JD, Tanaka TT. Temporomandibular disorders: Diagnosis, management, education, and research. J Am Dent Assoc 1990;120:253–260.
19. Mohl ND. Temporomandibular disorders: The role of occlusion, TMJ imaging, and electronic devices—A diagnostic update. J Am Coll Dent 1991;58:4–10.
20. Fernandez E, Turk DC. The utility of cognitive coping strategies for altering pain perception: A meta-analysis. Pain 1989;38:123–135.
21. Flor H, Birbaumer N. Comparison of the efficacy of electromyographic biofeedback, cognitive-behavioral therapy, and conservative medical interventions in the treatment of chronic musculoskeletal pain. J Consult Clin Psychol 1993;61:653–658.
22. Gardea MA, Gatchel RJ, Mishra KD. Long-term efficacy of biobehavioral treatment of temporomandibular disorders. J Behav Med 2001;24:341–359.

23. Mishra KD, Gatchel RJ, Gardea MA. The relative efficacy of three cognitive-behavioral treatment approaches to temporomandibular disorders. J Behav Med 2000;23:293–309.

24. Rudy TE, Turk DC, Kubinski JA, Zaki HS. Differential treatment response of TMD patients as a function of psychological characteristics. Pain 1995;61:103–112.

25. Turk D, Zaki H, Rudy T. Effects of intraoral appliance and biofeedback/stress management alone and in combination in treating pain and depression in TMD patients. J Prosthet Dent 1993;70:158–164.

26. Turk DC, Rudy TE, Kubinski JA, Zaki HS, Greco CM. Dysfunctional patients with temporomandibular disorders: Evaluating the efficacy of a tailored treatment protocol. J Consult Clin Psychol 1996;64:139–146.

27. Griffiths RH. Report of the president's conference on the examination, diagnosis and management of temporomandibular disorders. J Am Dent Assoc 1983;106:75–77.

28. Rinchuse DJ, Kandasamy S, Sciote J. A contemporary and evidence-based view of canine protected occlusion. Am J Orthod Dentofacial Orthop 2007;132:90–102.

29. D'Amico A. The canine teeth: Normal functional relation of the natural teeth of man. J S Cal Dent Assoc 1958;26:6–23.

30. Okeson JR. Management of Temporomandibular Disorders and Occlusion, ed 5. St Louis: Mosby, 2005:121–122.

31. Woda A, Vigneron P, Kay D. Non-functional and functional occlusal contacts: A review of the literature. J Prosthet Dent 1979;42:335–341.

32. McNamara Jr JA, Seligman DA, Okeson JP. Occlusion, orthodontic treatment, and temporomandibular disorders: A review. J Orofac Pain 1995;9:73–89.

33. The Academy of Prosthodontics. Glossary of prosthodontic terms, ed 8. J Prosthet Dent 2005;94:10–92.

34. Rinchuse DJ. Counterpoint: A three-dimensional comparison of condylar position changes between centric relation and centric occlusion using the mandibular position indicator. Am J Orthod Dentofacial Orthop 1995;107:319–328.

35. Pameijer JH, Brion M, Glickman I, Roeber FW. Intraoral occlusal telemetry. V. Effect of occlusal adjustment upon tooth contacts during chewing and swallowing. J Prosthet Dent 1970;24:492–497.

36. Pameijer JH, Glickman I, Roeber FW. Intraoral occlusal telemetry. 3. Tooth contacts in chewing, swallowing, and bruxism. J Periodontol 1969;40:253–258.

37. Glickman JI, Martigoni M, Haddad A, Roeber FW. Further observation on human occlusion monitored by intraoral telemetry [abstract 612]. IADR 1970:201.

38. Seligman DA, Pullinger AG. The role of functional occlusal relationships in temporomandibular disorders: A review. J Craniomandib Disord 1991;5:265–279.

39. Luecke PE, Johnston LE Jr. The effect of maxillary first premolar extraction and incisor retraction on mandibular position: Testing the central dogma of "functional orthodontics." Am J Orthod Dentofacial Orthop 1992;101:4–12.

40. Cordray FE. Centric relation treatment and articulator mountings in orthodontics. Angle Orthod 1996;66:153–158.

41. Cordray FE. Three-dimensional analysis of models articulated in the seated condylar position from a deprogrammed asymptomatic population: A prospective study. Part 1. Am J Orthod Dentofacial Orthop 2006;29:619–630.

42. Karl PJ, Foley TF. The use of a deprogramming appliance to obtain centric relation. Angle Orthod 1999;69:117–125.

43. Kulbersh R, Dhutia M, Navarro M, Kaczynski R. Condylar distraction effects of standard edgewise therapy versus gnathologically based edgewise therapy. Semin Orthod 2003;9:117–127.

44. Utt TW, Meyers CE Jr, Wierzba TF, Hondrum SO. A three-dimensional comparison of condylar position changes between centric relation and centric occlusion using the mandibular position indicator. Am J Orthod Dentofacial Orthop 1995;107:298–308.

45. Kulbersh R, Kaczynski R, Freeland T. Orthodontics and gnathology. Semin Orthod 2003;9:93–95.

46. Posselt U. Studies in the mobility of the human mandible. Acta Odontol Scand 1952:10(suppl 10):1–160.

47. Lindauer SJ, Sabol G, Isaacson RJ, Davidovitch M. Condylar movement and mandibular rotation during jaw opening. Am J Orthod Dentofacial Orthop 1995;105:573–577.

48. Alexander SR, Moore RN, DuBois LM. Mandibular condyle position: Comparison articulator mountings and magnetic resonance imaging. Am J Orthod Dentofacial Orthop 1993;104:230–239.

49. Rinchuse DJ. Kandasamy S. Articulators in orthodontics: An evidence-based perspective. Am J Orthod Dentofacial Orthop 2006;129:299–308.

50. Buschang P, Santos-Pinto A. Condylar growth and glenoid fossa displacement during childhood and adolescence. Am J Orthod Dentofacial Orthop 1998;113:437–42.

51. Ellis PE, Benson PE. Does articulating study casts make a difference to treatment planning? J Orthod 2003;30:45–49.

52. de Leeuw R. Internal derangements of the temporomandibular joints. Oral Maxillofac Surg Clin North Am 2008;20:159–168.

53. Kircos L, Ortendahl D, Mark AS, Arakawa M. Magnetic resonance imaging of the TMJ disc in asymptomatic volunteers. J Oral Maxillofacial Surg1987;45:852–854.

54. Larheim TA, Westesson PL, Sano T. Temporomandibular joint disk displacement: Comparison in asymptomatic volunteers and patients. Radiol 2001;218:428–432.

55. Tallents RH, Katzberg RW, Murphy W, Proskin H. Magnetic resonance imaging findings in asymptomatic volunteers and symptomatic patients with temporomandibular disorders. J Prosthet Dent 1996;75:529–533.

56. Klasser GD, Greene CS. Role of oral appliances in the management of sleep bruxism and temporomandibular disorders. Alpha Omegan 2007;100:111–119.

57. Dolwick LF. Intra-articular disc displacement. Part I: Its questionable role in temporomandibular joint pathology. J Oral Maxillofacial Surg 1995;53:1069–1072.

58. Kurita K, Westesson PL, Yuasa H, Toyama M, Machida J, Ogi N. Natural course of untreated symptomatic temporomandibular joint disc displacement without reduction. J Dent Res 1998;77:361–365.

59. de Leeuw R, Boering G, Stegenga B, de Bont LG. Clinical signs of TMJ osteoarthrosis and internal derangement 30 years after nonsurgical treatment. J Orofac Pain 1994;8:18–24.

60. Sato S, Nasu F, Motegi K. Natural course of nonreducing disc displacement of the temporomandibular joint: Changes in chewing movement and masticatory efficiency. J Oral Maxillofac Surg 2002;60:867–872.

61. Farrar WB. Differentiation of temporomandibular joint dysfunction to simplify treatment. J Prosthet Dent 1972;28:629–636.

62. Farrar WB. Disk derangement and dental occlusion: Changing concepts. Int J Periodontics Restorative Dent 1985;33:713–721.

63. Farrar WB, McCarty WL Jr. The TMJ dilemma. J Ala Dent Assoc 1979;63:19–26.

64. Choi BH, Yoo JH, Lee WY. Comparison of magnetic resonance imaging before and after nonsurgical treatment of closed lock. Oral Surg Oral Med Oral Pathol 1994;78:301–305.

65. Clark GT. The TMJ repositioning appliance: A technique for construction, insertion, and adjustment. J Craniomand Pract 1986;4:37–46.

66. Clark GT. Classification, causation and treatment of masticatory myogenous pain and dysfunction. Oral Maxillofac Surg Clin North Am 2008;20:145–157.

67. Moloney F, Howard JA. Internal derangements of the temporomandibular joint: Anterior repositioning splint therapy. Aust Dent J 1986;31:30–39.

68. Greene CS, Laskin DM. Long-term evaluation of treatment for myofascial pain-dysfunction analysis. J Am Dent Assoc 1983;107:235–238.

69. Rinchuse DJ, Kandasamy S. Orthodontics and TMD management. In: Manfredini D (ed). Current Concepts on Temporomandibular Disorders. Chicago: Quintessence, 2010:429–446.

70. Turp JC, Greene CS, Strub JR. Dental occlusion: A critical reflection on past, present and future concepts. J Oral Rehabil 2008;35:446–453.

71. Greene CS. The etiology of temporomandibular disorders: Implications for treatment. J Orofac Pain 2001;15:93–105.
72. Thurman MM, Huang GJ. Insufficient evidence to support the use of stabilization splint therapy over other active interventions in the treatment of temporomandibular myofascial pain. J Am Dent Assoc 2009;140:1524–1525.
73. Greco CM, Rudy TE, Turk DC, Herlich A, Zaki HH. Traumatic onset of temporomandibular disorders: Positive effects of a standardized conservative treatment program. Clin J Pain 1997;13:337–347.
74. Dworkin SF, Massoth DL. Temporomandibular disorders and chronic pain: Disease or illness? J Prosthet Dent 1994;72:29–38.
75. Dworkin SF, LeResche L. Research diagnostic criteria for temporomandibular disorders: Review, criteria, examinations, and specifications, critique. J Craniomandib Disord 1992;6:301–355.

Daniel J. Rinchuse
DMD, MS, MDS, PhD

Peter G. Miles
BDS, MDS

John J. Sheridan
DDS, MSD

CHAPTER

12 | Orthodontic Retention and Stability

Retention and treatment stability are important goals of orthodontics. Nonetheless, despite decades of research, the consensus is still that the stability of aligned teeth is variable and largely unpredictable.[1] In this respect the frustrations of orthodontists have not changed much since Dr Calvin Case argued that the permanent retention of adjusted teeth was the part of orthodontics most indispensable to its success, iterating these words in 1920: "What does this temporary pleasure and satisfaction to ourselves and our patients amount to, if we find in a few years that the very cases which create in us the greatest pride are going back to their former malpositions and disharmonies, in spite of everything we have been able to do with retaining appliances."[2] Similarly, Vanarsdall and White[3] maintained that the public (and dentists themselves) were misled in the early years of orthodontics to think that the results of orthodontic treatment could last a lifetime. Citing a friend, Hawley stated, "If anyone would take my cases when they are finished, retain them, and be responsible for them afterward, I would gladly give him half the fee."[4] Not surprisingly, retention is a difficult component of orthodontics because of the unpredictable nature of stability and patient compliance.

In a Cochrane systematic review resulting in five trials that satisfied their inclusion criteria, Littlewood et al[5] concluded that there are insufficient data regarding orthodontic retention to guide clinical practice and that there is need of high-level randomized controlled trials (RCTs) in this area of orthodontic practice. Therefore, this chapter focuses on an evaluation of the best available evidence, serving as an update of what the authors previously published in 2007 on retention and stability.[6]

Retention for Life

As a result of extensive research at the University of Washington, Little et al[7] concluded that the orthodontist should not assume that stability will occur but rather that instability will likely be the pattern. They stated that the only way to ensure continued satisfactory alignment after orthodontic treatment is most likely retention for life. As a clinical point, it is best not to promise perfectly stable results postretention, even with diligent wear of retainers, but to advocate reasonable alignment postretention.

In a comprehensive review of the orthodontic literature regarding relapse, Shah[8] reported the pejorative aspects of postretention relapse of the mandibular incisors. Moreover, he argued that this relapse could be fallaciously interpreted as a misdiagnosis, the wrong treatment, or inappropriate treatment mechanics. However, mandibular incisor relapse is almost inevitable, regardless of the timing of orthodontic treatment and the treatment techniques employed. Even extraction of premolars to alleviate crowding in conjunction with orthodontic treatment does not appear to make the results any more stable.[1,9,10]

Arch Perimeter and Intercanine Width

The main reason for this propensity for relapse or crowding is the tendency for the dental arch perimeter and the intercanine width to decrease, constricting over time in treated as well as untreated subjects.[11] As early as 1959, Moorrees[12] published his findings, which demonstrated this pattern of dental arch reduction over time from mixed dentition through the transitional dentition and into early adulthood.

Gianelly[13,14] and others[15–18] have argued that the stability of orthodontic treatment can be enhanced by preservation of mandibular pretreatment intercanine width. Therefore, any increase in mandibular intercanine dimension is not stable.[15,17,19,20] A meta-analysis by Burke et al[19] of mandibular intercanine width in treatment and postretention found that mandibular intercanine width tends to expand during treatment by 0.8 to 2.0 mm irrespective of pretreatment classification or whether treatment was extraction or nonextraction. Furthermore, postretention, mandibular intercanine width tends to constrict by 1.2 to 1.9 mm, regardless of the pretreatment classification or whether the treatment was extraction or nonextraction. The results of this study support the concept of maintaining the original pretreatment intercanine width. Unfortunately, some orthodontists still believe in mandibular arch expansion and expanded intercanine width. Dr Lysle Johnston, Jr commented that "once lower canine expansion became an accepted treatment, clinical anarchy became the rule of the day."[21]

Blake and Bibby[22] made six suggestions in regard to enhancing stability of finished orthodontic cases:

1. The patient's pretreatment mandibular arch form should be maintained during orthodontic treatment as much as possible.
2. Original mandibular intercanine width should be maintained as much as possible because expansion of mandibular intercanine width is the most predictable of all orthodontic relapse.
3. Mandibular arch length decreases with time.
4. The most stable position of the mandibular incisor is its pretreatment position. Advancing the mandibular incisors is unstable and should be considered to seriously compromise stability.
5. Fiberotomy is an effective means of reducing rotational relapse.
6. Mandibular incisor reproximation (reducing the tooth width) shows long-term improvements in posttreatment stability.

Circumferential Supracrestal Fiberotomy and Interproximal Force

When evaluating the effectiveness of fiberotomy in the long term, Edwards[23] found it to be somewhat more effective in alleviating pure rotational relapse than labiolingual relapse. Fiberotomy was shown to be more successful in

reducing relapse in the maxillary anterior segment than in the mandibular anterior segment. Furthermore, significant and unpredictable individual tooth movement was still observed. Reorganization of the periodontal ligament occurs over a 3- to 4-month period after treatment,[24,25] while the gingival collagen fiber network typically takes 4 to 6 months to be remodeled, and the elastic supracrestal fibers remain deviated for more than 232 days.[26]

A continuous, compressive interproximal force (IPF), originating in the periodontium and acting on adjacent teeth at their contact points, may be responsible for some long-term arch constriction.[27] Southard et al[28] found a significant correlation between mandibular anterior malalignment and IPF. It has been suggested that if IPF does have an influence on dental alignment, it probably acts in conjunction with lip and cheek forces to collapse the arch. These forces are opposed by the tongue, which tends to expand the arch.

It follows that the influence of IPF should be more evident in the anterior segment of the arch, where the contact points are narrower, the crowns more tapered, and the expansive force of the tongue more intermittent compared with the posterior regions. Perhaps for this reason, mandibular incisor reproximation can counteract IPF by slightly narrowing the teeth and by broadening their contacts to resist contact slippage.

Boese[29] found an improvement in posttreatment stability of the mandibular anterior segment, without retention, when fiberotomy and reproximation were used in combination with overcorrection and selective root torque. This protocol often included serial posttreatment reproximation. Boese's cases all involved extractions, however, and the impact of individual treatment variables could not be isolated.

The effect of the amount and structure of mandibular bone on mandibular incisor stability has recently been investigated in a case-control study at the University of Washington. After measuring trabecular bone structure and cortical bone thickness in both relapsed and stable subjects, Rothe[30] concluded that patients with thinner mandibular cortices are at increased risk of dental relapse.

Third Molars

Mandibular incisor relapse

Kandasamy et al[31] did a comprehensive review of third molars and incisor crowding. Besides the eruption of mandibular third molars, other factors have been associated with mandibular incisor crowding: anterior growth, rotations and remodeling of the mandible,[32–34] mesial migration of posterior teeth,[35] anterior component of force on the occlusion,[36–38] lack of attrition,[39] effects of soft tissue maturation on the position of the teeth,[40,41] differences between the evolutionary reduction of tooth size and jaw size,[42] and tooth size and shape.[43,44]

The justification often stated for extraction of third molars is prevention of mandibular incisor relapse and irregularity. However, Southard[45] and others[46] have argued against the prophylactic extraction of disease-free third molars for the sole purpose of relieving interdental pressure and prevention of incisor crowding. An RCT by Harradine et al[47] on the effect of mandibular third molar extractions on late incisor crowding also failed to demonstrate that removal of third molars prevented mandibular incisor irregularity. According to these findings, orthodontic retention may be more efficacious and cost-effective than third molar extractions.

As a result of a systematic review,[48] the Cochrane group has taken a more conservative view. Based on only three trials that met their selection criteria, they found that there was no evidence to support or refute routine prophylactic removal of asymptomatic impacted third molars in adults. Furthermore, of the three trials, two were RCTs, which suggested that the prophylactic removal of third molars in adolescents does not lessen or prevent late incisor crowding.

Morbidity associated with third molars

Silvestri and Singh[49] have further contended that the morbidity data supporting third molar removal is suspect because most studies have been short-term and retrospective, cross-sectional, and focused mainly on radiographic evidence of disease with sparse or no histopathologic data. Also, with many asymptomatic, disease-free impacted third molars extracted prophylactically early in life, assessing morbidity is problematic. One can even take the contrary point of view that surgical extraction of third molars can be a risk factor for future temporomandibular disorder symptoms.[50]

One example of a possible need for third molar extraction is periodontal pockets in the second and third molar area. Blakey et al[51] reported that 38% of their patients with pocket depth of ≥ 4 mm in the second/third molar region at the beginning of the study worsened over time, increasing morbidity. Therefore, periodontal pockets and other factors need to be considered when evaluating extraction of third molars.

AAOMS Third Molar Multidisciplinary Conference

On October 19, 2010, the American Association of Oral and Maxillofacial Surgeons (AAOMS) held a press conference[52] to present morbidity data for proactive removal of asymptomatic impacted or potentially problematic third molars. In a "point/counterpoint" debate in the *American Journal of Orthodontics and Dentofacial Orthopedics (AJODO)* in July 2011, White and Proffit[53] made similar arguments. An important foundational point made at the conference is that, contrary to what is lumped together in many studies and papers, the designation "asymptomatic or disease free" is unsound because many patients with asymptomatic third molars may have disease, periodontal and/or systemic, and an absence of symptoms does not equal the absence of disease.

The evidence presented at this conference focused on research in three areas:

1. Analyses of outcomes with patients who retained third molars
2. Analyses of the impact of third molar surgery on the patients' quality of life
3. Analyses of third molar data from population and clinical studies conducted for other purposes

The findings reported at this conference recommended third molar removal during young adulthood for enhanced quality of life relating to dental and oral health and reduced risk of illness later in life. Some key findings reported at this conference and on the AAOMS website (http://www.aaoms.org/third_molar_news.php) are as follows:

- An absence of symptoms does not equal the absence of disease.
- Eighty percent of young adult patients who retained previously healthy third molars developed problems within 7 years.
- Extraction of third molars in young adults produces less pain and shorter healing times compared with extraction in older patients.
- Monitoring retained third molars may be more expensive than extraction over a lifetime.
- Most patients (60%) with asymptomatic third molars prefer extraction to retention.
- Retaining third molars can increase the risk for broader conditions, including preterm birth and cardiovascular disease.

A counterargument to these findings was made by Kandasamy[54] in the July *AJODO* debate, in which he advocated a more conservative, low-risk alternative approach. His argument in regard to asymptomatic third molars is one of watchful monitoring and not immediate extraction.

In respect to age and sex, a recent study from the University of North Carolina by Phillips et al[55] involving 958 patients treated at nine academic centers and twelve community practices found that recovery after third molar surgery is faster for younger patients. Specifically, patients younger than 21 years of age (especially females), including adolescents completing an orthodontic treatment regimen, recovered more quickly for quality-of-life outcomes, pain, lifestyle, and oral functions compared to cohorts 21 years and older.

In summary, from a practice-management perspective, because mandibular third molars are not associated with mandibular incisor crowding, orthodontists should distance themselves from involvement. In other words, orthodontists should not write extraction orders for third molar removal for the purpose of preventing incisor crowding because they would therefore have a legal obligation to obtain informed consent from the patient, parent, or legal guardian even though they are not the person removing the teeth.[56] Orthodontists can tell their patients that there may be morbidity data supporting the removal of third molars, but because this is rarely (if ever) related to future crowding, particularly mandibular anterior crowding, the patient's family dentist or oral surgeon should take responsibility for the decision to extract those teeth.

Types of Retention: Rationale

Fixed bonded retainers

Fixed or bonded retainers are most commonly attached canine to canine in the mandibular arch. These can be fabricated from 0.030- to 0.036-inch stainless steel wire and bonded only to the canine teeth, the principle being that they prevent loss of intercanine width and prevent lingual movement of the incisors. Similarly, they can be made of round beta-titanium wire, which has the added advantage of a greater range, acting somewhat like a shock absorber, and is therefore less likely to distort or debond if inadvertently knocked.

Alternatively, a 0.0175-inch, twisted, flexible wire can be bonded to every mandibular tooth, canine to canine. This wire is heat treated to "dead" soft to remove shape memory; otherwise, canine teeth may reposition facially as the wire ends straighten. These can be bonded with conventional composites, although it is easier to place them with the less viscous retainer composite adhesives or a flowable restorative composite. The advantage of bonding to each individual tooth, canine to canine (Fig 12-1), is that it reduces the occasional labial movement or rotation of incisors that can occur if the rigid type is bonded only to the two canines.

A five-stranded 0.0215-inch twisted wire, which is not heat treated and can be shaped to the arch form with a fine, three-pronged plier, has been recommended by Zachrisson.[57] The wire must be completely passive when bonded into position on the teeth. The author reported no side effects from wire distortion,[57] but ideally this would be the subject of a clinical trial to assess any differences in the short and long term. Additionally, the author also suggested a short labial bonded retainer to maintain closed extraction sites in adults.[57]

If fixed bonded retainers are used in the maxillary arch, removable thermoplastic retainers can also be fabricated to fit over these fixed appliances if desired. However, if the bonded retainer creates an interference with the occlusion and mandibular function, Topouzelis and Diamantidou[58] recommend cutting a groove on the palatal surfaces of the maxillary anterior teeth where the retention wire can be bonded, thus eliminating any interference. This is generally not the recommendation of the authors.

Woven, plasma-treated, polyethylene ribbon–reinforced material has been promoted as an alternative to multistranded wire as a bonded fixed retainer. However, in a prospective study, Rose et al[59] concluded that multistranded wire was superior to the ribbon-composite when bonded canine to canine.

The consequences of long-term fixed retainer wear have been a concern. Over a 6-month retention period, Heier et al[60] found limited gingival inflammation with either Hawley-type removable or bonded lingual retainers. Although they found slightly more plaque and calculus on the lingual surfaces in the fixed retainer group, this did not result in more significant gingival inflammation. Pertaining to longer-term use (up to 8 years), the presence of a bonded lingual retainer and the occasional accumulation of plaque and calculus gingival to the retainer wire caused no apparent damage to the hard and soft tissues.[61]

In comparing both short-term (3 to 6 months), and long-term (mean period of 9.65 years) wear of mandibular fixed retention, Pandis et al[62] found no significant difference in plaque and gingival indices and bone level between the two groups. However, the long-term group showed higher calculus accumulation, greater marginal recession, and increased probing depth. Therefore, this study raised some concerns about the morbidity associated with long-term fixed retention. However, the authors pointed out that these findings should be evaluated on an individual basis depending on the anatomy of tissues and oral hygiene. A confounding factor in this study may be time. With increased age, you might expect some of the findings in the long-term group regardless of fixed retainer wear compared with the short-term group. So how much of the result was associated with long-term wear of the fixed retainers and how much was associated with aging?

In a retrospective case-control retention study comparing permanent bonded retainers and removable retainers, Cerny at el[63] reported on 46 patients in their sample that had worn permanent bonded retainers for more than 15 years and 43 patients who had worn removable retainers for 2 years. Most removable retainer patients quit wearing their retainers before 2 years expired. The results of the study showed greater stability in alignment in the permanent bonded retainer group, and gingival recession, periodontal disease, and alveolar bone loss did not differ significantly between the two groups. The authors also found the permanent bonded retainers to be quite robust and durable and reported that the time usually required to repair a fractured permanent bonded retainer was less than 15 minutes per unit bond/wire.

With a sample of 221 consecutively treated patients, Renkema et al[64] evaluated the robustness and stability of a fixed bonded flexible spiral wire to the mandibular six anterior teeth over a 5-year posttreatment period. The effectiveness of maintaining alignment in a very high percentage of patients was reported. However, they recommended regular checkups of patients to detect bonding failures, posttreatment changes, or complications as early as pos-

Fig 12-1 Maxillary bonded lateral-to-lateral fixed retainer *(a)* and mandibular bonded canine-to-canine fixed retainer *(b)*.

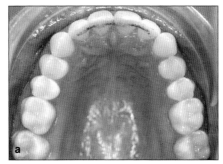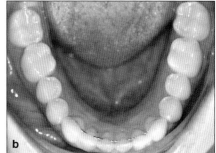

Fig 12-2 *(a and b)* This patient failed to wear the prescribed removable vacuum formed retainer, and the occlusion has altered even with a fixed wire retainer in place. This is possibly due to distortion of the wire during function or stress relaxation of the wire.

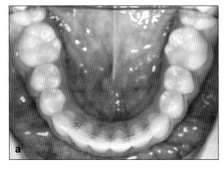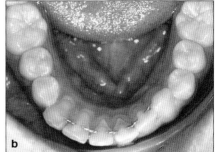

sible. In 21 patients, alignment was mostly compromised by bond failure of the retainers.

Advantages

It has been contended in the orthodontic literature that orthodontic patients with reduced periodontium may be better off with fixed retainers because removable retainers may produce "jiggling" forces, compromising healing and bone regeneration, while a fixed retainer can serve as a periodontal splint during orthodontic retention.[54,65,66] In addition, there is not a compliance issue with fixed retainers like there is with removable retainers, and minor settling of the posterior occlusion can occur.

Disadvantages

The patient is obviously responsible for cleaning the teeth and the retainer, but who takes responsibility if a fixed retainer breaks and the teeth subsequently relapse? Obviously the failure of the fixed retainer can occur at any time, and the material will eventually fail. So even with diligent recalls and supervision by the orthodontist, a broken fixed retainer may not be detected by the patient, and relapse, decalcification, and caries may result. A bonded wire retainer can also be distorted by occlusal or outside forces. Katsaros et al[67] reported significant unexpected changes such as torque changes of individual teeth or changes in canine position, which may necessitate retreatment (Fig 12-2). With this in mind, a removable appliance may be best suited for lifetime retention.

Removable Hawley-type retainers

The Hawley-type retainer is still commonly used in the maxillary arch. To enhance mechanical retention, acrylic can be added to the labial bow from canine to canine.

Hawley full- or part-time wear?

In a master's thesis (under Dr Sheridan's supervision), Butler measured the stability of orthodontic results over the first 9 months after the delivery of removable Hawley retainers (Sheridan JJ, personal communication, 2006). Full-time wear was compared with night-only wear in both extraction and nonextraction cases. Sixty percent of the full-time patients lost or broke their retainers, as opposed to only 13% of the night-only patients. There were no significant differences between the two groups in any of the retention parameters, including incisal stability, intercanine width, arch length, and intermolar width.

Likewise, an RCT by Shawesh et al[68] compared two different orthodontic retention protocols: night-only wear of maxillary and mandibular Hawley retainers for 1 year compared with 6 months of full-time wear followed by 6 months of night-only wear. Study casts were made at the start (T0) and end (T1) of treatment and 1 year after debonding (T2). Little's irregularity index was used to measure maxillary and mandibular labial segment crowding. There were no statistically significant differences between the two retention regimens at T2 for labial segment irregularity or crowding. Therefore, because both retention regimens were equally effective during the 1-year reten-

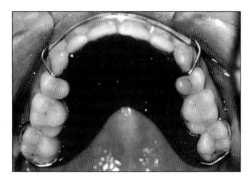

Fig 12-3 Hawley retainer with C-clasp around the maxillary second molars.

tion period, it appears reasonable to instruct orthodontic patients to wear their retainers only at night.

When microsensors were implanted in maxillary Hawley retainers to accurately monitor patient compliance, there was a significant difference between the amount of actual and prescribed retainer usage in a small sample (9 patients in the test group and 10 in the control group) of teenage orthodontic patients. Orthodontic patients who were aware that they were actively being monitored demonstrated better compliance than those who were unaware of the monitoring. However, even though they were being monitored, very few in the test group demonstrated full-time retainer wear. Therefore, it was concluded that a more reasonable compliance protocol in this sample of teenagers would be to wear their maxillary Hawley retainers half-time, or 12 hours per day. Limitations of this study were the small sample size and the duration of the study (only 30 days).[69]

Advantages

Sauget et al[70] noted that a traditional Hawley retainer allows occlusal settling, and thus an improvement in posterior occlusal contacts, compared to full-coverage thermoplastic retainers. Furthermore, a Hawley retainer is quite robust, some lasting longer than 15 years in the authors' practices.

Disadvantages

Settling cannot occur where wires cross the occlusion, and iatrogenic problems may arise in these areas. There is often sufficient clearance for a crossover wire between the canine and premolar, however, and the posterior wire can be fabricated as a distally approaching ring or C-clasp rather than an Adams clasp to avoid occlusal interference (Fig 12-3). An alternative design is the Begg-style wraparound retainer with the labial bow crossing distal to the molars. Thin stabilizing wires can be added in the anterior region to keep the labial section from moving vertically, incisally, or gingivally.

Of course, compliance is always a concern with removable appliances. In addition, contrary to expectation, removable retainers may still challenge patient oral hygiene. For instance, there is some evidence to suggest that removable partial dentures can promote plaque accumulation.[71,72]

Removable thermoplastic retainers/vacuum formed retainers

Thermoplastic retainers, or vacuum formed retainers (VFRs), can generally be made from two classes of material: copolyester (Essix type A) and polypropylene or ethylene copolymer (Essix type C+). An attachment such as a button can be bonded with acrylic to type A retainers (Fig 12-4) but not to the more robust type C+ material. The procedure for bonding an attachment is as follows: roughen the area to be bonded, then apply a monomer acrylic to the area and let it stand for 2 to 5 minutes; then reapply the monomer, place the acrylic on the attachment, and cure it either chemically or with a light source; then let the retainer set for 30 minutes.

Type A materials are generally more esthetic because of better clarity, but they have a propensity to tear and crack (Fig 12-5). Type C+ materials are more robust, but their mechanical retention is not as good. Manufacturers are creating a new generation of thermoplastic materials, including Essix ACE (Denstply) and Duraclear (Dentsply), in an attempt to combine the benefits of the A and C+ materials: durability, retention, clarity, and bondability to acrylic. In the authors' experience, however, these new materials and other VFRs are not durable, tend to crack easily, and discolor. Testing by Karam and Rinchuse[73] showed that VFRs that cover surfaces of teeth restored with dental amalgam become tarnished and confine amalgam corrosion products, including mercury and zinc (Fig 12-6).

In a study by Lindauer and Shoff[74] at the Medical College of Virginia, 56 patients were randomly assigned to Essix and Hawley retention groups, 28 patients in each group. The patients in the Essix group, canine-to-canine type, were instructed to wear their mandibular retainers full-time and their maxillary retainers half-time for the first 4 weeks, followed by both retainers only at night thereafter. The thermoplastic retainers were as effective as the Hawley retainers in maintaining orthodontic corrections, and there was no incidence of anterior open bite in the Essix group.

In a prospective RCT comparing the clinical effectiveness of Hawley retainers (n = 196) and VFRs (n = 201), Rowland et al[75] found after 6 months that more incisor irregularity occurred in the Hawley group than in the VFR group. In another study,[76] 389 patients who were about to have their fixed appliances removed were randomly assigned to Hawley (n = 192) or VFR (n = 197) groups. Participants were less satisfied with Hawleys than VFRs in terms of speech and esthetics. Moreover, VFRs were considered more cost-effective in controlling irregularity.

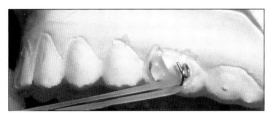

Fig 12-4 Type A thermoplastic material with a bonded metal attachment for elastics.

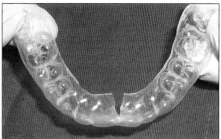

Fig 12-5 Torn and cracked thermoplastic retainer showing the fragility of plastic.

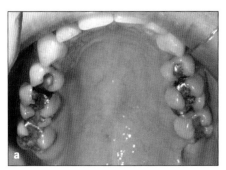

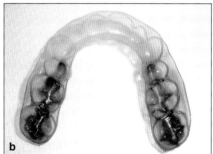

Fig 12-6 (a) Note the large posterior amalgam restorations. (b) The VFR for the same patient, which was only worn for 6 months. Note the corresponding discoloration where the patient's amalgam restorations have leached into the thermoplastic material.

VFR full- or part-time wear?

An RCT by Thickett and Power[77] evaluated the efficacy of wearing VFRs full-time or part-time in patients that had four first premolars extracted. Study casts were compared at the start of active treatment (T1), at debonding (T2), 6 months into retention (T3), and 1 year after debonding (T4). Variables measured were irregularity index, intercanine width, intermolar width, arch length, overbite, overjet, and Peer Assessment Rating Index. Although there were some subtle differences such as in overbite, overall there were no statistically significant differences in the full-time group compared with the part-time group. Therefore, the authors recommended that VFRs can be worn at nighttime only. This regimen will minimize the chance of VFRs being lost at school or at restaurants or left out and chewed on by family pets. The VFRs can be stored in a bathroom cabinet when not worn during the day.

Advantages

Some additional advantages of VFRs are that the responsibility of retention resides with the patient and that minor tooth movement can be accomplished as described by Sheridan et al,[78,79] Rinchuse and Rinchuse,[80] and Rinchuse et al.[81] Canine-to-canine thermoplastic retainers, as advocated by Sheridan in nonextraction cases, may enhance posterior occlusal contacts without causing an anterior open bite if worn only at night or part-time.

These clear and inexpensive plastic devices can also be used as habit appliances, molar uprighting appliances, bleaching trays, space maintainers, and bite planes. As a retainer after orthodontic treatment, it offers precise adaptation to the teeth. Because it is light and less visible, many patients prefer this type of retainer compared with the conventional Hawley retainer, whose esthetic characteristics and comfort may be compromised by acrylic and metal.

VFRs can be sectioned to allow settling of the posterior occlusion if desired. The patient presented in Fig 12-7a had some disocclusion of the molars, so the VFR material was sectioned to permit settling of the teeth in this area. Figure 12-7b shows the sectioned VFRs in the mouth to permit occlusal settling. Figure 12-7c shows the occlusion after 9 weeks, with the posterior teeth in good occlusion.

In a deep bite case, a maxillary 3×3 VFR may help maintain bite opening and prevent relapse. Conversely, an open bite patient will need full-coverage VFRs to minimize the risk of bite opening during retention.

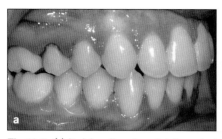
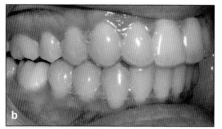
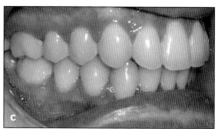

Fig 12-7 *(a)* At debonding, there is infraocclusion at the first molar area. *(b)* VFRs were sectioned to allow settling of the posterior occlusion. *(c)* Occlusion after 9 weeks of settling with segmented VFRs.

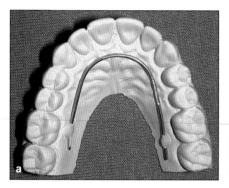
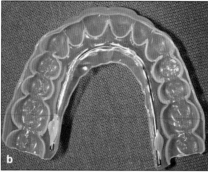

Fig 12-8 *(a)* A U-shaped wire (0.032-inch) is placed adjacent to the gingival margin. The distal tips of the wire are held off the cast with a 0.05-inch mound of composite. *(b)* After thermoforming, the transarch stability wire is securely incorporated into the appliance.

Disadvantages

The material is not as robust and durable as a Hawley-type retainer. Therefore, there is a need for more remakes. They do not allow occlusal settling if they extend back to the molars (full coverage). Obviously another disadvantage compared with a fixed retainer is compliance.

Because of their minimal thickness and U-shape configuration, VFRs are not rigid enough for transarch stability. This discrepancy was described by Gill et al[82] when they reported that, in cases that required significant expansion techniques, a rigid Hawley-type retainer rather than an Essix appliance was considered more efficient for the maintenance of arch expansion.

However, Sheridan[83] introduced a procedure to make it possible to induce formidable transarch stability into a VFR by simply incorporating a stable metal strut into the appliance when it is thermoformed by bending a thick round wire (0.032-inch is recommended) into a U shape and placing it on the lingual surface of the cast a few millimeters below the cervical line (Fig 12-8a). When the plastic thermoforms over the cast, it will completely encapsulate the wire, making it an integral part of the retainer (Fig 12-8b). To ensure said encapsulation, a 0.05-inch mound of composite should be placed under the distal tips of the stability wire (see Fig 12-8a). Additionally, the incorporation of the lateral stability gives the clinician the option of using different thicknesses and types of plastic when transarch stability is assured.

Combination of removable and fixed retainers

A Hawley-style maxillary retainer with labial acrylic coverage to control rotations and distally approaching C-clasps rather than Adams clasps is an excellent all-purpose maxillary retainer that allows minor occlusal settling. Because the mandibular arch is more prone to relapse, a fixed retainer bonded to six anterior teeth reduces this risk.

In Class II, division 2 treatment or a case with substantial maxillary anterior rotations or spacing, a bonded maxillary retainer may also be desirable. For added security and long-term retention, a thermoplastic retainer can be made over the fixed bonded retainer for nighttime wear (see Fig 12-2), as some have described as wearing both "belt and suspenders."

Bonded retainers can be left in place for a predetermined period of 1 to 2 years and then replaced by removable retainers.

In an RCT[84] designed to evaluate three retention protocols for 1 year—VFR in the maxilla and canine-to-canine bonded mandibular retainer, VFR in the maxilla and interproximal enameloplasty (IPR) of the 10 proximal surfaces of the mandibular anterior teeth, and prefabricated positioner covering both maxillary and mandibular teeth—no clinically significant differences were found among the three groups for Little irregularity index, intercanine and intermolar width, arch length, overjet, and overbite after 1 year of retention.

Stability

From an original sample of 1,641 randomly selected primary school children observed from ages 7 to 17 years, Jonsson and Magnusson[85] reported on 308 patients who were available 25 years later for reexamination. They evaluated the long-term changes in anterior crowding and spacing in orthodontically treated and untreated patients. Their findings were as follows: The long-term nonextraction group developed unfavorable maxillary and mandibular anterior crowding. Maxillary spacing was universally reduced in untreated and treated patients. They recommended prolonged or permanent bonded retainers, especially in the nonextraction and untreated groups. However, some limitations or confounders in this study were small sample sizes of subgroups, varying premolar extraction patterns, and vague sample descriptions.

Using American Board of Orthodontics cases, Greco et al[86] looked at posttreatment "settling" from 9 months to 9 years, 8 months; the average was 3 years, 4 months posttreatment. They found that although alignment deteriorates during "settling," all other parameters such as marginal ridges, overjet, occlusal contacts, occlusal relationships, and interproximal contacts do not. The most significant enhancement of occlusal contacts happens prior to 4 years posttreatment. They also noticed little difference in the magnitude of change in occlusal contacts between fixed and removable retainers. Lastly, using the irregularity index, they found significant anterior changes with both Hawley retainers and multistranded, bonded lingual wires.

One approach evaluated by Aasen and Espeland[87] to maintain alignment of mandibular incisors without the use of retainers was IPR, both during and after orthodontic treatment, and overcorrection of rotated teeth early in treatment. Good stability was noted up to 3 years posttreatment, with a mean increase in irregularity index of only 0.6 mm. During active orthodontic treatment, diligence was taken to maintain dental arch form and to avoid lateral expansion of the mandibular arch and proclination of the incisors.

One long-held tenet in orthodontics is that stability of extraction space closure is enhanced by root parallelism of adjacent teeth. A recent retrospective study of 56 patients treated with four first premolar extractions looked at the effect of the degree of root parallelism on relapse of extraction spaces.[88] The findings showed that there were no differences in root angulation at the end of treatment in patients with and without relapse of the extraction spaces. Therefore, the angulation between the canines and the second premolars after treatment had no influence on the relapse of the extraction spaces.

Regarding the stability of orthodontic treatment, Proffit et al[89] argue for stability from the frame of reference of a "soft tissue paradigm" instead of the outdated "Angle's paradigm." In the "soft tissue paradigm," stability is related primarily to soft tissue pressure and equilibrium effects and not primarily to dental occlusion. According to Proffit et al,[89] the adaptations of the soft tissue to tooth position—not tooth position itself—is what determines the stability of the orthodontic treatment.

In a study of 87 Class I malocclusion patients treated with four premolar extractions and edgewise appliances, de Freitas et al[90] concluded that the quality of the finished occlusion is not a determinant for postretention stability; similarly, high-quality orthodontic finishing does not guarantee postretention stability. This conclusion is supported by Ormiston et al,[91] who also found that the quality of finishing does not necessarily relate to postretention stability. Considering these studies and the evidence presented in this chapter, lifetime retention is indicated irrespective of the severity of the pretreatment malocclusion and the quality of the treatment results.

Conclusion

The authors believe that it is essential to establish a retention protocol based on the needs and concerns of each individual patient. With conflicting views and lack of scientific evidence regarding the causes of relapse, the most predictable and cost-effective way to ensure the stability of orthodontic treatment is probably a lifetime of retainer wear. Therefore, patient compliance is of the utmost importance. With this goal in mind, the authors have their patients (even minor children) and parents sign both pretreatment and posttreatment agreements acknowledging that they will have to wear retainers for an extended period of time—a lifetime. Patients thus share the responsibility with orthodontists of keeping their teeth straight.

Summary points

- Retention should be for a lifetime.
- It appears that half-time (night-only) wear of removable retainers may be as good as full-time wear.
- High-quality orthodontic results may not be related to posttreatment stability.
- If using mandibular 3 × 3 bonded retainers, continued monitoring is necessary to detect breakage as soon as possible. Even with diligent recalls and supervision by the orthodontist, a broken fixed retainer may not be detected by the patient, and relapse, decalcification, and caries may result.
- Pretreatment mandibular intercanine width should be maintained.
- Prophylactic extraction of third molars to prevent mandibular incisor relapse and irregularity is not founded.
- For third molars, an absence of symptoms does not necessarily equate to the absence of disease. Therefore, seemingly asymptomatic, disease-free third molars should be evaluated for extraction before the age of 21 years, preferably by the family dentist or oral surgeon.

- From a practice-management perspective, because mandibular third molars are not associated with mandibular incisor crowding, orthodontists should distance themselves from involvement, not writing extraction orders for third molar removal.

References

1. Freitas KM, de Freitas MR, Henriques JF, Pinzan A, Janson G. Postretention relapse of mandibular anterior crowding in patients treated without mandibular premolar extraction. Am J Orthod Dentofacial Orthop 2004;125:480–487.
2. Case CS. Principles of retention in orthodontia. Am J Orthod Dentofacial Orthop 2003;124:352–361.
3. Vanarsdall RL, White RP Jr. Relapse and retention: Professional and public attitudes. Am J Orthod Dentofacial Orthop 1990;98:184.
4. Hawley CA. "A removable retainer." Dental Cosmos 1919;61:449–554.
5. Littlewood SJ, Millett DT, Doubleday B, Bearn DR, Worthington HV. Retention procedures for stabilising tooth position after treatment with orthodontic braces. Cochrane Database Syst Rev 2006;(1):CD002283.
6. Rinchuse DJ, Miles PG, Sheridan JJ. Orthodontic retention and stability: A clinical perspective. J Clin Orthod 2007;41:125–132.
7. Little RM, Reidel RA, Artun J. An evaluation of changes in mandibular anterior alignment from 10 to 20 years post retention. Am J Orthod Dentofacial Orthop 1988;93:423–428.
8. Shah AA. Postretention changes in mandibular crowding: A review of the literature. Am J Orthod Dentofacial Orthop 2003;124:298–308.
9. Heiser W, Niederwanger A, Bancher B, Bittermann G, Neunteufel N, Kulmer S. Three-dimensional dental arch and palatal form changes after extraction and nonextraction treatment. Part 1. Arch length and area. Am J Orthod Dentofacial Orthop 2004;126:71–81.
10. Erdinc AE, Nanda RS, Isiksal E. Relapse of anterior crowding in patients treated with extraction and nonextraction of premolars. Am J Orthod Dentofacial Orthop 2006;129:775–784.
11. Sinclair R, Little R. Maturation of untreated normal occlusions. Am J Orthod Dentofacial Orthop 1983;83:114–123.
12. Moorrees C. The dentition of the growing child. A longitudinal study of dental development between 3 and 18 years of age. Cambridge, MA: Harvard University Press, 1959.
13. Gianelly A. Rapid palatal expansion in the absence of crossbites: Added value? Am J Orthod Dentofacial Orthop 2003;124:362–365.
14. Gianelly A. Evidence-based therapy: An orthodontic dilemma. Am J Orthod Dentofacial Orthop 2006;129:596–598.
15. Artun J, Garol JD, Little RM. Long-term stability of mandibular incisors following successful treatment of Class II, Division 1, malocclusion. Angle Orthod 1996;66:229–238.
16. Glenn G, Sinclair PM, Alexander RG. Nonextraction orthodontic therapy: Posttreatment dental and skeletal stability. Am J Orthod Dentofacial Orthop 1987;92:321–328.
17. Rossouw PE, Preston CB, Lombard DJ, Truter JW. A longitudinal evaluation of the anterior border of the dentition. Am J Orthod Dentofacial Orthop 1993;104:146–152.
18. Strang RH. The fallacy of denture expansion as a treatment procedure. Angle Orthod 1949;19:12–22.
19. Burke SP, Silveira AM, Goldsmith LJ, Yancey JM, Van Stewart A, Scarfe WC. A meta-analysis of mandibular intercanine width in treatment and postretention. Angle Orthod 1998;68:53–60.
20. Yavari J, Shrout MK, Russel CM, Haas AJ, Hamilton EH. Relapse in Angle Class II division 1 malocclusion treated by tandem mechanics without extraction of permanent teeth: A retrospective analysis. Am J Orthod Dentofacial Orthop 2000;118:34–42.
21. Bowman SJ. Educator profile. An interview with Dr. J Lysle E. Johnston, Jr., DDS, MS, PhD: Part 1. Orthod Pract US 2011;2:6–9.
22. Blake M, Bibby K. Retention and stability: A review of the literature. Am J Orthod Dentofacial Orthop 1998;114:299–306.
23. Edwards JG. A long-term prospective evaluation of the circumferential supracrestal fiberotomy in alleviating orthodontic relapse. Am J Orthod Dentofacial Orthop 1988;93:380–387.
24. Reitan K. Tissue rearrangement during retention of orthodontically rotated teeth. Angle Orthod 1959;29:105–113.
25. Reitan K. Clinical and histologic observations on tooth movement during and after orthodontic treatment. Am J Orthod 1967;53:721–745.
26. Reitan K. Principles of retention and avoidance of posttreatment relapse. Am J Orthod 1969;55:776–790.
27. Southard TE, Southard KA, Tolley EA. Periodontal force: A potential cause of relapse. Am J Orthod Dentofacial 1992;101:221–227.
28. Southard TE, Behrents RG, Tolley EA. The anterior component of occlusal force. Part 2: Relationship with dental malalignment. Am J Orthod Dentofacial Orthop 1990;97:41–44.
29. Boese LR. Fibrotomy and reproximation without lower retention 9 years in retrospect: Part II. Angle Orthod 1980;50:169–178.
30. Rothe LE. Trabecular and cortical bone as risk factors for orthodontic relapse. Am J Orthod Dentofacial Orthop 2006;130;476–484.
31. Kandasamy S, Rinchuse DJ, Rinchuse DJ. The wisdom behind third molar extractions. Aust Dent J 2009;54:284–292.
32. Björk A, Skieller V. Facial development and tooth eruption. An implant study at the age of puberty. Am J Orthod Dentofacial Orthop 1972;62:339–383.
33. Björk A, Skieller V. Normal and abnormal growth of the mandible. A synthesis of longitudinal cephalometric implant studies over a period of 25 years. Eur J Orthod 1983;5:1–46.
34. Broadbent BH. Ontogenic development of occlusion. Angle Orthod 1941;11:223–241.
35. Moss JP, Picton DC. Experimental mesial drift in adult monkeys (Macaca irus). Arch Oral Biol 1967;12:1313–1320.
36. Southard KA, Behrents RG, Tolley EA. The anterior component of force. Part 1. Measurement and distribution. Am J Orthod Dentofacial Orthop 1989;96:493–500.
37. Southard TE, Southard KA, Weeda LW. Mesial force from unerupted third molars. Am J Orthod Dentofacial Orthop 1991;99:220–225.
38. van Beek H, Fidler VJ. An experimental study of the effect of functional occlusion on mesial tooth migration in Macaque monkeys. Arch Oral Biol 1977;22:269–271.
39. Begg PR, Kesling PC. Begg orthodontic theory and technique. Philadelphia: Saunders, 1971.
40. van der Linden FP. Genetic and environmental factors in dentofacial morphology. Am J Orthod Dentofacial Orthop 1966;52:576–583.
41. Wood DP, Floreani KJ, Galil KA, Teteruck WR. The effect of incisal bite force on condylar seating. Angle Orthod 1994;64:53–61.
42. Björk A. Some biological aspects of prognathism and occlusion of the teeth. Acta Odontol Scand 1950;8:1–40.
43. Nordeval K, Wisth PJ, Boe OE. Mandibular anterior crowding in relation to tooth size and craniofacial morphology. Scand J Dent Res 1975;83:267–273.
44. Peck S, Peck H. Orthodontic aspects of dental anthropology. Angle Orthod 1975;45:95–102.
45. Southard TE. Third molars and incisor crowding: When removal is unwarranted. J Am Dent Assoc 1992;23:75–79.
46. Song F, O'Meara S, Wilson P, Golder S, Kleijnen J. The effectiveness and cost-effectiveness of prophylactic removal of wisdom teeth. Health Technol Assess 2000;4(15):1–43.
47. Harradine NW, Pearson MH, Toth B. The effect of extraction of third molars on late lower incisor crowding: A randomized controlled trial. Br J Orthod 1998;25:117–122.
48. Mettes TG, Nienhuijs ME, van der Sanden WJ, Verdonschot EH, Plasschaert AJ. Interventions for treating asymptomatic impacted wisdom teeth in adolescents and adults. Cochrane Database Syst Rev 2005;18(2):CD003879.
49. Silvestri Jr R, Singh I. The unresolved problem of the third molar: Would people be better off without it? J Am Dent Assoc 2003;134:450–455.

50. Threlfall AG, Kanaa MD, Davies SJ, Tickle M. Possible link between extraction of wisdom teeth and temporomandibular disc displacement with reduction: Matched case control study. Br J Oral Maxillofac Surg 2005;43:13–16.

51. Blakey GH, Jacks MT, Offenbacher S, et al. Progression of periodontal disease in the second/third molar region in subjects with asymptomatic third molars. J Oral Maxillofac Surg 2006;64:189–193.

52. Wisdom Tooth Research Press Event. Presented at the AAOMS Third Molar Interdisciplinary Conference, Washington DC, 19 October 2010. http://www.aaoms.org/third_molar_news.php. Accessed 9 April 2012.

53. White RP, Proffit WR. Evaluation and management of asymptomatic third molars: Lack of symptoms does not equate to lack of pathology. Am J Orthod Dentofacial Orthop 2011;140:10–16.

54. Kandasamy S. Evaluation and management of asymptomatic third molars: Watchful monitoring is a low-risk alternative to extraction. Am J Orthod Dentofacial Orthop 2011;140:11–17.

55. Phillips C, Gelesko S, Proffit WR, White RP Jr. Recovery after third-molar surgery: The effects of age and sex. Am J Orthod Dentofacial Orthop 2010;138:700.e1–700.e8.

56. Jerrold L. A matter of degrees. Am J Orthod Dentofacial Orthop 1998;114:606–608.

57. Zachrisson BU. Long-term experience with direct-bonded retainers: Update and clinical advice. J Clin Orthod 2007;41:728–737.

58. Topouzelis N, Diamantidou A. Orthodontic treatment in patients with reduced periodontium. Hellenic Orthod Rev 2003;6:175–192.

59. Rose E, Frucht S, Jonas IE. Clinical comparison of a multistranded wire and a direct-bonded polyethylene ribbon-reinforced resin composite used for lingual retention. Quintessence Int 2002;33:579–583.

60. Heier EE, De Smit AA, Wijgaerts IA, Adriaens PA. Periodontal implications of bonded versus removable retainer. Am J Orthod Dentofacial Orthop 1997;112:607–616.

61. Årtun J. Caries and periodontal reactions associated with long-term use of different types of bonded lingual retainers. Am J Orthod 1984;86:112–118.

62. Pandis N, Vlahopoulos K, Madianos P, Eliades T. Long-term periodontal status of patients with mandibular lingual fixed retention. Eur J Orthod 2007;29:471–476.

63. Cerny R, Cockrell D, Lloyd D. Long-term results of permanent bonded retention. J Clin Orthod 2010;44:611–616.

64. Renkema AM, Renkema A, Bronkhorst E, Katsaros. Long-term effectiveness of canine-to-canine bonded flexible spiral wire lingual retainers. Am J Orthod Dentofacial Orthop 2011;139:614–621.

65. Zachrisson BU. Clinical implications of recent orthodontic-periodontic research findings. Semin Orthod 1996;2:4–12.

66. Zachrisson BU. Orthodontics and periodontics. In: Lindhe J, Karring T, Lang NP (eds). Clinical Periodontology and Implant Dentistry, ed 3. Copenhagen: Munksgaard, 1997:741–793.

67. Katsaros C, Liva C, Renkema AM. Unexpected complications of bonded mandibular lingual retainers. Am J Orthod Dentofacial Orthop 2007;132:838–841.

68. Shawesh M, Bhatti B, Usmani T, Mandall N. Hawley retainers full- or part-time? A randomized clinical trial. Eur J Orthod 2010;32:165–170.

69. Ackerman MB, Thornton B. Posttreatment compliance with removable maxillary retention in a teenage population: A short-term randomized clinical trial. Orthodontics (Chic) 2011;12:22–27.

70. Sauget E, Covell DA, Boero RP, Lieber WS. Comparison of occlusal contacts with use of Hawley and clear overlay retainers. Angle Orthod 1997;67:223–230.

71. American Academy of Periodontology. Parameter on plaque-induced gingivitis. J Periodontol 2000;71:851–852.

72. Zlatarić DK, Celebić A, Valentić-Peruzović M. The effect of removable partial dentures on periodontal health of abutment and non-abutment teeth. J Periodontol 2002;73:137–144.

73. Karam J, Rinchuse DJ. Dental amalgam corrosion in vacuum-formed retainers. Orthodontics 2011;12:70–74.

74. Lindauer SJ, Schoff RC. Comparison of Essix and Hawley retainers. J Clin Orthod 1998;32:95–97.

75. Rowland H, Hichens L, Williams A, et al. The effectiveness of Hawley and vacuum-formed retainers: A single-center randomized controlled trial. Am J Orthod Dentofacial Orthod 2007;132:730–737.

76. Hichens L, Rowland H, Williams A, et al. Cost-effectiveness and patient satisfaction: Hawley and vacuum-formed retainers. Eur J Orthod 2007;29:372–378.

77. Thickett E, Power S. A randomized clinical trial of thermoplastic retainer wear. Eur J Orthod 2010;32:1–5.

78. Sheridan JJ, LeDoux W, McMinn R. Essix appliances: Minor tooth movement with divots and windows. J Clin Orthod 1994;28:659–663.

79. Sheridan JJ, McMinn R, LeDoux W. Essix thermosealed appliances: Various orthodontic uses. J Clin Orthod 1995;29:108–113.

80. Rinchuse DJ, Rinchuse DJ. Active tooth movement with the Essix appliance. J Clin Orthod 1997;3:109–112.

81. Rinchuse DJ, Rinchuse DJ, Dinsmore C. Elastic traction with Essix-based anchorage. J Clin Orthod 2002;36:46–48.

82. Gill D, Naini F, Jones A, Tredwin C. Part-time versus full-time retainer wear following fixed appliance therapy: A randomized prospective controlled trial. World J Orthod 2007;6:300–306.

83. Sheridan JJ. Incorporating formidable transarch stability into an Essix retainer. J Clin Orthod (in press).

84. Tynelius GE, Bondemark L, Lilja-Karlander E. Evaluation of orthodontic treatment after 1 year of retention—A randomized controlled trial. Eur J Orthod 2010;32:542–547.

85. Jonsson T, Magnusson TE. Crowding and spacing in the dental arches: Long-term development in treated and untreated subjects. Am J Orthod Dentofacial Orthop 2010;138:384.e1–384.e7.

86. Greco PM, English JD, Briss BS, et al. Posttreatment tooth movement: For better or for worse. Am J Orthod Dentofacial Orthop 2010;138:552–558.

87. Aasen TO, Espeland L. An approach to maintain orthodontic alignment of lower incsiors without the use of retainers. Eur J Orthod 2005;27:209–214.

88. Chiqueto K, Janson G, de Almeida CT, Storniolo JM, Barros SE, Henriques JF. Influence of root parallelism on the stability of extraction-site closures. Am J Orthod Dentofacial Orthop 2011;139:e505–e510.

89. Proffit WR, Fields HW Jr, Sarver DM. Orthodontic treatment planning: From problem list to specific plan. In: Contemporary Orthodontics, ed 4. St Louis: Mosby, 2007:237.

90. de Freitas KM, Janson G, de Freitas MR, Pinzan A, Henriques JF, Pinzan-Vercelino CR. Influence of the quality of the finished occlusion on postretention occlusal relapse. Am J Orthod Dentofacial Orthop 2007;132:428.e9–428.e14.

91. Ormiston JP, Huang GJ, Little RM, Decker JD, Seuk GD. Retrospective analysis of long-term stable and unstable orthodontic treatment outcomes. Am J Orthod Dentofacial Orthop 2005;128:568–574.

Eric Liou
DDS, MS

CHAPTER 13

Accelerated Orthodontic Tooth Movement

Orthodontic treatment is tedious and often takes 2 to 3 years in adult patients. While the acceleration of orthodontic tooth movement to shorten treatment time is a challenging task in orthodontics, several efforts have been made. Research in this area can be codified into the following five categories:

1. Biomechanical approach, such as self-ligating bracket systems
2. Physiologic approach, such as direct electric current stimulation or low-level laser therapies (LLLTs)
3. Pharmacologic approach, such as local injection of cytokines/hormones
4. Surgical-assisted approach, such as periodontal ligament (PDL) distraction osteogenesis, dentoalveolus distraction osteogenesis, selective decortication, piezoincision, corticision, or piezopuncture
5. Surgery-simulated approach, such as the submucosal injection of platelet-rich plasma (PRP)

Biomechanical Approach

Self-ligating bracket system

Self-ligating brackets have been gaining popularity in recent years. They are not new to orthodontics. The first self-ligating bracket, the Russell attachment, was introduced by Stolzenberg[1] in 1935 to enhance clinical efficiency by reducing ligation time. Subsequently, some early self-ligating brackets were introduced such as the Edgelock (Ormco) in 1972, Mobil-Lock (Forestadent) in 1980, SPEED (Orec) in 1980, and Activa ("A" Company) in 1986.[2,3] Self-ligating brackets can be divided into two main categories—active and passive—according to their mechanisms of closure. Active self-ligating brackets have a spring clip that stores energy to press against the archwire for rotation and torque

control. On the other hand, passive self-ligating brackets usually have a slide that can be closed, which does not encroach on the slot lumen. It has been claimed that self-ligating brackets enable a tooth to slide along an archwire with lower and more predictable net forces and yet under complete control, with almost none of the undesirable effects of a deformable mode of ligation, such as elastomeric ties.[4]

Mechanism

The claim of reduced friction with self-ligating brackets is often cited as a primary advantage over conventional brackets.[4–8] This occurs because the usual steel or elastomeric ligatures are not necessary, and it is claimed that passive designs generate even less friction than active ones.[8,9] The frictional force of an elastomeric tied in place in an O configuration was reported at 50 g.[10] Many in vitro studies have shown that less friction is generated with self-ligating brackets compared with conventional brackets,[5–8,11,12] and therefore less force is required to produce tooth movement.[13] Kapur et al[14] found that the friction per bracket with nickel-titanium (Ni-Ti) archwires was 41 g with Minitrim (Dentaurum) brackets under conventional ligation and 15 g with Damon brackets (Ormco); with the stainless steel wires, these values were 61 g and 3.6 g, respectively. With reduced friction and hence less force needed to produce tooth movement,[15] self-ligating brackets are proposed to have the potential advantages of producing more physiologically harmonious tooth movement by not overpowering the musculature and interrupting the periodontal vascular supply.[4] Therefore, more alveolar bone generation, greater amounts of expansion, less proclination of anterior teeth, and less need for extractions are claimed to be possible. It was recommended that in the case of rectangular wires, the Damon bracket was significantly better than any of the other brackets and should be preferred if sliding mechanics is the technique of choice.[12]

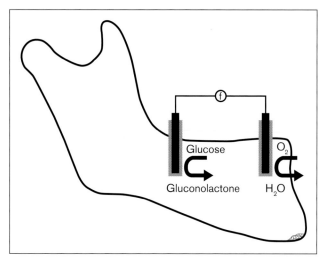

Fig 13-1 A schematic illustration of an oral biocatalytic fuel cell. (Reprinted from Kolahi et al[33] with permission.)

Current and future developments

Despite the findings that the in vitro friction of self-ligating brackets is extremely low, several systematic reviews,[16,17] randomized clinical trials,[18] and prospective cohort studies[19–23] have revealed that self-ligating brackets do not accelerate alignment or space closure in a clinical setting. This apparent paradox is likely due to the effects of binding because when the teeth tip, rotate, or torque, the edges of the slot engage the archwire, creating binding so that the resistance to sliding increases. Because many self-ligating bracket designs are narrower than conventional twin brackets, the effect of binding due to tipping is greater, resulting in increased resistance to sliding compared with conventional twin brackets. Shortened chair time and slightly less incisor proclination (1.5 degrees) appear to be the only significant advantages of self-ligating systems over conventional systems that are supported by the current evidence. Friction does not seem as critical as previously believed, and other factors such as binding may have a greater role in determining the rate of orthodontic tooth movement. Tooth movement is primarily a metabolic process of alveolar bone resorption on the pressure side and bone formation on the tension side,[24–28] regardless of what type of brackets are used. Therefore, acceleration of orthodontic tooth movement may have more promise from biologic and surgical perspectives.

Physiologic Approach

Direct electric current stimulation

The use of minute direct electric current for orthodontic tooth movement was first proposed by Beeson et al[29] and then Davidovitch et al.[30,31] By placing the electrodes at a noticeable distance from the moving teeth, Beeson at al[29] failed to demonstrate the effect of direct electric current in accelerating orthodontic tooth movement. In contrast, by placing the electrodes on the gingival tissues as near as possible to the moving teeth, Davidovitch et al[31] reported successful results in accelerating orthodontic tooth movement through direct electric current.

Mechanism

The direct electric current used was 7 volts and 15 microamperes (mA).[31] The anode was placed at the pressure side, and the cathode was placed at the tension side of the moving teeth. The degree of new bone formation at the electrically treated tension sites and bone resorption at the electrically treated pressure side were found to be higher than those of the corresponding sites of teeth treated by orthodontic force alone. There was also increased numbers of alveolar bone osteoblasts, PDL cells, and osteoclasts.[30,31] The mechanism is the direct electric current generating a local response to increase alveolar bone turnover.

Current and future developments

The use of minute direct electric current for accelerating orthodontic tooth movement has only been applied experimentally in cats.[29–31] No clinical application has been reported. One of the major problems with this approach is that the device and battery providing the electric current were too cumbersome and bulky to be used clinically. The clinical application of direct electric current stimulation for accelerating orthodontic tooth movement may not be possible until the development of microfabricated biocatalytic fuel cells (enzyme batteries) that function similar to a power supply for microsurgery robots or artificial organs.

In 2007, Sony announced the development of a biobattery that generates electricity from carbohydrates (sugar) using enzymes as their catalyst.[32] Another enzymatic microbattery using glucose as a fuel and immobilized microorganisms or enzymes as catalysts was invented in 2009 (Fig 13-1).[33] It could be placed on the gingiva near the alveolar bone and provide an electrical power source for accelerating orthodontic tooth movement. Furthermore, because of the very small size of these enzyme batteries, the procedure for delivering them into the human body can be done with no or minimal tissue injury.[32,34] Nevertheless, short lifetime and poor power density are the two major problems of these enzyme batteries as a clinical source of direct electric current for accelerating orthodontic tooth movement.

Endogenous piezoelectric stimulation

Electrical potentials can be created by applying a force to a tooth, which results in bending of the surrounding bone and the generation of piezoelectric charges.[35] It has been suggested that these forces should not be continuous because the piezoelectric charges are created when stress to the bone is applied and released.[35] Theoretically, vibration could be used to apply and release forces at a rapid rate, which could create these stress-induced electrical charges.

Animal studies involving rabbits[36,37] and rats[38] have demonstrated that applying cyclic forces to craniofacial bones enhances sutural growth. When investigating orthodontic tooth movement in rats, Nishimura et al[39] found that approximately 15% more tooth movement was achieved in 21 days when using resonance vibration for 8 minutes per day (on days 0, 7, and 14) when compared with a control group with only static forces. Similarly, when applying a vibrational force in *Macaca fuscata* monkeys for 1.5 hours per day over a period of 3 weeks, 1.3- to 1.4-times greater tooth movement (25% to 30% faster) was reported compared with the application of static force.[40]

The first report involving human subjects had patients use a vibrational appliance for 20 minutes per day and reported "promising rates of tooth movement."[41] Another study by the same author found approximately 2 to 3 mm of tooth movement per month in both arches.[42] However, both of these studies lacked control groups, and although 2 to 3 mm of movement may seem impressive, it must be remembered that this was a reduction in Little's Irregularity Index and not a translational movement, such as retracting a canine into an extraction site.

A prospective RCT examined 45 subjects requiring extraction of maxillary first premolars for crowding.[43] The patients were randomly allocated to use either the AcceleDent appliance (output force of 25 g with a frequency of 30 Hz) or a sham appliance for 20 minutes per day. A nickel-titanium coil spring was attached from the canine bracket and distally to a temporary skeletal anchorage device (TSAD) (Tomas Pin, Dentaurum). Every 4 weeks, the distance between the TSAD and the distal aspect of the canine bracket was measured to assess the rate of space closure. Thirty-nine of the subjects completed the trial, and the reported rate of tooth movement during space closure was 38% faster ($P = .02$) in the AcceleDent group (0.29 mm/week) when compared with the control group (0.21 mm/week). However, other published trials evaluating the rate of canine retraction using coil springs also found space closure rates of 0.28 to 0.29 mm/week without the use of vibration.[20,44]

The AcceleDent RCT is not reported in sufficient detail to fully assess the quality of the trial, but the lack of blinding and measurement methods could potentially affect the outcome. Although a TSAD may be expected to be a stable landmark, TSADs can drift up to 1.5 mm under orthodontic loading,[45] which can affect the measured rate of movement. There is the potential that vibration actually results in an accelerated drift of the TSAD, making the rate of space closure appear to have increased. The paper also reported accelerated tooth movement during initial alignment (2.06 times or 106% faster). However, this was assessed by measuring mandibular arch perimeter, which does not necessarily equate with a reduction in crowding or irregularity.

A more recent prospective RCT on another vibration appliance randomly assigned 66 patients to a vibration appliance (Tooth Masseuse) or a control group (Miles P, personal communication, 2012). The experimental group was instructed to use the vibrational appliance for a minimum of 20 minutes per day. This study evaluated the change in alignment or irregularity during the first 10 weeks of treatment and also assessed discomfort during the first week. In this study, the recorders of the irregularity index were blinded to the groups, and no significant differences in irregularity or pain levels were observed at any of the time points between groups. However, this appliance used a different vibrational frequency (111 Hz) and force level (about 6 g) when compared with the AcceleDent appliance (30 Hz and 25 g), so the results may not be generalized. Because there is a biologic basis for a potential effect from vibration, future research with the AcceleDent appliance would ideally address the previous study's shortcomings, with more reliable and valid measurement systems in addition to blinding.

Low-level laser therapy

The most frequently used LLLT for the purpose of potentially accelerating orthodontic tooth movement is gallium-aluminum-arsenide (GaAlAs) laser irradiation. The LLLT is applied on the mucosa buccally, distally, and palatally to the tested tooth. The wavelength of LLLT ranges from 630 to 860 nm, and the energy ranges from 4.5 to 6.0 J/cm^2.[46–61]

Mechanism

Similar to the application of electric stimulation, LLLT has been suggested to increase alveolar turnover.[46] The effects of low-level lasers on bone cellular activity, bone structures, bone healing, fibroblast activity, and the inflammatory process have already been investigated. LLLT caused significant histologic changes in the alveolar bone, including an increase in the number and differentiation of osteoclasts and accelerated bone resorption.[47–53] The increase in the numbers of osteoclasts could be the result of the light, which is known to be capable of stimulating or inhibiting both enzymatic and photochemical activities in living tissues.[54,55] It also has the capacity to stimulate both secretion and proliferation of fibroblasts, consequently increasing collagen matrix deposition,[29,30] and to increase the number of osteoblasts on the tension side of orthodontic tooth movement.[49]

Current and future developments

The effect of LLLT on accelerating orthodontic tooth movement is still controversial both experimentally and clinically. For instance, some reported positive results,[47] some reported no effects,[58,59] and some even reported that it retards orthodontic tooth movement.[60]

The wavelength has been shown not to be a key factor in determining the effects of acceleration.[60] It seems that the energy of the laser determines the effects of acceleration, and the optimal magnitude of energy needed for the acceleration varies accordingly in different experimental species. In a clinical study, Limpanichkul et al[58] used 25 J/cm² of GaAlAs low-level laser in 12 young adult patients who required retraction of the maxillary canine into the first premolar extraction space and reported that 25 J/cm² of LLLT at the surface level was too low to express either stimulatory effect or inhibitory effect on the rate of orthodontic tooth movement. In a similar clinical study, Youssef et al[47] used 54 J/cm² of low-level laser in 15 adult patients who required maxillary and mandibular canine retraction and concluded that LLLT can highly accelerate tooth movement during orthodontic tooth movement and can also effectively reduce pain levels.

In contrast, in a double-blind study in dogs, Goulart et al[61] demonstrated a biphasic effect of GaAlAs laser irradiation on the speed of orthodontic tooth movement. The 5.25–J/cm² dosage accelerated orthodontic movement during the first observation period (from 0 to 21 days [$P < .05$]), whereas the 35.0–J/cm² dosage retarded the orthodontic movement in the treated group when compared with the control group during both the first and second observation periods (from 0 to 42 days [$P < .05$]). Their results suggested that photoradiation may accelerate orthodontic movement at a dosage of 5.25 J/cm², whereas a higher dosage (35.0 J/cm²) may retard it.

More experimental and clinical studies on the level of energy density are needed before LLLT can be used as a routine clinical procedure to accelerate orthodontic tooth movement and shorten treatment duration.

Pharmacologic Approach

Certain endogenous agents, such as inflammatory mediators like cytokines and prostaglandins, and hormones have been used exogenously in an attempt to accelerate tooth movement. Cytokines and hormones that have been tested and tried for accelerating orthodontic tooth movement include corticosteroids, prostaglandins (PGs), growth hormone, parathyroid hormone, and relaxin. However, the local injection of most of these agents was only tested experimentally and not used clinically because of their adverse and systemic effects and the need for frequent injection. Among these agents, only PGs and relaxin have been tested clinically without obvious adverse and systemic effects.

Prostaglandins

PGs are a group of chemical messengers belonging to a family of hormones called *eicosanoids*. These are paracrine hormones, ie, they act only on cells near the point of hormone synthesis instead of being transported via blood to act on cells in other tissues or organs. They have a variety of dramatic effects on vertebrate tissues. Some of the effects of PGs are as follows[62–67]:

- They stimulate contraction of the smooth muscle of the uterus.
- They affect blood flow, sleep cycle, and response to hormones such as adrenaline and glucagon.
- They elevate body temperature and cause inflammation and pain.
- PG has been proven to be effective for significantly increasing tooth movement.

Mechanism

Both fibroblasts and osteoblasts within the PDL are sensitive to mechanical stimulation. Mechanosensing of osteoblasts was demonstrated by the release of signaling molecules such as PGs by human osteoblasts after direct and indirect deformation.[68,69]

It has been suggested that cytokines and other inflammatory markers, such as prostaglandin E₂ (PGE₂), may activate bone remodeling characterized by bone resorption in the compression region and bone deposition in the tension region of the PDL.[70–72] The mechanism of action of PGE₂ can be explained by the pressure-tension theory of tooth movement, which assumes chemical signals to be cell stimulants that lead to tooth movement.[73] According to this theory, pressure causes changes in the PDL blood circulation and the resultant release of chemical mediators. Inflammatory mediators may act in concert and produce synergistic potentiation of prostanoid formation in cells of the human PDL.[74] Furthermore, PGE₂ plays an important role as a mediator of bone remodeling under mechanical forces.[62,63,65] Several in vitro models have implicated PGs as mediators of mechanical stress in a number of cell types, including mechanically deformed osteoblasts,[75] gingival fibroblasts,[76] and PDL fibroblasts.[77]

Yamasaki et al[62] were among the earliest researchers to investigate the role of PGs in bone resorption associated with orthodontic tooth movement, using the rat molar model. In an interesting practical application of the findings of Harell et al,[78] they conducted experiments on rats to investigate whether the synthesis of PGs is induced by orthodontic force and whether exogenous PGs can produce bone resorption similar to that of orthodontic force. They reported that the application of orthodontic force did indeed cause increased synthesis of PGs, which in turn stimulated osteoclastic bone resorption. Furthermore, they found that indomethacin produced a dose-related inhibition in the appearance of osteoclasts and bone resorption that was limited to the first 12 hours of tooth movement. This explains why tooth movement is slower in patients taking nonsteroidal anti-inflammatory drugs. Injections of PGE₁ and PGE₂ into the gingival tissues near the maxillary first molar also stimulated osteoclast formation and bone resorption, which led to the conclusion that local PG injections could increase the rate of tooth movement.[63,64]

Current and future developments

There are only two clinical studies[64,79] that have been reported. Local injection of PGE_1, instead of PGE_2, into the gingival tissue was used for accelerating the rate of orthodontic tooth movement.[64,79] Following local anesthesia, 0.1 mL of a 0.01% PGE_1 solution in saline was injected submucosally or under the mucoperiosteum in the pressure side of the tooth movement. Injections were repeated at weekly intervals. For the palatal movement of the maxillary premolars that were scheduled to be extracted, the rate of tooth movement was two to three times faster than the control, which received vehicle injections.[64,79] The rate of canine retraction in premolar extraction cases was increased almost 1.6-fold on the side of PGE_1 injections compared with the vehicle-injected side.[64] Clinical and radiographic examinations of the teeth involved in the study as well as the surrounding tissues showed no evidence of pathologic changes. However, the rate of orthodontic tooth movement accelerated by the local injection of PGE_1 varied individually.[79]

Although the local injection of PGE_1 has demonstrated its clinical effectiveness in accelerating orthodontic tooth movement, its clinical application is still limited because of the need for weekly injections and the severe pain caused after the injection. Additionally, there is the mystery of why the rate of orthodontic tooth movement accelerated by the local injection of PGE_1 varied individually, which remains unresolved.

Relaxin

Relaxin is in the insulin/relaxin family of structurally related hormones. It is produced in many mammals during pregnancy; it promotes cervical softening and elongation of interpubic ligaments in mice and cattle.[80] Relaxin influences many other physiologic processes such as collagen turnover, angiogenesis, and antifibrosis. Relaxin can be found in many tissues of male and female rats—eg, kidneys, heart, lungs, liver, skin, and brain.[80] Some evidence suggests that relaxin can also be found in cranial sutures and PDL.[81] Moreover, there is a link between relaxin, matrix metalloproteinases, and matrix degradation; relaxin was found to induce degradative mediators in the nonreproductive, fibrocartilaginous synovial discs of temporomandibular joints.[82] Because of the role of relaxin in remodeling soft tissue, the use of relaxin in investigations of increasing orthodontic tooth movement rates and preventing relapse has been studied.[83–90]

Mechanism

Instead of increasing the alveolar bone turnover, the main action of relaxin is to increase the rate of degradation (turnover) of extracellular fibrous connective tissues. Increased collagen deposition in response to tensional forces and decreases in type I collagen and fibronectin protein in response to compressional forces were reported in orthodontic tooth movement.[83] Relaxin was found to stimulate collagenase production in a beagle dog study through localized relaxin receptors on gingival and PDL fibroblasts.[82] An increase in collagen synthesis during orthodontic tooth movement on the compression side also has been documented.[84] Interestingly, relaxin might have effects on osteoclastic behavior resulting in increased bone resorption through an increase of tumor necrosis factor and interleukin-1β secretion, although there is no direct evidence for this effect.[85] Based on these effects, relaxin was assumed to increase the amount and rate of tooth movement[86] and reduce rotational orthodontic relapse[87] through its effect on the PDL.

Current and future developments

Whether human relaxin accelerates orthodontic tooth movement and prevents orthodontic relapse is still unknown. The current experimental and clinical studies are few and not substantive enough to answer the question yet. More investigations are needed for the future development of relaxin in accelerating orthodontic tooth movement and preventing orthodontic relapse.

Experimentally, tooth relapse was studied in dogs, and it was found that the local injection of human relaxin reduced the relapse of rotation after orthodontic tooth movement compared to the control group.[87] The rate of orthodontic tooth movement was also studied in rats. Three groups of young rats received human relaxin through a miniosmotic pump, subcutaneous injection, or placebo (pump), and tooth movement was assessed.[88] Because of large individual variability and small sample sizes, statistically significant differences were not found for sagittal tooth movement over 14 days. Both relaxin-treated groups had increased tooth movement at day 3 compared with the controls, and postmortem measurement of molar lengths and intermolar spaces differed significantly for the control and relaxin groups. However, in another study,[89] relaxin did not accelerate orthodontic tooth movement in rats, although it reduced the level of PDL organization and mechanical strength and increased tooth mobility at an early time point.

In a single-center, blinded, placebo-controlled, randomized clinical trial, twenty subjects received weekly injections of 50 µg of relaxin and another 20 subjects received placebo for 8 weeks.[90] Aligners programmed to move a target tooth 2 mm during treatment were dispensed at weeks 0, 2, 4, and 6 to assess the rate of orthodontic tooth movement. All of the subjects were then followed through week 12 to assess relapse. The results revealed that, in comparing the patients who received relaxin injections weekly for 8 weeks with those who received placebo injections, the pattern and amount of tooth movement did not differ, nor did it relapse over 4 weeks. The local doses of relaxin might have been too low to affect tooth movement or short-term relapse, which may have contributed to the negative results.

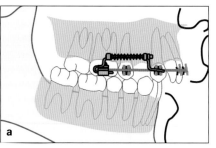 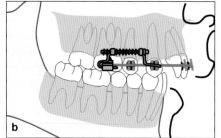 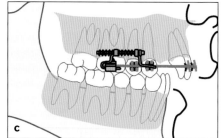

Fig 13-2 *(a to c)* Schematic illustrations of maxillary rapid canine retraction through distraction of the PDL with an intraoral distraction device.

Surgical-Assisted Approach

Surgical-assisted accelerated orthodontic tooth movement is currently the most effective technique experimentally and clinically in accelerating orthodontic tooth movement. This approach includes the techniques of rapid canine retraction through distraction of the PDL,[91–95] rapid canine retraction through distraction of the dentoalveolus,[96–98] corticotomy-assisted rapid orthodontic tooth movement,[99,100] and corticision.[101]

Rapid canine retraction through distraction of the PDL

This technique is beneficial in treating adult patients, for whom treatment duration may be a deciding factor toward the acceptance of treatment. The rate of orthodontic tooth movement in adults, particularly in the beginning of treatment, is slower than in adolescents.[102–104] Two basic components, the alveolar bone and PDL, are encountered during orthodontic tooth movement and affect its rate based on factors such as cellular activity,[105,106] mechanical strength of the PDL,[107] and bony resistance of alveolar bone.[108–110] In the initial stage of tooth movement, Young's modulus (stiffness) of the PDL is higher in adults than in adolescents, and this might produce a reduction in the biologic response of the PDL, leading to a delay in the early stage of tooth movement.[107] However, Young's modulus decreases markedly 4 to 7 days after application of orthodontic force and does not last through the entire period of orthodontic tooth movement.[111] The rate of tooth movement is shown to depend on the state of alveolar bone resistance, and it is faster in alveolar bone with loose bone trabeculae.[108–110,112]

Mechanism

By incorporating a surgical procedure on the interseptal bone distal to the canine at the time of extraction of the first premolar, the resistance on the pressure side of canine retraction is reduced, thus enhancing rapid canine retraction through distraction of the PDL[91] (Fig 13-2). This approach is based on the bifocal distraction osteogenesis technique. On the pressure side, the canine–interseptal bone complex is transported distally inside of the extraction socket. On the tension side, it is a distraction of the PDL followed by osteogenesis and ossification.[91]

Clinical and surgical procedures

Bonding and banding are performed before extraction of the first premolars. The first molars and second premolars are the anchor units. A triple tube is welded on the buccal side of the canine band and the molar band. No archwire or active appliance is placed on the anchor units before extraction, but a segment of Ni-Ti archwire is placed in the anterior teeth for the initial alignment and activation of the periodontal cells. The period of predistraction preparation is 1 to 2 months.

At the time of the first premolar extractions, surgery is performed with surgical burs to undermine and reduce the thickness of the interseptal bone distal to the canine. The surgery is then performed inside the extraction socket of the first premolar without a mucoperiosteal flap and osteotomy. The length of the canine can be either obtained directly from cone beam computed tomography (CBCT) or estimated by applying the ratio of the premolar length (which can be measured after extraction) to the canine length on the periapical film.

The socket of the first premolar is deepened to the same depth as that of the canine with a 4-mm carbide surgical round bur (Figs 13-3a and 13-3b). Then a cylinder carbide surgical bur is used to reduce the thickness of the interseptal bone distal to the canine. This procedure is critical to the distraction results. The interseptal bone is better reduced to 1.0 to 1.5 mm in thickness. The last step is to undermine the interseptal bone distal to the canine. A 1-mm carbide fissure bur is used to make two vertical grooves, running from the socket bottom to the alveolar crest, on the mesiobuccal and mesiolingual corners inside the extraction socket. These two vertical grooves extend and join obliquely toward the base of the interseptal bone (Figs 13-3c and 13-3d).

A custom-made intraoral distraction device (Fig 13-4) is delivered immediately after the extraction and surgical procedures. It is activated 0.5 mm/day right after the surgery until the canine is distracted into the desired position (Fig 13-5). Patients are seen once a week during the distraction procedure.

Fig 13-3 Schematic illustrations of the surgical procedure for undermining the interseptal bone distal to the canine in rapid canine retraction through distraction of the PDL. *(a and b)* The socket of the first premolar is deepened to the same depth as that of the canine with a 4-mm carbide surgical round bur. *(c and d)* A 1-mm carbide fissure bur is used to make two vertical grooves, running from the socket bottom to the alveolar crest, on the mesiobuccal and mesiolingual corners inside the extraction socket, and these two vertical grooves extend and join obliquely toward the base of the interseptal bone.

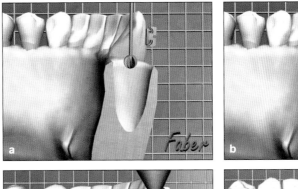
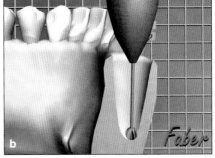
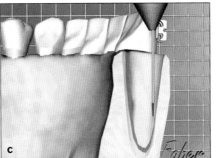
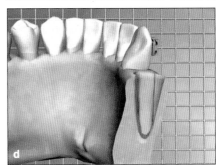

Fig 13-4 The intraoral distraction device for rapid canine retraction through distraction of the PDL.

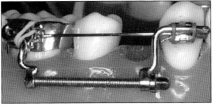

Fig 13-5 The clinical progress of maxillary rapid canine retraction through distraction of the PDL in a 23-year-old woman. The canine retraction was completed in 3 weeks. *(a and b)* Before distraction. *(c and d)* After 2 weeks of distraction. *(e and f)* After 3 weeks of distraction.

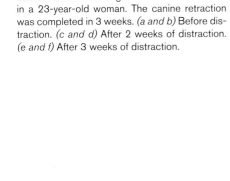
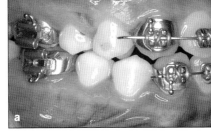
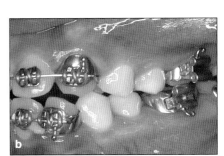
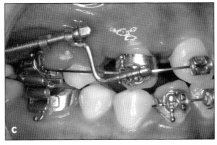
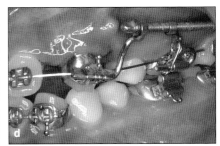
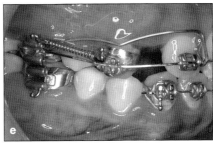
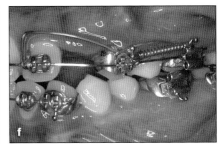

Rapid canine retraction through distraction of the dentoalveolus

Rapid canine retraction through distraction of the dento-alveolus[96,97] is a modified form of rapid canine retraction through distraction of the PDL, with the distraction osteogenesis in the osteotomy sites rather than in the PDL.

In this technique, a mucoperiosteal flap is reflected, and cortical holes are made in the alveolar bone with a small, round carbide bur from the canine to the second premolar, curving apically to pass 3 to 5 mm from the apex. A thin, tapered fissure bur is used to connect the holes around the root. Fine osteotomes are advanced in the coronal direction. The first premolar is then extracted and the buccal bone removed between the outlined bone cut at the distal canine region anteriorly and the second premolar region posteriorly. Larger osteotomes are used to fully mobilize the alveolar segment, which includes the canine, by fracturing the surrounding spongy bone around its root off the lingual or palatal cortex. The buccal and apical bone through the extraction socket and the possible bony interferences at the buccal aspect that might be encountered during the distraction process are eliminated or smoothed between the canine and the second premolar, preserving palatal or lingual cortical shelves. The palatal shelf is preserved, but the apical bone near the sinus wall is removed, leaving the sinus membrane intact to avoid interferences during the active distraction process. Osteotomes along the anterior aspect of the canine are used to split the surrounding bone around its root from the palatal or lingual cortex and neighboring teeth. The transport dentoalveolar segment includes the canine, the buccal cortex, and the underlying spongy bone that envelops the canine root, leaving an intact lingual or palatal cortical plate and the bone around the apex of the canine. The distraction is initiated within 3 days after surgery. The distractor is activated twice per day, in the morning and in the evening, for a total of 0.8 mm per day.

Current and future developments

Rapid canine retraction through both PDL distraction and dentoalveolar distraction has minimal loss of anchorage, and similar distractors are used. The anchorage loss in the maxillary and mandibular first molars was reported at 0.1 mm and 0.2 mm, respectively.[91,92] This could be because the retraction of the canine has been completed while the first molar is still in its lag period or just initiating its mesial movement. The subsequent anterior retraction or relief of the anterior crowding would be faster.[92]

However, rapid canine retraction through distraction of either the PDL or dentoalveolus can only accelerate the orthodontic tooth movement of one tooth. These two techniques are not able to accelerate orthodontic movement of a group of teeth or an entire dentition. Also, they can only be applied in cases of extraction of the first premolars. The surgery for distraction of the dentoalveolus is more extensive, aggressive, and complicated than that of the PDL. The rapid tooth movement achieved by both of these techniques cannot be accomplished by using only regular orthodontic appliances such as brackets and archwires. Both techniques need a special distractor, and the distractor is custom-made and bulky.

Selective alveolar decortication

Selective alveolar decortication, or corticotomy, is a technique of intentional injury of alveolar cortical bone to accelerate orthodontic tooth movement. It was first described in 1892 and then in 1959 as a surgical approach to correct malocclusion with incisions to the cortical alveolar bone while leaving the spongiosa intact to splint teeth into new positions.[113–115] This technique was later adapted to a dog model[116] and used in clinical cases.[117–119] In 1978, Generson et al[118] described rapid orthodontic treatment for open bite malocclusion using alveolar decortication without subapical osteotomy. Treatment of a large group of adult patients using this modified surgical procedure was reported in 1991 and was referred to as "corticotomy-facilitated orthodontics."[119] By adding bioabsorbable grafting material, Wilcko et al further developed this technique into a patented technique called *accelerated osteogenic orthodontics (AOO)*[99] or *periodontally accelerated osteogenic orthodontics (PAOO)*.[120]

Mechanism

It has been postulated clinically that selective alveolar decortication would manifest as a part of the regional acceleratory phenomenon (RAP) that involves the alveolar bone after being exposed to injury (corticotomy) and during active tooth movement.[99,100] It was further illustrated experimentally that the selective alveolar decortication enhances the rate of tooth movement during the initial tooth displacement phase through a transient burst increase of severe alveolar bone resorption followed by bone formation.[121,122]

RAP potentiates tissue reorganization and healing by way of a transient burst of localized severe bone resorption and remodeling.[123,124] The term *regional* refers to the demineralization of both the cut site and adjacent bone.[125] The term *acceleratory* refers to an exaggerated or intensified bone response in cuts that extend to the marrow. Several mechanisms have been postulated and proposed for the osteopenic effect in RAP, including shifts in the number of osteoclast and osteoblast cell populations,[123–126] neovascularization and local and systemic mediators,[123,124] and calcium depletion.[99,100]

RAP occurring in jaw bone could be induced by flap surgery,[127] corticotomy[99,100,112,128] or orthodontic tooth movement alone.[128,129] In rats, Yaffe et al[127] reflected mucoperiosteal flaps that were allowed to readapt without sutures. Evidence of RAP was first observed after 10 days of healing, and there was almost complete recovery after 120 days. The authors suggested that RAP in humans begins within a few days of surgery, typically peaks in the first and second month, and may take from 6 to more than 24 months to subside. They characterized the initial phase of RAP as an increase in cortical bone porosity because of increased osteoclastic activity and speculated that bone dehiscence might occur after periodontal surgery in an area where cortical bone is initially thin. They surmised that RAP might be a contributing factor to increased mobility of the teeth after periodontal surgery, a supposition consistent with a report by Pfeifer[130] of increased osteoclastic activity along the PDL surface following surgery. Orthodontic tooth movement also induced mild RAP in the adjacent alveolar bone in rats,[128,129] although its intensity is much less than that of corticotomy.[128]

Clinical techniques of AOO/PAOO

Full-thickness flaps are reflected labially and lingually using sulcular releasing incisions[131] (Figs 13-6 and 13-7). The releasing incision can also be made within the thickness of the gingival attachment or at the base of the gingival attachment (mucogingival junction). Vertical releasing incisions can be used, but they should be positioned at least one tooth away from the "bone activation." Flaps should be carefully reflected beyond the apices of the teeth to avoid damaging the neurovascular complexes exiting the alveolus and to allow adequate decortication around the apices. Selective alveolar decortication is performed in the form of decortication cuts and at points up to 0.5 mm in depth, combined with selective medullary penetration to enhance bleeding on both labial- and lingual-side cortical plates. The pattern of decortication is not critical; it could be dots, lines, or a combination of dots and lines. It is the decortications or injury of the cortical bone that is critical.

The major modification from the original approach is the placement of bioabsorbable grafting material over the injured bone. This is to compensate for the initial phase of RAP (an increase in cortical bone porosity because of increased osteoclastic activity) and to prevent potential bone dehiscence, which can occur after periodontal surgery in an area where cortical bone is initially thin. Flaps are then repositioned and sutured into place. Sutures should be left in place for a minimum of 2 weeks. Tooth movement should start 1 or 2 weeks after surgery. Unlike conventional orthodontics, the orthodontic appliance should be activated every 2 weeks until the end of treatment after PAOO. The clinical applications of PAOO are illustrated in Fig 13-6 and 13-7.

The impact of the injury is localized to the area immediately adjacent to the decortication injury. Selective alveolar decortication induced increased turnover of alveolar spongiosa, and the activity was localized; dramatic escalation of demineralization-remineralization dynamics is the likely biologic mechanism underlying rapid tooth movement following selective alveolar decortication.[121]

Current and future developments

The surgical technique of corticotomy-assisted orthodontics was reported to be effective in reducing clinical orthodontic treatment time by resolving anterior crowding,[99,100] retracting canines after premolar extraction,[132,133] facilitating eruption of impacted teeth,[134] facilitating slow expansion of the maxilla,[135,136] intruding molars and correcting open bite,[137,138] and decompensating for augmentation of the mandibular anterior ridge before orthognathic surgery.[139]

This technique has several advantages, including faster tooth movement, shorter treatment time, safer expansion of constricted arches, and enhanced postorthodontic treatment stability. Stability was reported as one of the major advantages of corticotomy-assisted orthodontics, and the corticotomy-facilitated orthodontic treatment was found to result in better retention compared with conventional orthodontic treatment.[140] The improved stability was attributed to the increase in alveolar bone turnover and the extended envelope of the alveolus by bone graft. Unfortunately, there is still no strong evidence for enhanced stability after corticotomy-assisted orthodontics in the literature, and definitive conclusions cannot be made unless prospective controlled studies are conducted.[131]

The major drawbacks of this technique are its invasive and aggressive nature, increasing postoperative discomfort, and the risk of complications. The patients have to be seen frequently—every 2 weeks—and this means that the duration of the increase in alveolar turnover induced by the selective alveolar decortications does not last long enough for the necessary orthodontic adjustments on a monthly visit basis. The duration of accelerated orthodontic tooth movement is only 3 to 4 months.

Several modifications, including single-sided partial corticotomy,[141] piezocision,[142,143] and corticision,[101] therefore have been developed to reduce the invasive nature and drawbacks of the traumatic conventional corticotomy procedures. It has been reported that single-sided partial corticotomy in the mandible appeared to be sufficient to stimulate rapid tooth movement.[141] *Piezocision* is a minimally invasive flapless procedure combining microincisions, piezoelectric incisions, and selective tunneling that allows for hard or soft tissue grafting. This approach was reported to lead to shortened orthodontic treatment time, minimal discomfort, and great patient acceptance, as well as enhanced periodontium because of the added grafting (bone and/or soft tissue).[141,142] However, the duration and intensity of RAP are proportional to the extent of injury and soft tissue involvement in the injury.[144]

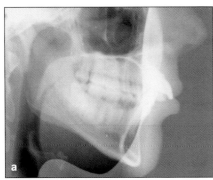

Fig 13-6 PAOO for accelerating orthodontic tooth alignment, leveling, and forward movement of the mandibular anterior teeth in a 22-year-old woman with a 14-mm overjet, 8-mm mandibular curve of Spee, and 8-mm mandibular anterior crowding. The period of active orthodontic treatment was 8 months. *(a to d)* Cephalogram and intraoral photos before orthodontic treatment. *(e to g)* Alveolar decortication and augmentation grafting in the labial and lingual aspects of the mandibular anterior teeth, including canines. *(h and i)* Rapid relief of the mandibular anterior crowding and leveling of the curve of Spee. *(j to l)* After 8 months of orthodontic treatment. (Courtesy of Dr D. J. Ferguson, Dubai Healthcare City, UAE.)

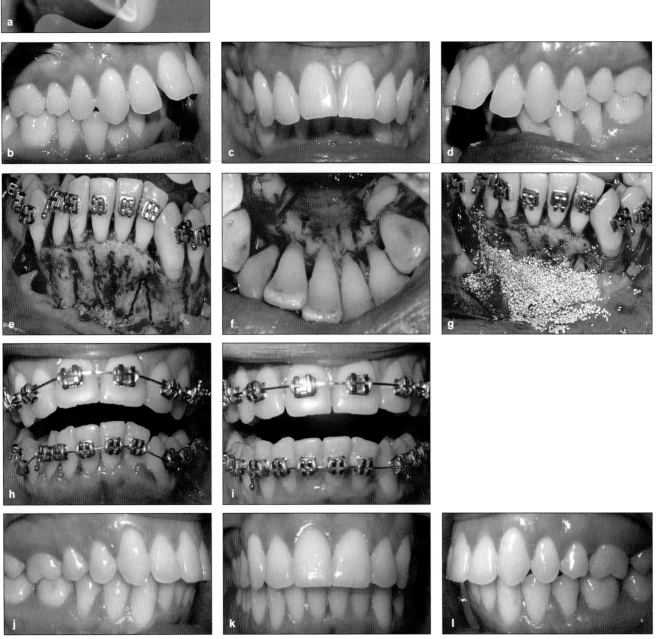

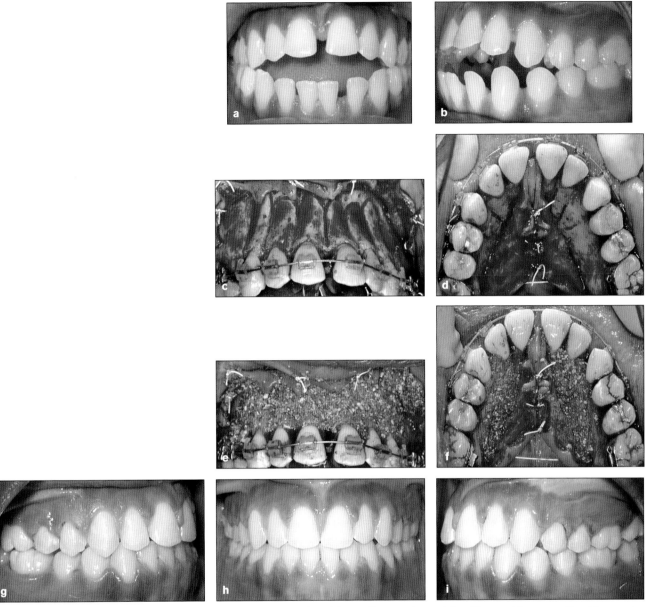

Fig 13-7 PAAO for accelerating orthodontic space closure and extrusion of the maxillary anterior teeth in a 23-year-old woman with a 10-mm anterior open bite and multiple spacings in the maxillary and mandibular anterior teeth. The period of active treatment was 8 months. *(a and b)* Intraoral photos before orthodontic treatment. *(c to f)* Alveolar decortication and augmentation grafting in the labial and palatal aspects of the maxillary anterior teeth. *(g to i)* After 8 months of orthodontic treatment. (Courtesy of Dr D. J. Ferguson, Dubai Healthcare City, UAE.)

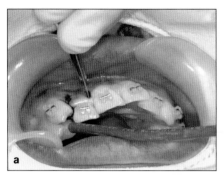 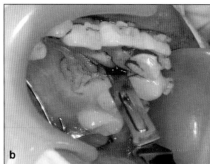

Fig 13-8 The clinical technique of corticision in the labial (a) and palatal (b) sides of the maxillary incisors. The surgical incision is kept 2 mm apically away from the papillary gingival margin in order to preserve the alveolar crest. (Courtesy of Dr Y. K. Park, Seoul, South Korea.)

Corticision

Similar to piezocision, *corticision* was introduced as a supplemental dentoalveolar surgery in orthodontic therapy to achieve accelerated tooth movement with minimal surgical intervention. Corticision minimized the degree of the surgical injury by excluding the flap reflection and bone graft in AOO/PAOO and the selective tunneling for hard or soft tissue grafting in piezocision.[101] This technique is based on the fact that only mucoperiosteal flap reflection without any decortication could serve the RAP, resulting in widening of the PDL space and tooth mobility without any force application but also reducing the complications of crestal bone resorption and bone dehiscence.[127]

Mechanism

Corticision has been shown histologically to accelerate both the catabolic and anabolic alveolar remodeling activities while not decreasing the alveolar bone density.[101] This was represented by extensive direct resorption of bundle bone with less hyalinization and more rapid removal of hyalinized tissue in the pressure side of tooth movement, and the bone apposition was 3.5-fold higher in the tension side. Histologic findings revealed neither pathologic changes in the paradental tissues nor root resorption following the corticision.

Clinical techniques

In order to avoid the complications of crestal bone resorption and bone dehiscence, corticision uses a reinforced scalpel to separate the interproximal cortices transmucosally without reflecting a flap. The reinforced surgical blade (No. 15T, Paragon) is capable of making a surgical incision with a minimum thickness of 400 μm. The blade is positioned on the interradicular attached gingiva at an inclination of 45 to 60 degrees to the long axis of the anterior teeth and is inserted gradually into the bone marrow by malleting the blade holder penetrating the overlying gingiva, cortical bone, and cancellous bone (Fig 13-8). The surgical incision is kept 2 mm apically away from the papillary gingival margin in order to preserve the alveolar crest and is extended 1 mm beyond the mucogingival junction (see Fig 13-8a). The blade is then pulled out by a swing motion.

Additional manual manipulation by twisting the incision sites labially and lingually, intended to lengthen the duration of the bone injury, is initiated immediately after the corticision and repeated every 2 weeks thereafter. This manual manipulation involves the interception of the lamellation process of woven bone at the incision site and provides repeated microdamage. However, the effect of periodic manual manipulation on the remodeling of alveolar bone proper and on the rate of tooth movement could not be elucidated.[101]

Current and future developments

Corticision could be indicated in resolving anterior crowding (Fig 13-9) or anterior open bite (Fig 13-10). Although corticision was developed as a replacement dentoalveolar surgery for selective alveolar decortication, it is still stressful for the patients when the surgical blade is being malleted into alveolar bone. Similar to selective alveolar decortication, the patient has to be seen every 2 weeks, and this means that the duration of the increase in alveolar turnover induced by the corticision does not last long enough for monthly orthodontic adjustments. The duration of the window of opportunity of accelerated orthodontic tooth movement is only 3 to 4 months. It does not include the advantage of expanding the alveolar envelope as with the piezocision and AOO/PAOO.

Corticision has recently advanced into "piezopuncture."[145] The surgical blade is replaced by piezoelectric puncture. Punctures rather than incisions penetrating the overlying gingiva, cortical bone, and cancellous bone are performed. This not only decreases tissue damage but also is more patient friendly compared with the use of a surgical blade and mallet. Whether the piezopuncture increases the intensity and duration of alveolar turnover still requires further investigation.

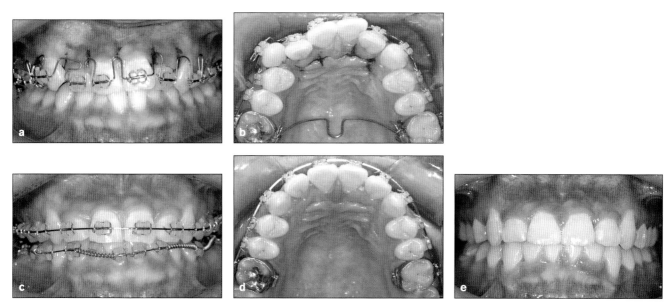

Fig 13-9 Corticision for accelerating tooth alignment in a 21-year-old woman with maxillary anterior crowding. The corticision was in the maxillary anterior teeth, the maxillary anterior alignment was completed in 9 weeks, and the total treatment period was 12 months. *(a and b)* Right after the maxillary corticision. *(c and d)* After 9 weeks of orthodontic alignment. *(e)* After 12 months of treatment. (Courtesy of Dr Y. K. Park, Seoul, South Korea.)

Fig 13-10 Corticision for accelerating maxillary anterior alignment and extrusion in a 22-year-old woman with maxillary and mandibular anterior crowding and open bite. The corticision was in the maxillary anterior teeth, the maxillary alignment and open bite were resolved in 3 months, and the total treatment period was 11 months. *(a and b)* One day after the corticision. *(c and d)* After 3 months of alignment and leveling. *(e and f)* After 11 months of treatment. (Courtesy of Dr Y. K. Park, Seoul, South Korea.)

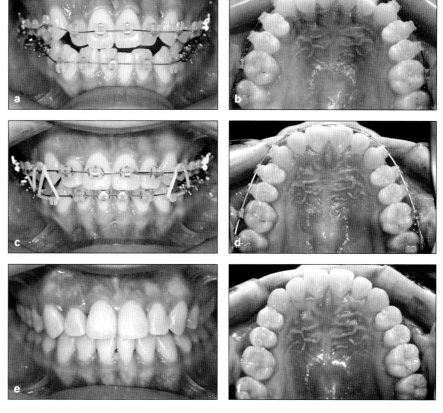

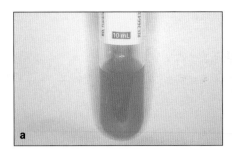
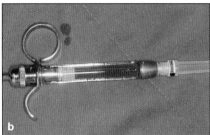

Fig 13-11 *(a and b)* The autologous PRP is loaded in an empty local anesthesia cartridge in a dental syringe for the submucosal injection. A 27-gauge dental needle is used for preventing the PRP from leaking out of the injection hole.

Submucosal Injection of PRP

The theory behind surgical-assisted accelerated tooth movement, currently the most effective technique, is that the bone surgery, no matter if it is orthognathic surgery,[146] AAO/PAOO,[99,100] piezocision,[142,143] corticision,[101] or piezopuncture,[145] triggers higher osteoclastic activity and/or lower alveolar bone density, which in turn accelerates orthodontic tooth movement. However, bone surgery is invasive and aggressive. Yet how can the effects of bone surgery be simulated without surgery? The local injection of cytokines/hormones has a similar effect as that of bone surgery, but it is not clinically practical because of its systemic effects and the need for frequent injections. Autologous PRP could be a substitute for local injection of cytokines/hormones to simulate the effects induced by bone surgery.[147]

Platelets are the initiator of both soft and hard tissue wound healing processes. Platelets contain growth factors such as platelet-derived growth factor (PDGF), transforming growth factor (TGF), endothelial growth factors (EGFs), and other components. These growth factors are critical in the regulation and stimulation of the wound healing process, and they play an important role in regulating cellular processes such as mitogenesis, chemotaxis, differentiation, and metabolism.[148] Peripheral blood contains 94% red blood cells (RBCs), 6% platelets, and less than 1% white blood cells (WBCs), while PRP contains 5% RBCs, 1% WBCs, and 94% platelets that accelerate the soft tissue healing and amplify osteogenesis. PRP has been extensively applied in dental implantology for its ability to enhance osseointegration of the dental implant and augment alveolar bone height in maxillary sinus elevation.[149–155]

Conventionally, PRP is applied to the region of interest through a flap operation and mixed and activated by calcium chloride ($CaCl_2$) and thrombine for the ease of application and release of growth factors. However, the flap surgery is aggressive in nature, and the activation of the PRP by mixing with $CaCl_2$ and thrombine initiates a transient burst release of growth factors all at once. To pro-

long the effects of PRP, an innovative approach is to inject PRP submucosally without mixing with $CaCl_2$ and thrombine.[147] It was surmised that the platelets first adhere and aggregate layer by layer on the surfaces of collagen, the intrinsic and extrinsic pathways of hemostasis initiate to generate thrombin, platelet clots lay down layer by layer above the periosteum, and then growth factors release and infiltrate into the periosteum gradually. The method for preparing autologous PRP has been well reported.[147] The platelet count in PRP ranges from 5 to 10 times that of the baseline platelet count. The PRP can be loaded in a dental syringe for the submucosal injection (Fig 13-11).

The technique and effects of submucosal injection of autologous PRP without mixing with $CaCl_2$ and thrombine for accelerating orthodontic tooth alignment in cases of anterior crowding was reported recently in a clinical study.[147] It could be applied for accelerating orthodontic alignment in extraction (Fig 13-12) or nonextraction cases (Fig 13-13). It was a single-dose injection. Before the injection of PRP, 0.9 mL of local anesthesia was injected in the labial and lingual mucosa of the anterior teeth for pain control. Subsequently, 0.7 mL of PRP was injected in the labial and lingual attached gingiva and oral mucosa from canine to canine at the same appointment when the brackets were bonded. Acetaminophen (500 mg) was prescribed for the postinjection pain control. Eighty-five percent of the patients reported 6 to 12 hours of acceptable postinjection discomfort including an itching sensation and mild to moderate pain, but 15% of the patients reported severe pain after the effect of the local anesthesia wore off. The results demonstrated that the rate of orthodontic tooth alignment of the maxilla and mandible in patients who had submucosal injection of autologous PRP was significantly faster compared with that in patients who had no injection of PRP. However, the rate of orthodontic tooth alignment was variable in the maxilla and mandible in all patients. Future research on the injection of PRP to accelerate orthodontic tooth alignment should include assessment of the individual differences in alveolar bone metabolism and density and the dose-dependent effects of submucosal injection of PRP.

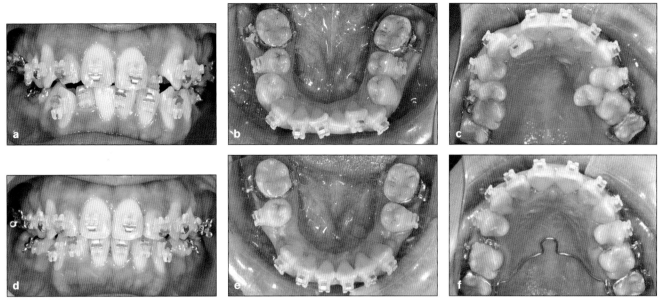

Fig 13-12 The submucosal injection of PRP in the case of a 22-year-old patient. The injection was in the maxillary and mandibular anterior teeth, and the maxillary and mandibular dentitions were well aligned 3 months after the injection. *(a to c)* Right before the injection. *(d to f)* Three months after the injection.

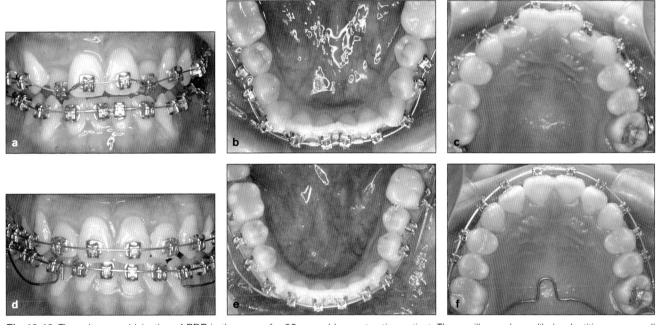

Fig 13-13 The submucosal injection of PRP in the case of a 28-year-old nonextraction patient. The maxillary and mandibular dentitions were well aligned 3 months after the injection. *(a to c)* Right before the injection. *(d to f)* Three months after the injection.

Future Concepts and Feasibility

The effectiveness of surgical-assisted approaches in accelerating orthodontic tooth movement is more consistent and has much less individual variation than the nonsurgical or regular approaches. The major problem of the surgical-assisted approaches is the invasive nature of surgery. On the other hand, the nonsurgical approaches are not reliable because of individual variability. The current nonsurgical approaches toward accelerating orthodontic tooth movement are mostly based on an arbitrary application of a certain agent, technique, or device without considering different individual responses. This explains why most orthodontists have experienced that the rate of orthodontic tooth movement and treatment duration vary greatly among cases with similar malocclusion, case difficulty, and treatment mechanics. The individual differences have a role in the rate of orthodontic tooth movement and need to be investigated further.[156,157]

What are the individual differences that determine the rate of orthodontic tooth movement? This question has been somewhat elucidated, and it seems to be related to the alveolar bone density and the baseline bone metabolism.[158]

Roles of alveolar bone density in situ and baseline bone metabolism

The impacts of the baseline bone metabolism and bone density on the rate of orthodontic tooth movement should be differentiated. One way to differentiate the impact of baseline bone metabolism and bone density on the rate of orthodontic tooth movement is to compare the rate of orthodontic tooth alignment between the maxillary and mandibular anterior teeth in the same individual. The baseline bone metabolism should be similar between the maxillary and mandibular alveoli within the same individual, and when the rate of orthodontic tooth alignment is different between the maxillary and mandibular anterior teeth, the difference must be related to a factor other than the baseline bone metabolism, such as the physical differences between the maxillary and mandibular alveoli. By using this methodology, Liou et al[158] illustrated that the rate of orthodontic tooth alignment in the maxillary and mandibular anterior teeth is different, and it is faster in the maxilla than in the mandible because the alveolar bone density is significantly lower in the maxillary anterior teeth than in the mandibular anterior teeth. Although some other physical factors might also contribute to the difference among individuals, the alveolar bone density in situ (alveolar bone density where the teeth reside) is a factor determining the rate of orthodontic tooth alignment. This means that the different sites of a jaw bone have different bone density and different rates of orthodontic tooth movement.

The assessment of baseline bone metabolism should include osteoblastic and osteoclastic activities, which could be illustrated clinically or experimentally by alkaline phosphatase (ALP) and C-terminal telopeptide of type I collagen (ICTP).[146,147,158] ALP is a bone enzyme secreted by osteoblasts for bone formation. It has been suggested that ALP activity in gingival crevicular fluid reflects the biologic activity in the periodontium during orthodontic movement and therefore should be further investigated as a diagnostic tool for monitoring orthodontic tooth movement in clinical practice.[159–161] ICTP is a metabolite of type I collagen of bone by osteoclasts. ICTP has been used to assess the risk and time course of oral bisphosphonate–induced osteonecrosis of the jaws,[162] and it has been suggested to be one of the best candidate markers to detect the activity and severity of periodontal disease.[163] Serum ALP and ICTP have been used clinically as the osteoblastic and osteoclastic markers for assessing the changes of baseline bone metabolism after orthognathic surgery.[146]

By assessing the ALP and ICTP markers for the baseline osteoblastic and osteoclastic activities, Liou at al[158] further showed that the rate of orthodontic tooth movement in both of the maxillary and mandibular anterior teeth significantly correlated to the baseline bone metabolism, especially the osteoclastic activity, but it did not correlate to the alveolar bone density when controlling for the baseline bone metabolism. This means that the baseline alveolar metabolism dominates over the alveolar bone density in determining the rate of orthodontic tooth alignment. Although the alveolar bone density in situ is a predetermined factor for the rate of orthodontic tooth alignment within an individual, it is the baseline bone metabolism that dominates the rate of orthodontic tooth alignment among different individuals (Fig 13-14).

Bone metabolism–density guided orthodontics

In consideration of the evidence on the baseline bone metabolism and alveolar bone density in situ, the concept of "bone metabolism–density guided orthodontics" for accelerating orthodontic tooth movement has been proposed.[158] The "anchorage value" of root surface area[164] or even the root volume that could be obtained from CBCT is another important factor to be included. For example, in a patient who will receive first premolar extraction for the correction of dentoalveolar protrusion, the baseline bone metabolism should be analyzed to evaluate whether the rate of tooth movement will be slow or fast. Next the alveolar bone in situ and dental root volume of the anterior teeth and posterior teeth should be analyzed to predict the relative rate and amount of anterior retraction and anchorage loss of posterior teeth so that a reinforced appliance for anchorage preparation, such as the orthodontic miniscrews, or a reinforced technique for accelerating en-masse anterior retraction, such as the submucosal injection of PRP,

Fig 13-14 Comparison of the rate of maxillary orthodontic tooth alignment in two women of similar age (50 and 54 years old) and with similar maxillary irregularity indices (14.6 and 14.5 mm). *(a and c)* Right after bonding. *(b and d)* After alignment. Although the alveolar bone density in situ of the maxillary anterior teeth of the patient shown in *a* and *b* is 33% higher than that of the patient shown in *c* and *d*, the period of the maxillary orthodontic alignment in the former patient was 2.7-fold faster (2.5 vs 7.0 months) than that of the latter patient because of the 2.6-fold higher baseline osteoclastic activity of the former patient.

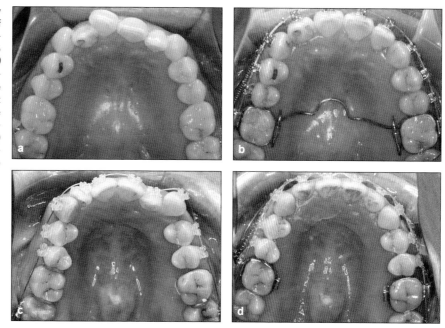

selective corticotomy, corticision, piezopuncture, or even gene therapy, for inducing higher levels of receptor activator of nuclear factor kappa B ligand (RANKL)[165] could be prescribed before the orthodontic treatment.

In the future, not only traditional records such as two- and three-dimensional cephalometric analyses but also baseline bone metabolism, alveolar bone density in situ of different sites of jaw bone, dental root volume, gene analysis, and so on, may be integrated in orthodontic treatment planning. Although one can only guess what the future may hold, the intent of this chapter was to give a provocative and evidence-based perspective on clinically feasible and patient-friendly techniques that may enhance a better future for accelerated tooth movement in orthodontics.

Summary Points

- Despite the low friction of self-ligating brackets in vitro, evidence has revealed that self-ligating brackets do not perform faster alignment or space closure in a clinical setting than conventional brackets. Shortened chair time and 1.5 degrees less incisor proclination appear to be the only significant advantages of self-ligating systems over conventional systems that are supported by the current evidence.

- The use of minute direct electric current for accelerating orthodontic tooth movement was only applied experimentally, and no clinical application has been reported.

- The effect of LLLT on accelerating orthodontic tooth movement is still controversial both experimentally and clinically.

- Although the local injection of PGE$_1$ has demonstrated its clinical effectiveness in accelerating orthodontic tooth movement, its clinical application is still limited because of the need for weekly injections and the severe pain caused after the injection.

- The question of whether human relaxin accelerates orthodontic tooth movement and prevents orthodontic relapse is still in dispute. The current experimental and clinical studies are limited and not substantive enough to answer the question yet.

- Surgical-assisted accelerated orthodontic tooth movement is currently the most effective technique experimentally and clinically in accelerating orthodontic tooth movement. These techniques include rapid canine retraction through distraction of the PDL or dentoalveolus, selective alveolar decortication, corticision, piezocision, and piezopuncture.

- The submucosal injection of PRP accelerates the original rate of orthodontic tooth alignment. However, research on the assessment of the dose-dependent effects of submucosal injection of PRP in accelerating orthodontic tooth alignment should be further investigated.

- Although the alveolar bone density in situ is a predetermined factor for the rate of orthodontic tooth alignment within an individual, baseline bone metabolism is the factor that dominates the rate of orthodontic tooth alignment among different individuals.

References

1. Stolzenberg J. The Russell attachment and its improved advantages. Int J Orthod Dent Child 1935;21:837–840.

2. Harradine NW. Self-ligating brackets and treatment efficiency. Clin Orthod Res 2001;4:220–227.

3. Rinchuse DJ, Miles PG. Self-ligating brackets: Present and future. Am J Orthod Dentofacial Orthop 2007;132:216–222.

4. Damon DH. The rationale, evolution and clinical application of the self-ligating bracket. Clin Orthod Res 1998;1:52–61.

5. Griffiths HS, Sherriff M, Ireland AJ. Resistance to sliding with 3 types of elastomeric modules. Am J Orthod Dentofacial Orthop 2005;127:670–675.

6. Henao SP, Kusy RP. Frictional evaluations of dental typodont models using four self-ligating designs and a conventional design. Angle Orthod 2005;75:75–85.

7. Khambay B, Millett D, McHugh S. Evaluation of methods of archwire ligation on frictional resistance. Eur J Orthod 2004;26:327–332.

8. Kim TK, Kim KD, Baek SH. Comparison of frictional forces during the initial leveling stage in various combinations of self-ligating brackets and archwires with a custom-designed typodont system. Am J Orthod Dentofacial Orthop 2008;133:187.e15–187.e24.

9. Budd S, Daskalogiannakis J, Tompson BD. A study of the frictional characteristics of four commercially available selfligating bracket systems. Eur J Orthod 2008;30:645–653.

10. Meling TR, Odegaard J, Holthe K, Segner D. The effect of friction on the bending stiffness of orthodontic beams: A theoretical and in vitro study. Am J Orthod Dentofacial Orthop 1997;112:41–49.

11. Shivapuja PK, Berger J. A comparative study of conventional ligation and self-ligation bracket systems. Am J Orthod Dentofacial Orthop 1994;106:472–480.

12. Pizzoni L, Ravnholt G, Melsen B. Frictional forces related to self-ligating brackets. Eur J Orthod 1998;20:283–291.

13. Sims AP, Waters NE, Birnie DJ, Pethybridge RJ. A comparison of the forces required to produce tooth movement in vitro using two self-ligating brackets and a pre-adjusted bracket employing two types of ligation. Eur J Orthod 1993;15:377–385.

14. Kapur R, Sinha PK, Nanda RS. Frictional resistance of the Damon SL bracket. J Clin Orthod 1998;32:485–489.

15. Berger JL. The influence of the SPEED bracket's self-ligating design on force levels in tooth movement: A comparative in vitro study. Am J Orthod Dentofacial Orthop 1990;97:219–228.

16. Chen SS, Greenlee GM, Kim JE, Smith CL, Huang GJ. Systematic review of self-ligating brackets. Am J Orthod Dentofacial Orthop 2010;137:726.e1–726.e18.

17. Fleming PS, Johal A. Self-ligating brackets in orthodontics. A systematic review. Angle Orthod 2010;80:575–584.

18. Pandis N, Polychronopoulou A, Eliades T. Self-ligating vs conventional brackets in the treatment of mandibular crowding: A prospective clinical trial of treatment duration and dental effects. Am J Orthod Dentofacial Orthop 2007;132:208–215.

19. Miles PG. SmartClip versus conventional twin brackets for initial alignment: Is there a difference? Aust Orthod J 2005;21:123–127.

20. Miles PG. Self-ligating vs conventional twin brackets during en-masse space closure with sliding mechanics. Am J Orthod Dentofacial Orthop 2007;132:223–225.

21. Miles PG, Weyant RJ, Rustveld L. A clinical trial of Damon 2 vs conventional twin brackets during initial alignment. Angle Orthod 2006;76:480–485.

22. Fleming PS, DiBiase AT, Sarri G, Lee RT. Efficiency of mandibular arch alignment with 2 preadjusted edgewise appliances. Am J Orthod Dentofacial Orthop 2009;135:597–602.

23. Scott P, DiBiase AT, Sherriff M, Cobourne MT. Alignment efficiency of Damon3 self-ligating and conventional orthodontic bracket systems: A randomized clinical trial. Am J Orthod Dentofacial Orthop 2008;133:470.e1–470.e8.

24. Schwarz AM. Tissue changes incidental to orthodontic tooth movement. Int J Orthod Oral Surg Rad 1932;18:331–352.

25. Storey E, Smith R. Force in orthodontics and its relation to tooth movement. Aust J Dent 1952;56:11–18.

26. Storey E. The nature of tooth movement. Am J Orthod 1973;63:292–314.

27. Reitan K. Some factors determining the evaluation of forces in orthodontics. Am J Orthod 1957;43:32–45.

28. Reitan K. Clinical and histological observations on tooth movement during and after orthodontic treatment. Am J Orthod 1967;53:721–745.

29. Beeson DC, Johnston LE, Wisotzky J. Effect of constant currents on orthodontic tooth movement in the cat. J Dent Res 1975;54:251–254.

30. Davidovitch Z, Finkelson MD, Steigman S, Shanfeld JL, Montgomery PC, Korostoff E. Electric currents, bone remodeling, and orthodontic tooth movement. I. The effect of electric currents on periodontal cyclic nucleotides. Am J Orthod 1980;77:14–32.

31. Davidovitch Z, Finkelson MD, Steigman S, Shanfeld JL, Montgomery PC, Korostoff E. Electric currents, bone remodeling, and orthodontic tooth movement. II. Increase in rate of tooth movement and periodontal cyclic nucleotide levels by combined force and electric current. Am J Orthod 1980;77:33–47.

32. Kakehi N, Yamazaki T, Tsugawa W, Sode K. A novel wireless glucose sensor employing direct electron transfer principle based enzyme fuel cell. Biosens Bioelectron 2007;22:2250–2255.

33. Kolahi J, Abrishami M, Davidovitch Z. Microfabricated biocatalytic fuel cells: A new approach to accelerating the orthodontic tooth movement. Med Hypotheses 2009;73:340–341.

34. Okuda-Shimazaki J, Kakehi N, Yamazaki T, Tomiyama M, Sode K. Biofuel cell system employing thermostable glucose dehydrogenase. Biotechnol Lett 2008;30:1753–1758.

35. Shapiro E, Roeber FW, Klempner LS. Orthodontic movement using pulsating force-induced piezoelectricity. Am J Orthod 1979;76:59–66.

36. Kopher RA, Mao JJ. Suture growth modulated by the oscillatory component of micromechanical strain. J Bone Miner Res 2003;18:521–528.

37. Peptan AI, Lopez A, Kopher RA, Mao JJ. Responses of intramembranous bone and sutures upon in vivo cyclic tensile and compressive loading. Bone 2008;42:432–438.

38. Vij K, Mao JJ. Geometry and cell density of rat craniofacial sutures during early postnatal development and upon in vivo cyclic loading. Bone 2006;38:722–730.

39. Nishimura M, Chiba M, Ohashi T, et al. Periodontal tissue activation by vibration: Intermittent stimulation by resonance vibration accelerates experimental tooth movement in rats. Am J Orthod Dentofacial Orthop 2008;133:572–583.

40. Shimizu Y. Movement of the lateral incisor of the Macaca fuscata as loaded by a vibrating force [in Japanese]. Nippon Kyosei Shika Gakkai Zasshi 1986;45:56–72.

41. Kau CH. A novel device in orthodontics. Aesthet Dent Today 2009;3:42–43.

42. Kau CH, Nguyen JT, English JD. The clinical evaluation of a novel cyclical force generating device in orthodontics. Orthod Pract US 2010;1:10–15.

43. AcceleDent website. http://acceledent.com/images/uploads/AcceleDent+Increases+the+Rate+of+Orthodontic+Tooth+Movement-Results+of+a+RCT+Final+for+Print+November+14+2011.pdf. Accessed 22 May 2012.

44. Burrow SJ. Canine retraction rate with self-ligating brackets vs conventional edgewise brackets. Angle Orthod 2010;80:626–633.

45. Liou EJ, Pai BC, Lin JC. Do miniscrews remain stationary under orthodontic forces? Am J Orthod Dentofacial Orthop 2004;126:42–47.

46. Yoshida T, Yamaguchi M, Utsunomiya T, et al. Low-energy laser irradiation accelerates the velocity of tooth movement via stimulation of the alveolar bone remodeling. Orthod Craniofac Res 2009;12:289–298.

47. Youssef M, Ashkar S, Hamade E, Gutknecht N, Lampert F, Mir M. The effect of low-level laser therapy during orthodontic movement: A preliminary study. Lasers Med Sci 2008;23:27–33.

48. Marquezan M, Bolognese AM, Araújo MT. Effects of two low-intensity laser therapy protocols on experimental tooth movement. Photomed Laser Surg 2010;28:757–762.

49. Habib FA, Gama SK, Ramalho LM, et al. Laser-induced alveolar bone changes during orthodontic movement: A histological study on rodents. Photomed Laser Surg 2010;28:823–830.

50. Altan BA, Sokucu O, Ozkut MM, Inan S. Metrical and histological investigation of the effects of low-level laser therapy on orthodontic tooth movement. Lasers Med Sci 2012;27:131–140.

51. Yamaguchi M, Hayashi M, Fujita S, et al. Low-energy laser irradiation facilitates the velocity of tooth movement and the expressions of matrix metalloproteinase-9, cathepsin K, and alpha(v) beta(3) integrin in rats. Eur J Orthod 2010;32:131–139.

52. Genovese MD, Olivi G. Use of laser technology in orthodontics: Hard and soft tissue laser treatments. Eur J Paediatr Dent 2010; 11:44–48.

53. Kim YD, Kim SS, Kim SJ, Kwon DW, Jeon ES, Son WS. Low-level laser irradiation facilitates fibronectin and collagen type I turnover during tooth movement in rats. Lasers Med Sci 2010;25:25–31.

54. Pinheiro AL, Gerbi ME. Photoengineering of bone repair processes. Photomed Laser Surg 2006;24:169–178.

55. Weber JB, Pinheiro AL, de Oliveira MG, Oliveira FA, Ramalho LM. Laser therapy improves healing of bone defects submitted to autologous bone graft. Photomed Laser Surg 2006;24:38–44.

56. Kreisler M, Christoffers AB, Willershausen B, d'Hoedt B. Effect of low-level GaAlAs laser irradiation on the proliferation rate of human periodontal ligament fibroblasts: An in vitro study. J Clin Periodontol 2003;30:353–358.

57. Jayasree RS, Gupta AK, Rathinam K, Mohanan PV, Mohanty M. The influence of photodynamic therapy on the wound healing process in rats. J Biomater Appl 2001;15:176–186.

58. Limpanichkul W, Godfrey K, Srisuk N, Rattanayatikul C. Effects of low-level laser therapy on the rate of orthodontic tooth movement. Orthod Craniofac Res 2006;9:38–43.

59. Fujita S, Yamaguchi M, Utsunomiya T, Yamamoto H, Kasai K. Low-energy laser stimulates tooth movement velocity via expression of RANK and RANKL. Orthod Craniofac Res 2008;11:143–155.

60. Seifi M, Shafeei HA, Daneshdoost S, Mir M. Effects of two types of low-level laser wave lengths (850 and 630 nm) on the orthodontic tooth movements in rabbits. Lasers Med Sci 2007;22:261–264.

61. Goulart CS, Nouer PR, Mouramartins L, Garbin IU, de Fátima Zanirato Lizarelli R. Photoradiation and orthodontic movement: Experimental study with canines. Photomed Laser Surg 2006;24: 192–196.

62. Yamasaki K, Miura F, Suda T. Prostaglandin as a mediator of bone resorption induced by experimental tooth movement in rats. J Dent Res 1980;59:1635–1642.

63. Yamasaki K, Shibata Y, Fukuhara T. The effect of prostaglandins on experimental tooth movement in monkeys (Macaca fuscata). J Dent Res 1982;61:1444–1446.

64. Yamasaki K, Shibuta Y, Ima S, Tan Y, Shibasaki Y, Fukuhara T. Clinical application of prostaglandin E_1 (PGE_1) upon orthodontic tooth movement. Am J Orthod 1984;85:508–518.

65. Chao CF, Shih C, Wang TM, Lo TH. Effects of prostaglandin E_2 on alveolar bone resorption during orthodontic tooth movement. Acta Anat (Basel) 1988;132:304–309.

66. Brudvik P, Rygh P. Root resorption after local injection of prostaglandin E_2 during experimental tooth movement. Eur J Orthod 1991;13:255–263.

67. Leiker BJ, Nanda RS, Currier GF, Howes RI, Sinha PK. The effects of exogenous prostaglandins on orthodontic tooth movement in rats. Am J Orthod Dentofacial Orthop 1995;108:380–388.

68. Lee KJ, Park YC, Yu HS, Choi SH, Yoo YJ. Effects of continuous and interrupted orthodontic force on interleukin-1β and prostaglandin E_2 production in gingival crevicular fluid. Am J Orthod Dentofacial Orthop 2004;125:168–177.

69. Mullender M, El Haj AJ, Yang Y, van Duin MA, Burger EH, Klein-Nulend J. Mechanotransduction of bone cells in vitro: Mechanobiology of bone tissue. Med Biol Eng Comput 2004;42:14–21.

70. Saito M, Saito S, Ngan PW, Shanfeld J, Davidovitch Z. Interleukin 1 beta and prostaglandin E are involved in the response of periodontal cells to mechanical stress in vivo and in vitro. Am J Orthod Dentofacial Orthop 1991;99:226–240.

71. Davidovitch Z, Nicolay OF, Ngan PW, Shanfeld JL. Neurotransmitters, cytokines, and the control of alveolar bone remodeling in orthodontics. Dent Clin North Am 1988;32:411–435.

72. Garlet TP, Coelho U, Silva JS, Garlet GP. Cytokine expression pattern in compression and tension sides of the periodontal ligament during orthodontic tooth movement in humans. Eur J Oral Sci 2007;115:355–362.

73. Rygh P, Bowling K, Hovlandsdal L, Williams S. Activation of the vascular system: A main mediator of periodontal fiber remodeling in orthodontic tooth movement. Am J Orthod 1986;89:453–468.

74. Ransjö M, Marklund M, Persson M, Lerner UH. Synergistic interactions of bradykinin, thrombin, interleukin 1 and tumor necrosis factor on prostanoid biosynthesis in human periodontal-ligament cells. Arch Oral Biol 1998;43:253–260.

75. Yeh CK, Rodan GA. Tensile forces enhance prostaglandin E synthesis in osteoblastic cells grown on collagen ribbons. Calcif Tissue Int 1984;36(suppl 1):S67–S71.

76. Ngan PW, Crock B, Varghese J, Lanese R, Shanfeld J, Davidovitch Z. Immunohistochemical assessment of the effect of chemical and mechanical stimuli on cAMP and prostaglandin E levels in human gingival fibroblasts in vitro. Arch Oral Biol 1988;33:163–174.

77. Ngan P, Saito S, Saito M, Lanese R, Shanfeld J, Davidovitch Z. The interactive effects of mechanical stress and interleukin-1 beta on prostaglandin E and cyclic AMP production in human periodontal ligament fibroblasts in vitro: Comparison with cloned osteoblastic cells of mouse (MC3T3-E1). Arch Oral Biol 1990;35:717–725.

78. Harell A, Dekel S, Binderman I. Biochemical effect of mechanical stress on cultured bone cells. Calcif Tissue Res 1977;22(suppl): 202–207.

79. Spielmann T, Wieslander L, Hefti AF. Acceleration of orthodontically induced tooth movement through the local application of prostaglandin (PGE_1). Schweiz Monatsschr Zahnmed 1989;99: 162–165.

80. Sherwood OD. Relaxin's physiological roles and other diverse actions. Endocr Rev 2004;25:205–234.

81. Nicozisis JL, Nah-Cederquist HD, Tuncay OC. Relaxin affects the dentofacial sutural tissues. Clin Orthod Res 2000;3:192–201.

82. Hsu SY, Nakabayashi K, Nishi S, et al. Activation of orphan receptors by the hormone relaxin. Science 2002;295:671–674.

83. He Y, Macarak EJ, Korostoff JM, Howard PS. Compression and tension: Differential effects on matrix accumulation by periodontal ligament fibroblasts in vitro. Connect Tissue Res 2004;45:28–39.

84. Bumann A, Carvalho RS, Schwarzer CL, Yen EH. Collagen synthesis from human PDL cells following orthodontic tooth movement. Eur J Orthod 1997;19:29–37.

85. Kristiansson P, Holding C, Hughes S, Haynes D. Does human relaxin-2 affect peripheral blood mononuclear cells to increase inflammatory mediators in pathologic bone loss? Ann N Y Acad Sci 2005;1041:317–319.

86. Masella RS, Meister M. Current concepts in the biology of orthodontic tooth movement. Am J Orthod Dentofacial Orthop 2006; 129:458–468.

87. Stewart DR, Sherick P, Kramer S, Breining P. Use of relaxin in orthodontics. Ann N Y Acad Sci 2005;1041:379–387.

88. Liu ZJ, King GJ, Gu GM, Shin JY, Stewart DR. Does human relaxin accelerate orthodontic tooth movement in rats? Ann N Y Acad Sci 2005;1041:388–394.

89. Madan MS, Liu ZJ, Gu GM, King GJ. Effects of human relaxin on orthodontic tooth movement and periodontal ligaments in rats. Am J Orthod Dentofacial Orthop 2007;131:8.e1–8.10.

90. McGorray SP, Dolce C, Kramer S, Stewart D, Wheeler TT. A randomized, placebo-controlled clinical trial on the effects of recombinant human relaxin on tooth movement and short-term stability. Am J Orthod Dentofacial Orthop 2012;141:196–203.

91. Liou EJ, Huang CS. Rapid canine retraction through distraction of the periodontal ligament. Am J Orthod Dentofacial Orthop 1998; 114:372–382.

92. Liou EJ. Distraction of the periodontal ligament: Rapid canine retraction. In: Samchukoy M, Cope J (eds). Craniofacial Distraction Osteogenesis. St Louis: Mosby, 2001.

93. Bilodeau JE. Dental distraction for an adult patient. Am J Orthod Dentofacial Orthop 2003;123:683–689.

94. Bilodeau JE. Nonsurgical treatment with rapid mandibular canine retraction via periodontal ligament distraction in an adult with a Class III malocclusion. Am J Orthod Dentofacial Orthop 2005;128:388–396.

95. Sayin S, Bengi AO, Gürton AU, Ortakoğlu K. Rapid canine distalization using distraction of the periodontal ligament: A preliminary clinical validation of the original technique. Angle Orthod 2004;74:304–315.

96. Kisniscu RS, Iseri H, Tuz HH, Altug AT. Dentoalveolar distraction osteogenesis for rapid orthodontic canine retraction. J Oral Maxillofac Surg 2002;60:389–394.

97. Iseri H, Kisnisci R, Bzizi N, Tuz H. Rapid canine retraction and orthodontic treatment with dentoalveolar distraction osteogenesis. Am J Orthod Denfacial Orthop 2005;127:533–541.

98. Sukurica Y, Karaman A, Gurel HB, Dolanmaz D. Rapid canine distalization through segmental alveolar distraction osteogenesis. Angle Orthod 2007;77:226–236.

99. Wilcko WM, Wilcko T, Bouquot JE, Ferguson DJ. Rapid orthodontics with alveolar reshaping: Two case reports of decrowding. Int J Periodontics Restorative Dent 2001;21:9–19.

100. Wilcko WM, Ferguson DJ, Booouquot JE, Wilcko T. Rapid orthodontic decrowding with alveolar augmentation: Case report. World J Orthod 2003;4:197–205.

101. Kim SJ, Park YG, Kang SG. Effects of Corticision on paradental remodeling in orthodontic tooth movement. Angle Orthod 2009;79:284–291.

102. Zeigler P, Ingervall B. A clinical study of maxillary canine retraction with a retraction spring and with sliding mechanics. Am J Orthod Dentofacial Orthop 1989;95:99–106.

103. Miyajima K, Nagahara K, Lizuka T. Orthodontic treatment for a patient after menopause. Angle Orthod 1996;66:173–180.

104. Darendeliler MA, Darendeliler H, Uner O. The drum spring (DS) retractor: Constant and continuous force for canine retraction. Eur J Orthod 1997;19:115–130.

105. Bridges T, King G, Mohammed A. The effect of age on tooth movement and mineral density in the alveolar tissues of the rat. Am J Orthod Dentofacial Orthop 1988;93:245–250.

106. Kyomen S, Tanne K. Influences of aging changes in proliferative rate of PDL cells during experimental tooth movement in rats. Angle Orthod 1997;67:67–72.

107. Tanne K, Yoshida S, Kawata T, Sasaki A, Knox J, Jones ML. An evaluation of the biomechanical responses of the tooth and periodontium to orthodontic forces in adolescent and adult subjects. Br J Orthod 1998;25:109–115.

108. Midgett RJ, Shaye R, Fruge JF. The effect of altered bone metabolism on orthodontic tooth movement. Am J Orthod 1981;80:256–262.

109. Goldie RS, King GJ. Root resorption and tooth movement in orthodontically treated, calcium deficient and lactating rats. Am J Orthod 1984;85:424–430.

110. Soma S, Iwamoto M, Higuchi Y, Kurisu K. Effects of continuous infusion of PTH on experimental tooth movement in rats. J Bone Miner Res 1999;14:546–554.

111. Fukui T. Analysis of stress-strain curves in the rat molar periodontal ligament after application of orthodontic force. Am J Orthod Dentofacial Orthop 1993;104:27–35.

112. Liou EJ, Polley JW, Figueroa AA. Distraction osteogenesis: The effects of orthodontic tooth movement on distracted mandibular bone. J Craniofac Surg 1998;9:564–571.

113. Kole H. Surgical operations on the alveolar ridge to correct occlusal abnormalities. Oral Surg Oral Med Oral Pathol 1959;12:515–529.

114. Kole H. Surgical operations on the alveolar ridge to correct occlusal abnormalities. Oral Surg Oral Med Oral Pathol 1959;12:413–420.

115. Kole H. Surgical operations on the alveolar ridge to correct occlusal abnormalities. Oral Surg Oral Med Oral Pathol 1959;12:277–288.

116. Anholm JM, Crites DA, Hoff R, Rathbun WE. Corticotomy-facilitated orthodontics. CDA J 1986;14:7–11.

117. Gantes B, Rathbun E, Anholm M. Effects on the periodontium following corticotomy-facilitated orthodontics. Case reports. J Periodontol 1990;61:234–238.

118. Generson RM, Porter JM, Zell A, Stratigos GT. Combined surgical and orthodontic management of anterior open bite using corticotomy. J Oral Surg 1978;36:216–219.

119. Suya H. Corticotomy in orthodontics. In: Hosl E, Baldauf A (eds). Mechanical and Biological Basics in Orthodontic Therapy. Heidelberg: Hütlig Buch, 1991:207–226.

120. Wilcko MT, Wilcko WM, Bissada NF. An evidence-based analysis of periodontally accelerated orthodontic and osteogenic techniques: A synthesis of scientific perspectives. Semin Orthod 2008;14:305–316.

121. Sebaoun JD, Kantarci A, Turner JW, Carvalho RS, Van Dyke TE, Ferguson DJ. Modeling of trabecular bone and lamina dura following selective alveolar decortication in rats. J Periodontol 2008;79:1679–1688.

122. Baloul SS, Gerstenfeld LC, Morgan EF, Carvalho RS, Van Dyke TE, Kantarci A. Mechanism of action and morphologic changes in the alveolar bone in response to selective alveolar decortication-facilitated tooth movement. Am J Orthod Dentofacial Orthop 2011;139(suppl):S83–S101.

123. Frost HM. The biology of fracture healing. An overview for clinicians. Part I. Clin Orthop Relat Res 1989;248:283–293.

124. Frost HM. The biology of fracture healing. An overview for clinicians. Part II. Clin Orthop Relat Res 1989;248:294–309.

125. Bogoch E, Gschwend N, Rahn B, Moran E, Perren S. Healing of cancellous bone osteotomy in rabbits—Part I: Regulation of bone volume and the regional acceleratory phenomenon in normal bone. J Orthop Res 1993;11:285–291.

126. Schilling T, Müller M, Minne HW, Ziegler R. Influence of inflammation-mediated osteopenia on the regional acceleratory phenomenon and the systemic acceleratory phenomenon during the healing of a bone defect in the rat. Calcif Tissue Int 1998;63:160–166.

127. Yaffe A, Fine N, Binderman I. Regional accelerated phenomenon in the mandible following mucoperiosteal flap surgery. J Periodontol 1994;65:79–83.

128. Lee W, Karapetyan G, Moats R, et al. Corticotomy-/osteotomy-assisted tooth movement microCTs differ. J Dent Res 2008;87:861–865.

129. Verna C, Dalstra M, Melsen B. The rate and the type of orthodontic tooth movement are influenced by bone turnover in a rat model. Eur J Orthod 2000;22:343–352.

130. Pfeifer JS. The reaction of alveolar bone to flap procedures in man. Periodontics 1965;3:135–140.

131. Hassan AH, Al-Fraidi AA, Al-Saeed SH. Corticotomy-assisted orthodontic treatment: Review. Open Dent J 2010;4:159–164.

132. Ren A, Lv T, Zhao B, Chen Y, Bai D. Rapid orthodontic tooth movement aided by alveolar surgery in beagles. Am J Orthod Dentofacial Orthop 2007;131:160.e1–160.e10.

133. Mostafa YA, Fayed MM, Mehanni S, ElBokle NN, Heider AM. Comparison of corticotomy-facilitated vs standard tooth-movement techniques in dogs with miniscrews as anchor units. Am J Orthod Dentofacial Orthop 2009;136:570–577.

134. Fischer TJ. Orthodontic treatment acceleration with corticotomy assisted exposure of palatally impacted canines. Angle Orthod 2007;77:417–420.

135. Vanarsdall RL Jr. Transverse dimension and long-term stability. Semin Orthod 1999;5:171–180.

136. Brin I, Ben-Bassat Y, Blustein Y, et al. Skeletal and functional effects of treatment for unilateral posterior crossbite. Am J Orthod Dentofacial Orthop 1996;109:173–179.

137. Moon CH, Wee JU, Lee HS. Intrusion of overerupted molars by corticotomy and orthodontic skeletal anchorage. Angle Orthod 2007;77:1119–1125.

138. Oliveira DD, de Oliveira BF, de Araújo Brito HH, de Souza MM, Medeiros PJ. Selective alveolar corticotomy to intrude overerupted molars. Am J Orthod Dentofacial Orthop 2008;133:902–908.

139. Kim SH, Kim I, Jeong DM, Chung KR, Zadeh H. Corticotomy-assisted decompensation for augmentation of the mandibular anterior ridge. Am J Orthod Dentofacial Orthop 2011;140:720–731.

140. Nazarov AD, Ferguson DJ, Wilcko WM, Wilcko MT. Improved retention following corticotomy using ABO objective grading system. J Dent Res 2004;83:2644.

141. Germec D, Giray B, Kocadereli I, Enacar A. Lower incisor retraction with a modified corticotomy. Angle Orthod 2006;76:882–890.

142. Dibart S, Sebaoun JD, Surmenian J. Piezocision: A minimally invasive, periodontally accelerated orthodontic tooth movement procedure. Compend Contin Educ Dent 2009;30:342–344,346, 348–350.

143. Sebaoun JD, Surmenian J, Dibart S. Accelerated orthodontic treatment with piezocision: A mini-invasive alternative to conventional corticotomies. Orthod Fr 2011;82:311–319.

144. Frost HM. The regional acceleratory phenomenon: A review. Henry Ford Hosp Med J 1983;31:3–9.

145. Park YG. Patient-friendly orthodontics to accelerate tooth movement. Presented at the 23rd Annual Conference of Taiwan Association of Orthodontists, 2011, Taichung, Taiwan.

146. Liou EJ, Chen PH, Wang YC. The surgery-first accelerated orthognathic surgery: Part II, The postoperative rapid orthodontic tooth movement. J Oral Maxillofac Surg 2011;69:781–785.

147. Liou EJ, Wang YC, Lee YC, Teng G, Chen YR. Submucosal Injection of platelet-rich plasma accelerates orthodontic tooth movement. Am J Orthod Dentofacial Orthop (in press).

148. Garg AK. The use of platelet-rich plasma to enhance the success of bone grafts around dental implants. Dental Implantol Update 2000;11:17–21.

149. Schlegel KA, Kloss FR, Kessler P, Schultze-Mosgau S, Nkenke E, Wiltfang J. Bone condition to enhance implant osseointegration: An experimental study in pigs. Int J Oral Maxillofac Implant 2003; 18:505–511.

150. Kim SG, Chung CH, Kim YK, Park JC, Lim SC. Use of particulate dentine-plaster of Paris combination with/ without platelet-rich plasma in the treatment of bone defects around implants. Int J Oral Maxillofac Implant 2002;17:86–94.

151. Kim SG, Kim WK, Park JC, Kim HJ. A comparative study of osseointegration of Avana implants in a demineralized freeze-dried bone alone or with platelet-rich-plasma. J Oral Maxillofac Surg 2002;60:1018–1025.

152. Rodriguez A, Anastassov GE, Lee H, Buchbinder D, Wettan H. Maxillary sinus augmentation with deproteinated bovine bone and platelet-rich plasma with simultaneous insertion of endosseous implants. J Oral Maxillofac Surg 2003;61:157–163.

153. Zechner W, Tangl S, Tepper G, et al. Influence of platelet-rich plasma on osseous healing of dental implants: A histologic and histomorphometric study in minipigs. Int J Oral Maxillofac Implant 2003;18:15–22.

154. Okuda K, Kawase T, Momose M, et al. Platelet-rich plasma contains high levels of platelet-derived growth factor and transforming growth factor-β and modulates the proliferation of periodontally related cells in vitro. J Periodontol 2003;74:849–857.

155. Sanchez AR, Sheridan PJ, Kupp LI. Is platelet-rich plasma the perfect enhancement factor? A current review. Int J Oral Maxillofac Implants 2003;18:93–103.

156. Iwasaki LR, Haack JE, Nickel JC, Reinhardt RA, Petro TM. Human interleukin-1 beta and interleukin-1 receptor antagonist secretion and velocity of tooth movement. Arch Oral Biol 2001;46:185–189.

157. Iwasaki LR, Crouch LD, Tutor A, et al. Tooth movement and cytokines in gingival crevicular fluid and whole blood in growing and adult subjects. Am J Orthod Dentofacial Orthop 2005;128:483–491.

158. Liou EJ, Wang YC, Lee YC, Sheng SL, Chen YR. Baseline osteoclastic activity dominates over alveolar bone density in situ in determining rate of orthodontic alignment. Am J Orthod Dentofacial Orthop (in press).

159. Insoft M, King GJ, Keeling SD. The measurement of acid and alkaline phosphatase in gingival crevicular fluid during orthodontic tooth movement. Am J Orthod Dentofacial Orthop 1996;109:287–296.

160. Last KS, Donkin C, Embery G. Glycosaminoglycans in human gingival crevicular fluid during orthodontic movement. Arch Oral Biol 1988;33:907–912.

161. Perinetti G, Paolantonio M, D'Attilio M, et al. Alkaline phosphatase activity in gingival crevicular fluid during human orthodontic tooth movement. Am J Orthod Dentofacial Orthop 2002;122:548–556.

162. Marx RE, Cillo JE Jr, Ulloa JJ. Oral bisphosphonate-induced osteonecrosis: Risk factors, prediction of risk using serum CTX testing, prevention, and treatment. J Oral Maxillofac Surg 2007;65:2397–2410.

163. Pellegrini GG, Gonzales CM, Somoza JC, Friedman SM, Zeni SN. Correlation between salivary and serum markers of bone turnover in osteopenic rats. J Periodontol 2008;79:158–165.

164. Freeman DC. Root Surface Area Related to Anchorage in Begg Technique [thesis]. Memphis: University of Tennessee Department of Orthodontics, 1965.

165. Iglesias-Linares A, Moreno-Fernandez AM, Yanes-Vico R, Mendoza-Mendoza A, Gonzalez-Moles M, Solano-Reina E. The use of gene therapy vs corticotomy surgery in accelerating tooth movement. Orthod Craniofac Res 2011;14:138–148.

Index

Page numbers followed by "f" indicate figures; those followed by "t" indicate tables; those followed by "b" indicate boxes